Handbook of Obstetrics and Gynecology

Edited by Annabelle Coleman

hayle medical

New York

Hayle Medical,
750 Third Avenue, 9th Floor,
New York, NY 10017, USA

Visit us on the World Wide Web at:
www.haylemedical.com

ISBN: 978-1-63241-621-6

Cataloging-in-Publication Data

Handbook of obstetrics and gynecology / edited by Annabelle Coleman.
 p. cm.
Includes bibliographical references and index.
ISBN 978-1-63241-621-6
1. Obstetrics. 2. Gynecology. 3. Generative organs, Female--Diseases.
I. Coleman, Annabelle.
RG524 .H36 2019
618.2--dc23

Table of Contents

Preface

Obstetrics is a medical field which concentrates on pregnancy, childbirth and the postpartum period. Prenatal care and postnatal care are the main areas which come under it. Prenatal care is important in the screening of pregnancy complications, whereas, postnatal care is the care provided to the mother following parturition. Gynecology deals with the health of the breasts and female reproductive organs, consisting of the vagina, uterus and ovaries. Women may suffer from a number of gynecological disorders such as cancer, amenorrhoea, menorrhagia, pelvic inflammatory diseases and UTI, infertility, prolapse, etc. The diagnosis of such conditions is aided by physical examination, diagnostic laparoscopy, hysteroscopy, exploratory laparotomy, etc. The topics included in this book on obstetrics and gynecology are of utmost significance and bound to provide incredible insights to readers. It presents researches and studies performed by experts across the globe. Students, researchers, experts and all associated with obstetrics and gynecology will benefit alike from this book.

After months of intensive research and writing, this book is the end result of all who devoted their time and efforts in the initiation and progress of this book. It will surely be a source of reference in enhancing the required knowledge of the new developments in the area. During the course of developing this book, certain measures such as accuracy, authenticity and research focused analytical studies were given preference in order to produce a comprehensive book in the area of study.

This book would not have been possible without the efforts of the authors and the publisher. I extend my sincere thanks to them. Secondly, I express my gratitude to my family and well-wishers. And most importantly, I thank my students for constantly expressing their willingness and curiosity in enhancing their knowledge in the field, which encourages me to take up further research projects for the advancement of the area.

Editor

Pneumocystis Pneumonia in Non-HIV Pregnant Women Receiving Chemotherapy for Malignant Lymphoma: Two Case Reports

Yuki Fukutani, Yoshitsugu Chigusa, Eiji Kondoh, Kaoru Kawasaki, Shingo Io, and Noriomi Matsumura

Department of Gynecology and Obstetrics, Kyoto University, 54 Shogoin Kawahara-cho, Sakyo-ku, Kyoto 606-8507, Japan

Correspondence should be addressed to Yoshitsugu Chigusa; chigusa@kuhp.kyoto-u.ac.jp

Academic Editor: Akihide Ohkuchi

Pneumocystis pneumonia (PCP) is a life-threatening opportunistic infection that sometimes occurs in immunocompromised patients with human immunodeficiency virus (HIV). Here, we report two extremely rare cases of PCP in non-HIV pregnant women who underwent chemotherapy for malignant lymphoma. Case 1 is a 34-year-old primigravida who was diagnosed with Hodgkin's lymphoma. She received ABVD chemotherapy and developed PCP at 37 weeks of gestation. After the onset of PCP, emergent cesarean section was performed due to a nonreassuring fetal status. Case 2 is a 31-year-old multigravida with diffuse large B-cell lymphoma who was administered R-CHOP chemotherapy. At 34 weeks of gestation, she complained of dyspnea and developed PCP. She delivered her baby vaginally immediately after the onset of symptoms. Both patients were treated with sulfamethoxazole-trimethoprim (ST) and recovered shortly thereafter. The babies' courses were also uneventful. PCP remains a serious cause of death, especially in non-HIV patients, and, therefore, appropriate prophylaxis and a prompt diagnosis are imperative.

1. Introduction

Pneumocystis pneumonia (PCP) is one of the most prevalent opportunistic infections in immunocompromised patients, especially in those infected with the human immunodeficiency virus (HIV). Lately, the incidence of PCP in non-HIV immunosuppressed patients has also been on the rise. These cases include hematological malignancies and patients who undergo chemotherapy for cancer or immunosuppressive drugs. In terms of PCP during pregnancy, most cases are HIV immunosuppressed patients, and non-HIV cases are extremely rare. Importantly, compared with HIV-positive patients, PCP in HIV-positive patients is associated with a higher mortality rate and poorer prognosis [1]. However, the standard prophylaxis and strategy for the treatment of PCP that develops in HIV-negative pregnant women have not yet been established.

This article describes two cases of PCP during pregnancy that occurred in patients receiving chemotherapy due to malignant lymphoma. We also reviewed the relevant literature to reveal the proper management of this life-threatening opportunistic infection in HIV-negative pregnant women.

2. Case Reports

2.1. Case 1. A 34-year-old woman, gravida 0, complained of a swollen lymph node on the left side of the neck and underwent a biopsy of the neck and mediastinal lymph nodes at 20 weeks of gestation. Pathological diagnosis was classical stage IIA (Ann Arbor staging system) Hodgkin's lymphoma, with involvement of the left supraclavicular and mediastinal nodes. ABVD (doxorubicin 25 mg/m^2, bleomycin 10 mg/m^2, vinblastine 6 mg/m^2, and dacarbazine 375 mg/m^2) chemotherapy was started at 23 weeks of gestation. After 4 cycles of ABVD, at 37 weeks and 0 days of gestation, she experienced a cough and slight dyspnea. Chest X-ray showed high density areas in both lower lobes, which were detected as diffuse ground-glass patterns on computed tomography (CT) (Figure 1(a)). We included interstitial pneumonia caused by bleomycin as well as PCP in the differential diagnosis, and oral prednisone was administered. We did not prescribe

(a)

(b)

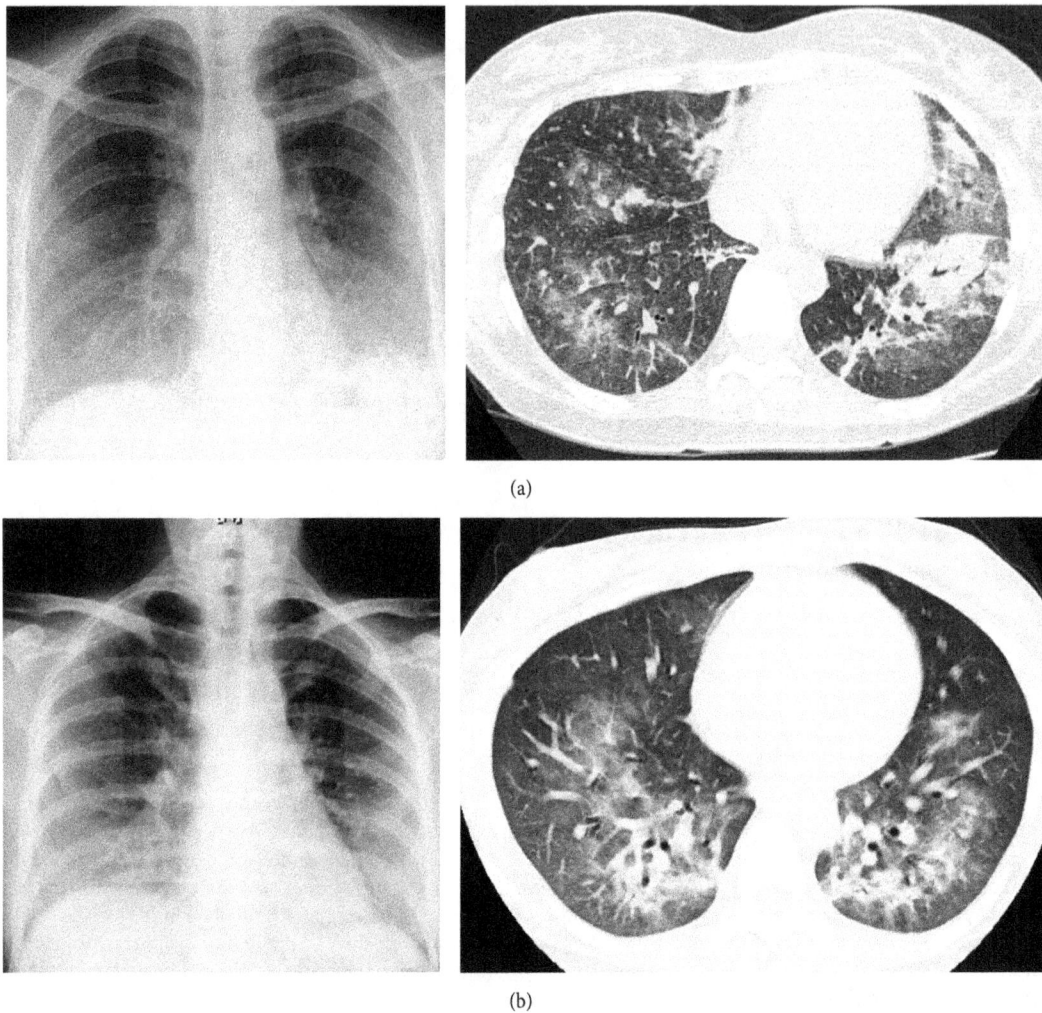

FIGURE 1: Chest X-ray (left) and computed tomography (CT) (right) images of case 1 (a) and case 2 (b). Chest X-ray showed a high density area in the lower lobes, which was detected as a diffuse ground-glass pattern on CT in both cases.

sulfamethoxazole-trimethoprim (ST) because the safety of ST in pregnancy was unclear at that time. At 37 weeks and 1 day of gestation, fetal movement was profoundly decreased, and repeated variable deceleration was observed on the fetal heart rate monitor. Consequently, emergent cesarean section due to nonreassuring fetal status and breech presentation was performed, and she delivered a 2596 g male baby. After surgery, she was treated with ST based on the clinical suspicion of PCP. Eventually, she was diagnosed with PCP by a PCR method that detects *Pneumocystis jirovecii*-specific DNA in the sputum. After a 3-week treatment with ST and prednisone, she recovered and thereafter received two additional cycles of ABVD. She has had no sign of disease relapse, and the subsequent clinical course of the baby has been uneventful.

2.2. Case 2. A 31-year-old woman, gravida 1, para 1, who had undergone conization due to stage IA1 uterine cervical cancer, noticed swelling of the right side of the pharynx shortly after she conceived; as a result, she visited an otolaryngologist. The tonsil biopsy at 13 weeks of gestation showed diffuse large

B-cell lymphoma (DLBCL). The patient had multiple swollen lymph node groups on the same side of the diaphragm and was therefore classified as stage II according to the Cotswold modification of the Ann Arbor staging system. In all, 6 cycles of R-CHOP (rituximab 375 mg/m^2, cyclophosphamide 750 mg/m^2, doxorubicin 50 mg/m^2, vincristine 1.4 mg/m^2, and prednisone 100 mg/body) every 3 weeks were administered. At 32 weeks of gestation, she was hospitalized due to rapidly shortening cervical length (15 mm), and tocolysis with ritodrine was started. At 34 weeks and 0 days of gestation, she suddenly complained of dyspnea and a nonproductive cough, and chest CT showed a ground-glass pattern on both sides of the lungs (Figure 1(b)). *Pneumocystis* pneumonia was highly suspected in view of her history and CT findings, and she was presumptively treated with sulfamethoxazole-trimethoprim (ST), azithromycin, and oral prednisone. Then, tocolysis was stopped and she delivered a 1939 g female baby at 34 weeks and 1 day of gestation. Although *Pneumocystis jirovecii* was not observed in bronchoalveolar lavage (BAL) fluid by Grocott stain, *Pneumocystis jirovecii*-specific DNA was detected by PCR using BAL fluid. She recovered and was discharged home 14 days later, and her baby's course was uneventful. She has shown no signs of DLBCL recurrence.

3. Discussion

In the present report, we described two cases of PCP during pregnancy. Numerous cases of PCP in HIV-infected pregnant individuals have been reported. However, our cases are extremely rare in that both occurred in pregnant women without HIV. To the best of our knowledge, only one similar case of PCP has been reported thus far, and, in that case, PCP developed in a pregnant woman who was infected with human T lymphotropic virus type 1 (HTLV-1) [2].

With increasing maternal age, the incidence of cancer and the opportunity to administer chemotherapy during pregnancy also increase. Malignant lymphoma, which is the fourth most common malignancy diagnosed in pregnancy, is estimated to occur in 1 : 6,000 pregnancies [3]. Basically, chemotherapy in pregnant women with lymphoma should be similar to that in nonpregnant individuals, although it remains unclear whether the increased plasma volume and renal clearance of drugs during pregnancy might necessitate different doses of chemotherapy. The available existing data suggest that ABVD for Hodgkin's disease and CHOP for non-Hodgkin's disease during the second and third trimester can be administered safely without severe fetal outcomes [4]. In addition, compared with CHOP, rituximab with CHOP (R-CHOP) was revealed to be more effective and to lead to a better prognosis in patients (aged 18 to 60 years) with DLBCL [5]. Rituximab, which is a monoclonal antibody against CD20, is considered to be relatively safe for pregnant women although it may be associated with preterm birth [6, 7]. Based on these views, ABVD was given from 23 weeks of gestation in case 1, and R-CHOP was given from 16 weeks of gestation in case 2. In terms of R-CHOP, however, to our knowledge, only nine patients thus far have received that particular therapy [6–8], and more cases are necessary to analyze the safety of R-CHOP in pregnancy.

Generally, chemotherapy treatment for cancer can cause opportunistic infections, and patients with hematologic malignancies are particularly susceptible to a different set of infections [9]. However, the occurrence of PCP in patients who are administered R-CHOP or ABVD is infrequent. Hardak et al. reported that the incidence of PCP among patients treated with R-CHOP was 2.6% [10] in spite of the finding that R-CHOP includes a high dose of prednisone. Moreover, the frequency of PCP in patients who are given ABVD is currently unknown. The only literature that we found involved five patients with PCP and Hodgkin's lymphoma who were treated with ABVD [11]. Nevertheless, we have encountered two cases of PCP following ABVD or R-CHOP therapy. Presumably, PCP is more likely to occur in pregnant women who undergo cancer chemotherapy since pregnancy itself can give rise to immunosuppression [12].

Although PCP during pregnancy in HIV-negative patients is very rare, it is notable that the mortality rate of patients with PCP in the absence of HIV is higher (30 to 60%) than that in patients with HIV (10 to 20%) [13].

Moreover, PCP in HIV-negative patients has an abrupt onset that consists of respiratory insufficiency, and patients can deteriorate rapidly. Therefore, the appropriate prophylaxis is necessary to reduce the risk of PCP, even among HIV-negative pregnant women. Sulfamethoxazole-trimethoprim (ST), also known as cotrimoxazole, has already been demonstrated to be effective for the prevention of PCP in patients with HIV [14], while ST has been recommended for HIV-infected pregnant women with a low CD4 cell count. According to the systematic review and meta-analysis regarding the safety of cotrimoxazole conducted by Ford et al., the overall prevalence of congenital abnormalities in those exposed to cotrimoxazole was not significantly higher than the reported rates in the general population [15]. Thus, patients with hematological cancers, such as lymphoma and leukemia, are at risk for PCP because they are treated with cytotoxic chemotherapy, which sometimes causes immunosuppression. In addition, chronic corticosteroid administration is one of the most common risk factors for PCP in patients without HIV infection. For nonpregnant women, therefore, it is recommended that prophylaxis with ST be considered for those with hematological malignancies who are treated with chemotherapy, and for those who are treated with more than 20 mg/day of prednisone for longer than 1 month [16]. This recommendation may be pertinent to pregnant women as well.

In addition to prophylaxis, prompt diagnosis and appropriate treatment are essential for a good prognosis of PCP. However, PCP is sometimes difficult to diagnose, as the patients present nonspecific symptoms such as fever, dyspnea, and nonproductive cough. Although the final diagnosis of PCP should be made based on the microscopic detection of *Pneumocystis* from specimens of sputum or bronchoalveolar fluid, the PCR method that is used to detect *Pneumocystis jirovecii*-specific nucleic acids has also become available, which has a higher diagnostic sensitivity. Moreover, chest CT is more sensitive and superior as a diagnostic tool compared with chest radiography. Indeed, in our two cases, expeditious CT revealed typical features of PCP, such as a ground-glass attenuation, which encouraged us to initiate treatment with sulfamethoxazole-trimethoprim. The fetal radiation doses from chest CT are very low, since this type of scan does not involve direct irradiation, but rather it results in scattered radiation. The maximum estimated conceptus radiation dose from chest CT is less than 1 mGy [17], and the average dose is 0.22 mGy [18]. Therefore, physicians should not hesitate to perform chest CT examination, even during pregnancy, when PCP is suspected.

In summary, we described two rare cases of PCP after chemotherapy was administered for lymphoma during pregnancy. PCP remains a serious cause of death in immunocompromised patients, and, therefore, appropriate prophylaxis and prompt diagnosis are imperative.

Consent

Written informed consent was obtained from both patients for the publication of this case report and its accompanying images.

References

[1] N. G. Mansharamani, R. Garland, D. Delaney, and H. Koziel, "Management and outcome patterns for adult *Pneumocystis carinii* pneumonia, 1985 to 1995: comparison of HIV-associated cases to other immunocompromised states," *Chest*, vol. 118, no. 3, pp. 704–711, 2000.

[2] Y. Tamaki, F. Higa, D. Tasato et al., "Pneumocystis jirovecii pneumonia and alveolar hemorrhage in a pregnant woman with human T cell lymphotropic virus type-1 infection," *Internal Medicine*, vol. 50, no. 4, pp. 351–354, 2011.

[3] B. Brenner, I. Avivi, and M. Lishner, "Haematological cancers in pregnancy," *The Lancet*, vol. 379, no. 9815, pp. 580–587, 2012.

[4] A. Avilés and N. Neri, "Hematological malignancies and pregnancy: A final report of 84 children who received chemotherapy in utero," *Clinical Lymphoma*, vol. 2, no. 3, pp. 173–177, 2001.

[5] M. Pfreundschuh, L. Trümper, A. Österborg et al., "CHOP-like chemotherapy plus rituximab versus CHOP-like chemotherapy alone in young patients with good-prognosis diffuse large-B-cell lymphoma: a randomised controlled trial by the MabThera International Trial (MInT) Group," *The Lancet Oncology*, vol. 7, no. 5, pp. 379–391, 2006.

[6] E. F. Chakravarty, E. R. Murray, A. Kelman, and P. Farmer, "Pregnancy outcomes after maternal exposure to rituximab," *Blood*, vol. 117, no. 5, pp. 1499–1506, 2011.

[7] E. J. Lee, K. H. Ahn, S. C. Hong, E. H. Lee, Y. Park, and B. S. Kim, "Rituximab, cyclophosphamide, doxorubicin, vincristine, and prednisone (R-CHOP) chemotherapy for diffuse large B-cell lymphoma in pregnancy may be associated with preterm birth," *Obstetrics & Gynecology Science*, vol. 57, no. 6, pp. 526–529, 2014.

[8] P. K. Mandal, T. K. Dolai, B. Bagchi, M. K. Ghosh, S. Bose, and M. Bhattacharyya, "B cell suppression in newborn following treatment of pregnant diffuse large B-cell lymphoma patient with rituximab containing regimen," *Indian Journal of Pediatrics*, vol. 81, no. 10, pp. 1092–1094, 2014.

[9] T. R. Zembower, "Epidemiology of infections in cancer patients," *Cancer Treatment and Research*, vol. 161, pp. 43–89, 2014.

[10] E. Hardak, I. Oren, E. J. Dann et al., "The increased risk for pneumocystis pneumonia in patients receiving rituximab-CHOP-14 can be prevented by the administration of trimethoprim/sulfamethoxazole: a single-center experience," *Acta Haematologica*, vol. 127, no. 2, pp. 110–114, 2012.

[11] M. Kalin, S. Y. Kristinsson, H. Cherif, M. Lebbad, and M. Björkholm, "Fatal pneumocystis jiroveci pneumonia in ABVD-treated Hodgkin lymphoma patients," *Annals of Hematology*, vol. 89, no. 5, pp. 523–525, 2010.

[12] P. Luppi, "How immune mechanisms are affected by pregnancy," *Vaccine*, vol. 21, no. 24, pp. 3352–3357, 2003.

[13] C. F. Thomas Jr. and A. H. Limper, "Pneumocystis pneumonia," *The New England Journal of Medicine*, vol. 350, no. 24, pp. 2487–2498, 2004.

[14] S. Bozzette, D. M. Finkelstein, and S. A. Spector, "A randomized trial of three antipneumocystis agents in patients with advanced human immunodeficiency virus infection," *The New England Journal of Medicine*, vol. 332, no. 11, pp. 693–699, 1995.

[15] N. Ford, Z. Shubber, J. Jao, E. J. Abrams, L. Frigati, and L. Mofenson, "Safety of cotrimoxazole in pregnancy: a systematic review and meta-analysis," *Journal of Acquired Immune Deficiency Syndromes*, vol. 66, no. 5, pp. 512–521, 2014.

[16] A. H. Limper, K. S. Knox, G. A. Sarosi et al., "An official American Thoracic Society statement: treatment of fungal infections in adult pulmonary and critical care patients," *American Journal of Respiratory and Critical Care Medicine*, vol. 183, no. 1, pp. 96–128, 2011.

[17] S. Goldberg-Stein, B. Liu, P. F. Hahn, and S. I. Lee, "Body CT during pregnancy: Utilization trends, examination indications, and fetal radiation doses," *American Journal of Roentgenology*, vol. 196, no. 1, pp. 146–151, 2011.

[18] E. Lazarus, C. DeBenedectis, D. North, P. K. Spencer, and W. W. Mayo-Smith, "Utilization of imaging in pregnant patients: 10-year review of 5270 examinations in 3285 patients - 1997–2006," *Radiology*, vol. 251, no. 2, pp. 517–524, 2009.

Subtotal Resection of an Anaplastic Ganglioglioma in Pregnancy

Matthew J. Bicocca ⓘ,[1] **Andrea R. Gilbert,**[2] **Saeed S. Sadrameli,**[3] **and Michael L. Pirics**[1,4]

[1]*Department of Obstetrics and Gynecology, Houston Methodist Hospital, Houston, TX, USA*
[2]*Department of Pathology and Genomic Medicine, Houston Methodist Hospital, Houston, TX, USA*
[3]*Department of Neurosurgery, Houston Methodist Hospital, Houston, TX, USA*
[4]*Department of Obstetrics and Gynecology, Weill Cornell Medical College, New York, NY, USA*

Correspondence should be addressed to Matthew J. Bicocca; mbicocca@gmail.com

Academic Editor: Akihide Ohkuchi

Background. Anaplastic ganglioglioma is a rare malignant brain tumor associated with high morbidity and mortality. The diagnosis of a central nervous system malignancy in the early 3rd trimester presents management challenges to both neurosurgeons and obstetricians. *Case.* A 33-year-old woman, gravida 2 para 1, presented at 28 6/7 weeks with four months of worsening headaches, nausea, vomiting, and mental status changes due to a 7.5 cm anaplastic ganglioglioma. Maternal deterioration necessitated subtotal tumor debulking allowing prolongation of the gestation to 34 6/7 weeks. After delivery, the patient underwent further resection, followed by chemotherapy and radiation. Both mother and infant are well. *Discussion.* This case underscores the importance of timely diagnostic imaging in pregnant women and demonstrates subtotal tumor debulking as a viable means of prolonging gestation.

1. Introduction

Primary brain tumors in pregnancy are a rare cause of maternal morbidity with an estimated incidence of 3.6 malignant brain tumors per one million live births [1]. Although the overall incidence of primary intracranial neoplasms in pregnant women is slightly decreased compared to age matched nonpregnant counterparts [1], the dramatic physiologic and hormonal changes of pregnancy are associated with a more complicated clinical course, exacerbated maternal symptoms, and increased velocity of diametric tumor expansion [2, 3]. Additionally, pregnant patients with malignant primary brain tumors have elevated rates of fetal growth restriction, maternal mortality, hyperemesis gravidarum, and cesarean delivery [4].

Ganglioglioma (GG), a rare glial-neuronal brain tumor characterized by dysplastic ganglion cells and neoplastic glial cells, accounts for about 0.4% of all tumors arising in the central nervous system (CNS) [5]. The malignant subtype of GG, called anaplastic ganglioglioma (AGG), comprises about 1–8% of all adult and pediatric GGs and has an estimated incidence of 0.02 cases per million per year [6]. Although

there are reported instances of a lower grade GG arising in a pregnant woman [7] and an AGG diagnosed during the postpartum period [8, 9], we are the first to document a case of an AGG diagnosed during pregnancy.

2. Case Presentation

The patient was a 33-year-old woman, gravida 2 para 1, with an intrauterine pregnancy dated by a 9-week ultrasound. She had an obstetrical history of one prior vaginal term delivery and a family history of breast cancer. Beginning at 11 weeks gestation, she reported headaches that were not relieved by acetaminophen, as well as a pulsing sensation in her left ear. Treatment was initiated with acetaminophen/butalbital/caffeine (Fioricet) for presumed migraine headaches. At 14 weeks, she complained of new onset jaw-tightness and a vibrating sensation in her ears, which prompted a referral to a primary care physician. At 20 weeks, the fetal anatomy scan showed appropriate growth with no fetal anomalies, but the patient's headaches had worsened and required frequent narcotic use. Four weeks later, the patient was referred to a neurologist who attributed her

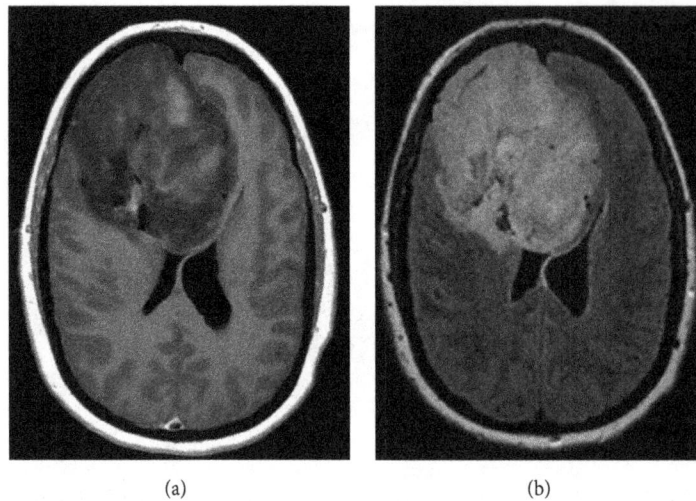

(a)   (b)

FIGURE 1: Axial MRI shows a 7.5 cm heterogenous mass in the right frontal lobe with T1-weighted sequences showing patchy enhancement following contrast administration (a) and hyperintensity with surrounding vasogenic edema on T2-weighted fluid attenuated inversion recovery sequences (b).

worsening symptoms to occipital neuralgia. Beginning at 26 weeks, her headaches were accompanied by anorexia, nausea, and vomiting. She also experienced two vasovagal episodes with questionable seizure activity. Psychiatric changes, which included severe depression and neglected hygiene, prompted two visits to the emergency department where she was diagnosed with migraine headaches and received opiates and antiemetics.

At 28 6/7 weeks, the patient underwent a workup for preeclampsia for which laboratory investigations were negative. However, magnetic resonance imaging (MRI) of the brain revealed a 7.5 cm heterogenous mass in the right frontal lobe (Figure 1) that showed patchy contrast enhancement, focal calcifications with blood products, and surrounding vasogenic edema with mild midline shift. At this time, the patient was transferred to our institution for the remainder of her care.

On admission, she was noted to have sluggishly reactive pupils and mild weakness in the left upper extremity. An ultrasound confirmed appropriate estimated fetal weight and amniotic fluid level. Levetiracetam was administered as well as dexamethasone, which was switched to methylprednisolone after 48 hours.

Three days following transfer of care, the patient showed evidence of clinical deterioration, including recurrent aphasia and a generalized atonic seizure. The decision was made to proceed with neurosurgical resection of the brain mass to relieve intracranial pressure. Given the extent of the mass, involvement of eloquent cortex, and safety concerns for the fetus and the mother, the operation was planned in a staged fashion, with the second stage scheduled after delivery. At 29 4/7 weeks, the patient underwent a bifrontal craniotomy and subtotal right frontal lobectomy with excision of a highly vascular tumor; the posterior aspect of the neoplasm encroached on the motor cortex and was not resected at that time. Estimated blood loss was 100 mL. Continuous fetal heart

monitoring performed throughout the operation showed a baseline of 135 beats per minute with minimal variability and no acceleration or deceleration. Once in recovery, the fetal heart tracing improved to moderate variability with 10×10 acceleration. Postoperatively, the patient recovered well. Her neurological status improved with resolution of her aphasia and cessation of seizure activity. She was discharged home on postoperative day two.

Hematoxylin and eosin (H&E) staining and immunohistochemistry were performed on sections prepared from formalin-fixed paraffin-embedded tissue. Microscopic examination showed hypercellular neuroglial tissue featuring GFAP-positive neoplastic astrocytes and clusters of dysplastic-appearing ganglion cells highlighted by NeuN and synaptophysin immunostains. The ganglioglioma was qualified as anaplastic due to increased cellularity, nuclear atypia, and mitotic activity in the glial component (Figure 2).

Due to the highly aggressive nature of AGG, a compromise was reached between prolonging gestation and delaying further treatment. At 34 6/7 weeks, a viable 2800 gram male infant was born via cesarean delivery with Apgar scores of 7 and 8 at one and five minutes, respectively. Eleven weeks after the initial resection and five weeks after delivery, the patient underwent the second operative phase consisting of an awake-craniotomy with neuronavigation. There was complete gross resection of residual tumor, except for a small portion attached to the anterior cerebral artery.

Intensity modulated radiotherapy to the brain was initiated two weeks after the operation. The patient underwent 2 Gy external beam radiotherapy in thirty sessions for a total of 60 Gy. She then completed twelve cycles of adjuvant temozolomide with excellent tolerability. The patient is now two years status post-initial tumor resection. She has no neurologic sequelae; however, her latest MRI showed continued slow growth of an enhancing 1.7 cm left frontal calvarium lesion. The clinical significance is yet undetermined. Her

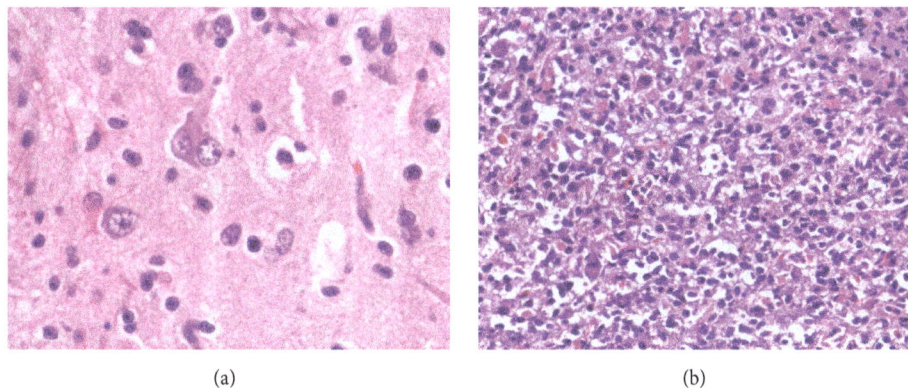

FIGURE 2: H&E stain shows a biphasic neoplasm characterized by dysplastic ganglion cells, including binucleate forms ((a) 400x magnification), and a hypercellular malignant glial component with nuclear atypia and increased mitotic activity ((b) 200x magnification).

infant required hospitalization in the neonatal intensive care unit for 19 days due to feeding difficulties prior to discharge but is currently doing well.

3. Discussion

Headache is a very common patient complaint, but new onset or worsening headaches in a pregnant woman should raise concern. A broad differential must be considered and include common etiologies, such as migraines, tension, or cluster type headaches, as well as pregnancy specific causes like preeclampsia. Other rarer and often grave etiologies should also be entertained, including intracranial hemorrhage, cerebral venous sinus thrombosis, infectious meningitis/encephalitis, and brain tumors.

Glial tumors diagnosed in pregnancy are rare, mostly being reported in case series or case reports, and have a decreased incidence compared to age matched nonpregnant counterparts [1]. Yust-Katz et al. performed a retrospective review at The MD Anderson Cancer Center over seventeen years and found only ten patients diagnosed with gliomas while pregnant and an additional five diagnosed in the immediate postpartum period, none of whom had AGG [10]. A 2017 case series reviewed 75 cases of pregnant women in whom new onset glioma developed: 42 women had high grade gliomas, none with AGG, and there were seven maternal deaths. They note that all types of antitumor therapy, including surgical resection, chemotherapy, and radiation, have been safely applied during pregnancy, but consideration must be given to the gestational age and maternal symptoms at time of presentation [11].

GG is a rare glial-neuronal brain tumor characterized by neoplastic glial cells and dysplastic neuronal cells. According to the recently revised fourth edition of the World Health Organization (WHO) Classification of Tumors of the CNS, GG is considered to be WHO Grade I neoplasm [5]. The criteria for Grade II designation are not well defined, but tumors that demonstrate overt malignant features like increased cellularity, nuclear atypia, and mitotic activity, typically in the glial component, are classified as a Grade III AGG [5].

There is a single report of a woman diagnosed with a WHO Grade I GG prior to becoming pregnant who had accelerated tumor growth during pregnancy [3]. Similar findings have been reported in women harboring gliomas, including one study, gathered from a multi-institutional database, of eleven women with Grade II diffuse gliomas who experienced significant increase in the velocity of diametric tumor expansion during pregnancy [2]. Complications secondary to accelerated tumor growth, compounded by dramatic physiologic changes of pregnancy, increase the risk of adverse outcomes and underscore the importance of timely diagnosis [4]. Pregnancy should not delay appropriate diagnostic testing in the workup of patients with headache nor should it delay management of pregnant patients diagnosed with a brain tumor.

To our knowledge, the English literature has only one report of a low grade GG initially diagnosed during pregnancy [7] and two cases of AGG diagnosed in the postpartum period [8, 9], but our patient is the first report of an AGG diagnosed during pregnancy. The patient presented with headaches, a common complaint with a broad differential. This case underscores the importance of timely diagnostic imaging in pregnant women and demonstrates subtotal tumor debulking as a viable means of prolonging gestation. As was the case in our patient, a collaborative approach to management of brain tumors in pregnancy should involve multiple specialties, such as maternal-fetal medicine, neurosurgery, and obstetrics, to optimize patient care and minimize risks to the fetus and mother.

Disclosure

Matthew J. Bicocca, M.D., lead author of this manuscript, affirms that this manuscript is an honest, accurate, and transparent account of the data being reported and that no important aspects of the literature have been omitted.

References

[1] J. F. Haas, W. Jänisch, and W. Staneczek, "Newly diagnosed primary intracranial neoplasms in pregnant women: A population-based assessment," *Journal of Neurology, Neurosurgery & Psychiatry*, vol. 49, no. 8, pp. 874–880, 1986.

[2] J. Pallud, E. Mandonnet, C. Deroulers et al., "Pregnancy increases the growth rates of World Health Organization grade II gliomas," *Annals of Neurology*, vol. 67, no. 3, pp. 398–404, 2010.

[3] S. Knafo, S. Goutagny, and J. Pallud, "Increased growth rate of a WHO grade i ganglioglioma during pregnancy," *British Journal of Neurosurgery*, vol. 27, no. 1, pp. 119–121, 2013.

[4] A. R. Terry, F. G. Barker, L. Leffert, B. T. Bateman, I. Souter, and S. R. Plotkin, "Outcomes of hospitalization in pregnant women with CNS neoplasms: A populationbased study," *Neuro-Oncology*, vol. 14, no. 6, pp. 768–776, 2012.

[5] D. N. Louis, A. Perry, G. Reifenberger et al., "The 2016 World Health Organization Classification of Tumors of the Central Nervous System: a summary," *Acta Neuropathologica*, vol. 131, no. 6, pp. 803–820, 2016.

[6] S. K. Selvanathan, S. Hammouche, H. J. Salminen, and M. D. Jenkinson, "Outcome and prognostic features in anaplastic ganglioglioma: Analysis of cases from the SEER database," *Journal of Neuro-Oncology*, vol. 105, no. 3, pp. 539–545, 2011.

[7] V. M. Ravindra, J. A. Braca, R. L. Jensen, and E. A. M. Duckworth, "Management of intracranial pathology during pregnancy: Case example and review of management strategies," *Surgical Neurology International*, vol. 6, no. 1, article no. 43, 2015.

[8] J. J. Rodríguez-Uranga, E. Franco-Macías, F. Delgado-López, and D. Chinchón-Espino, "The onset of an anaplastic ganglioglioma during the post-natal period with signs of toxemia of pregnancy," *Revista de Neurología*, vol. 37, no. 5, pp. 438–440, 2003.

[9] S. Pikis, T. Petrosyan, K. Diamantopoulou, and C. Kelesis, "Anaplastic ganglioglioma becoming symptomatic in the third trimester of pregnancy," *International Journal of Reproduction, Contraception, Obstetrics and Gynecology*, vol. 6, no. 3, p. 1158, 2017.

[10] S. Yust-Katz, M. D. Anderson, D. Liu et al., "Clinical and prognostic features of adult patients with gangliogliomas," *Neuro-Oncology*, vol. 16, no. 3, pp. 409–413, 2014.

[11] H. Zwinkels, J. Dörr, F. Kloet, M. J. B. Taphoorn, and C. J. Vecht, "Pregnancy in women with gliomas: A case-series and review of the literature," *Journal of Neuro-Oncology*, vol. 115, no. 2, pp. 293–301, 2013.

3

Uterine Rupture at 21 Weeks in Twin Pregnancy with TTTS and Previous C-Section

Gieta Bhikha-kori, Marieke Sueters, and Johanna M. Middeldorp

Fetal Therapy, Department of Obstetrics, Leiden University Medical Center, Leiden, Netherlands

Correspondence should be addressed to Gieta Bhikha-kori; bgieta@yahoo.com

Academic Editor: Michael Geary

Uterine rupture is a health problem in every country. The diagnosis is not always obvious and fetal and maternal morbidity and mortality can be high.

1. Introduction

Uterine rupture is defined as the complete disruption of all uterine layers, including the serosa. Undiagnosed and untreated, this is a life-threatening complication for mother and fetus. Other adverse outcomes related to uterine rupture are bladder laceration, severe hemorrhage, hysterectomy, and neonatal morbidity related to intrauterine hypoxia.

A large majority of uterine rupture occurs in the setting of a vaginal birth after caesarean (VBAC), resulting in intrapartum injury and spontaneous rupture of a gravid uterus. Out of hospital trauma represents the remainder of etiologies for uterine rupture. Motor vehicle accidents, domestic violence, and falls are the most common causes of blunt trauma during pregnancy.

The incidence of C-section in 2010 was 25.2% in North Europe and 32% in the United States. The C-section rate in the Netherlands increased from 7.4% in 1990 to 16.3% in 2012 [1, 2].

The incidence of uterine rupture in women with a previous C-section is 0.2–1.5% [3–9]. The incidence in the Netherlands was 0.64% in the period of 2004 till 2006 [10].

Several factors are known to increase the risk of uterine rupture. Contractions in spontaneous labor and the induction and augmentation of labor are the most important. Other known factors are maternal age, advanced gestational age, birth weight > 4000 gram, and interpregnancy interval < 18–24 months [9–12]. Twin pregnancy should also be considered a risk factor [13, 14].

Here we report a case of uterine rupture at 21 weeks of gestation in a patient with a previous C-section and currently pregnant with a monochorionic twin pregnancy complicated by twin to twin transfusion syndrome (TTTS) and premature contractions.

Besides TTTS polyhydramnion can be a risk factor for developing an uterine rupture.

2. Case

A 33-year-old woman was referred to our tertiary center (Leiden University Medical Center, the national referral center for fetal therapy in the Netherlands), because of a monochorionic pregnancy complicated by TTTS. In her obstetrical history she had a HELLP syndrome and intrauterine growth restriction and a C-section at 31 + 2 weeks of gestation.

In the current pregnancy she had prenatal screening with no associated high risk and an advanced structural echo with no abnormalities. For further summarization of the pregnancy, see Table 1.

At gestation of 21 + 5 the patient became anxious and hypotensive, with a blood pressure of 60/30 mm Hg and a pulse of 105 beats per minute.

At examination the uterus was tense on palpation with no signs of contractions. Ultrasound examination revealed two vital fetuses with a normal adjacent lying placenta. Again, some intraperitoneal free fluid was seen. At vaginal examination no vaginal blood loss was seen and the cervix

TABLE 1

Gestational age (weeks)	Symptoms	Physical/plan
12	Pain in her lower abdomen	Ultrasound examination: some free fluid was seen beside the uterus and a small hematoma in the fundus of the uterus. The explanation for the free fluid was thought to be a corpus luteum bleeding.
16	Trauma, fall on right side of her abdomen	In ultrasound examination some free fluid was seen intraperitoneally. Hemoglobin level was 8.85 g/dl.
21 + 2	Presentation with vaginal bleeding	The ultrasound was normal and no signs of TTTS were seen; the cervical length was 15–17 mm.
21 + 3	There was an increase in contractions and pain	A threatening TTTS Quintero stage 1 was diagnosed: fetus 1 showed a deepest vertical pocket (DVP) of amniotic fluid of 79 mm and fetus 2 a DVP 19 mm. Stomach and bladder filling were present in both fetuses and Dopplers were normal. The cervical length was 15 mm. There was not yet an indication for fetoscopic laser coagulation of the vascular anastomosis. Tocolysis with indomethacin was started.
21 + 4	There was minimum of painless brown vaginal bleeding	Ultrasound examination showed signs of TTTS Quintero stage 1, with a DVP of 10 cm in fetus 1 and a DVP of 1.9 cm in fetus 2. Stomach and bladder filling were normal in both fetuses as were the Dopplers. There was an anterior localization of the placenta. Because of TTTS Quintero 1 with cervical shortening a laser procedure was planned for the next day.
21 + 5		See further.

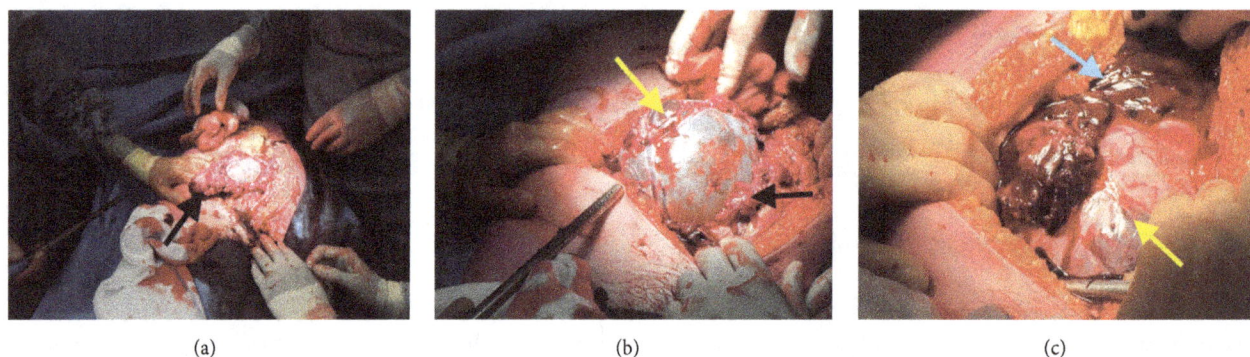

(a)   (b)   (c)

FIGURE 1: Laparotomy: after midline incision the uterus rupture on the right side with the bulging amniotic sac was visible (yellow arrows), the placenta partially protruding on the edges of the rupture wound (black arrows) with blood clots in the free abdominal cavity (blue arrow).

was 1 cm dilated. Also a fluid challenge of 2 liter ringers solution and natrium chloride was given. The hemoglobin count was 7.8 (9.1) g/dl, prothrombin time slightly prolonged (16.1 seconds), and fibrinogen was normal (3.3 g/L). The differential diagnosis was threatening labor or uterine rupture or abruption.

An epidural for pain relief was given and the dilatation progressed to 2 cm.

Hemodynamically the patient continued to be compromised (RR 100/60 and pulse 120); despite a fluid challenge (now in total 4,5 L ringers and natrium chloride solution alternately) the Glasgow coma scale (GCS) was 15/15. Furthermore she developed fever (38,1 Celsius), for which antibiotics were administered.

The differential diagnosis was broad: uterine rupture, infected hematoma, or intrauterine infection. A CT abdomen was planned. Before transportation to the radiology department the patient became acutely instable with loss of consciousness, a very low blood pressure of 60/30, and a high pulse rate of 150 beats per minute. Laparotomy was planned immediately.

Explorative laparotomy was conducted through a midline incision. A uterine rupture at the right side of the uterine scar was diagnosed with necrotic/fibrotic wound edges, the placenta was partially protruding on the edges, and two dead fetuses were born (Figures 1(a), 1(b), and 1(c)). The insertion of the placenta was not in the scar. There were no signs of placenta percreta.

The rupture was closed in 2 layers with a total blood loss of 4000 ml. Transfusion of 10 packed cells and 2 units of fresh frozen plasma was given. During the procedure platelet count was 131, the prothrombin time (PT) was 17.0 seconds (slightly prolonged) and the fibrinogen was 1.8 g/L (low).

After operation the patient recovered gradually. She was discharged seven days after laparotomy. Hemoglobin was 8.37 g/dl at dismission.

3. Discussion

In monochronic twin pregnancies there is a 10–15% chance of developing TTTS.

Very little has been published on uterine ruptures in TTTS pregnancies, as this is the third case since 2004. In 2004 Tutscheck [15] reported a uterine rupture in a twin pregnancy with TTTS at a gestational age of 19 weeks. This case report describes a uterine rupture in a patient with a C-section through a corporal incision in the obstetric history [15].

The second case report from Smid in 2015 describes a 42-year-old woman, with a C-section in her obstetric history, with a posterior uterine rupture at 21 weeks of gestation with stage 1 TTTS [16].

Also dichorionic twin pregnancies can be complicated by uterine rupture.

Greenwald et al. described a case of asymptomatic uterine dehiscence in the second trimester of a dichorionic twin pregnancy diagnosed at 19 weeks with ultrasound [17]. The other case report was from Lana Saciragic who described a postpartum diagnosed uterine rupture after vaginal delivery of a dichorionic twin at 32 weeks of an unscarred uterus [18].

In our case the hypothesis is that at the gestational age of 16 weeks there already was a small dehiscence, explaining the free fluid seen at ultrasound investigation. Also at 12 weeks there is a great suspicion that the dehiscence was present if we look at the free fluid at ultrasound investigation and complaint of pain in the lower abdomen. This dehiscence grew while the gestation progressed, and the premature contractions in combination with the polyhydramnion due to TTTS augmented this process into a uterine rupture.

The first signs were already present at 12 weeks. The first change in the maternal condition was the hypotension, progressing to shock in hours ahead.

The free fluid beside the uterus with a normal condition of fetuses did not raise the suspicion of a uterine rupture at first, although it was in our differential diagnosis. The reassuring condition of the fetuses especially did not plead for uterine rupture, and the focus was on threatening labour or an abruption placentae. Fever raised the suspicion of an infection. This created the delay in the diagnosis because of this peculiar presentation of this case. The acute hypotension with loss of consciousness was a clear indication of an acute incident very suspicious for an uterine rupture, followed by a laparotomy.

Multiple signs/symptoms can precede a uterine rupture; these are abdominal pain (69%), fetal heart rate abnormalities (67%) [9, 10], vaginal bleeding (27%), hypertonia of the uterus (20%), and abrupt cessation of contractions (14%) [10]. In most cases the combination of abdominal pain and fetal heart rate abnormalities is present [9–11].

In our case there was hypertonia of the uterus with 2 vital fetuses and signs of contractions and vaginal blood loss.

The risk factors for uterine rupture in our case were a C-section in the obstetric history at preterm gestation of 31 weeks, a twin pregnancy, and TTTS with polyhydramnion. With preterm C-section there would be probably a corporal incision because a lower uterine segment has not been developed. The necrotic/fibrotic wound edges indicate a chronic process, as we did not see signs of an infection. An explanation is that the scar defect was present for a longer time but not bleeding actively and that this scar defect got bigger as a result of TTTS and polyhydramnion.

What we have to learn from this case is that TTTS with polyhydramnion (with or without contractions) can be a risk factor for uterine rupture. We know that 80.5% of uterine ruptures occur in women with a trial of labour [10]. The presence of contractions (and the loss of it acutely) is not always necessary to consider uterine rupture as a diagnosis, as a "silent" rupture can occur in women with TTTS and polyhydramnion without contractions. In fact, in every case of spacious uterine distention we have to keep a uterine rupture in mind.

4. Conclusion

Uterine rupture is one of the rare complications of TTTS that can appear in a twin pregnancy, especially when other risk factors such as a uterine scar, with or without contractions, are present. Also polyhydramnion in the setting of the TTTS should be considered a risk factor. Furthermore, as we know of earlier reported cases [17], we also have to consider uterine dehiscence in women with a uterine scar and TTTS.

Consent

Patient consent was provided.

References

[1] Netherlands Perinatal Registry (PRN), "Perinatal care in the Netherlands 2007," Utrecht, Netherlands, 2009.

[2] H. A. A. Brouwers, H. W. Bruinse, J. Dijs-Elsinga et al., "The Netherlands perinatal registry trends 1999-2012".

[3] J. M. Guise, M. Berlin, M. Mc Donagh, P. Osterweil, and B. Chan, "Helfland M: safety of vaginal birth after cesarean: a systematic review," Obstet Gynacol, 2004.

[4] M. B. Landon, C. Y. Spong, E. Thom et al., "Risk of uterine rupture with a trial of labor in women with multiple and single prior cesarean delivery," Obstetrics and Gynecology, vol. 108, no. 1, pp. 12–20, 2006.

[5] M. B. Landon, J. C. Hauth, K. J. Leveno et al., "Maternal and perinataal outcomes associated with a trial of labor after prior cesarean delivery," The New England Journal of Medicine, vol. 351, no. 25, pp. 2581–2589, 2004.

[6] A. Kwee, M. L. Bots, G. H. Visser, and H. W. Bruinse, "Obstetric management and outcome of pregnancy in women with a history of caesarean section in the Netherlands," European Journal of Obstetrics & Gynecology and Reproductive Biology, vol. 132, no. 2, pp. 171–176, 2007.

[7] J. Jang, "P25.15: Uterine rupture following uterine artery embolisation due to retained placenta," Ultrasound in Obstetrics & Gynecology, vol. 44, no. S1, pp. 335-335, 2014.

[8] J. Guise, J. Hashima, and P. Osterweil, "Evidence-based vaginal birth after Caesarean section," Best Practice & Research Clinical Obstetrics & Gynaecology, vol. 19, no. 1, pp. 117–130, 2005.

[9] J. Guise, "Systematic review of the incidence and consequences of uterine rupture in women with previous caesarean section," BMJ, vol. 329, no. 7456, pp. 19–25, 2004.

[10] J. J. Zwart, J. M. Richters, F. Öry, J. I. P. De Vries, K. W. M. Bloemenkamp, and J. Van Roosmalen, "Uterine rupture in the Netherlands: a nationwide population-based cohort study," *BJOG*, vol. 116, no. 8, pp. 1069–1078, 2009.

[11] Green Top Guideline, no. 45, Oktober, 2015.

[12] M. B. Landon, "Predicting uterine rupture in women undergoing trial of labor after prior cesarean delivery," *Seminars in Perinatology*, vol. 34, no. 4, pp. 267–271, 2010.

[13] M. F. Mazzone and J. Woolever, "Uterine rupture in a patient with an unscarred uterus: A case study," *Wisconsin Medical Journal*, vol. 105, no. 2, pp. 64–66, 2006.

[14] C. M. Tarney, P. Whitecar, M. Sewell, and L. Grubish, "Hope E: rupture of an unscarred uterus in a quadruplet pregnancy," *Obstet Gynecol*, 2013.

[15] B. Tutschek, K. Hecher, T. Somville, and H. G. Bender, "Twin-to-twin transfusion syndrome complicated by spontaneous mid-trimester uterine rupture," *Journal of Perinatal Medicine*, vol. 32, no. 1, pp. 95–97, 2004.

[16] M. Smid, R. Waltner-Toews, and W. Goodnight, "Spontaneous posterior uterine rupture in twin-twin transfusion syndrome," *American Journal of Perinatology Reports*, vol. 06, no. 1, pp. 68–70, 2016.

[17] S. R. Greenwald, J. M. Gonzalez, R. G. Goldstein, and M. G. Rosenstein, "Asymptomatic uterine dehiscence in a second-trimester twin pregnancy," *American Journal of Obstetrics and Gynecology*, vol. 213, no. 4, pp. 590–590.e2, 2015.

[18] L. Saciragic, S. Mehdizadeh, Y. Amankwah, and S. Singh, "Spontaneous uterine rupture of an unscarred uterus in a twin pregnancy," *Journal of Obstetrics and Gynaecology Canada*, vol. 37, no. 5, p. 391, 2015.

4

A Case of Sevoflurane Use during Pregnancy in the Management of Persistent Status Asthmaticus

Jessica Parrott,[1] **Mitch Tener,**[2] **Katie Dennis,**[3] **Matthew Sharpe,**[2] **and Cecily Clark-Ganheart**[1]

[1]*Division of Maternal Fetal Medicine, Department of Obstetrics and Gynecology, University of Kansas School of Medicine, 3901 Rainbow Boulevard, Kansas City, KS 66160, USA*

[2]*Department of Pulmonary and Critical Care Medicine, University of Kansas School of Medicine, 3901 Rainbow Boulevard, Kansas City, KS 66160, USA*

[3]*Department of Pathology and Laboratory Medicine, University of Kansas School of Medicine, 3901 Rainbow Boulevard, Kansas City, KS 66160, USA*

Correspondence should be addressed to Jessica Parrott; jparrott3@kumc.edu

Academic Editor: Svein Rasmussen

Background. Sevoflurane is rarely used for the treatment of status asthmaticus. We report a case of sevoflurane hepatotoxicity in pregnancy with presentation similar to HELLP syndrome. *Case*. A G2P1001 at 23 weeks in status asthmaticus presented with pCO2 > 130 and pH < 7. She was nonresponsive to traditional therapy. Sevoflurane was added for a 24 hr period. Respiratory status improved. Extubation occurred on day 12. Workup for preeclampsia spectrum disorders occurred due to maternal hypertension. Given the atypical presentation and hepatotoxicity, a liver biopsy was performed. Histologic features suggested drug induced hepatic injury. Liver function subsequently normalized. She delivered a term neonate without short-term complications. *Conclusion*. The use of sevoflurane is a treatment option of status asthmaticus during pregnancy. Providers should be aware of the potential for hepatotoxicity.

1. Introduction

Status asthmaticus is a severe asthma exacerbation that is refractory to bronchodilator and corticosteroid treatment. Standard treatment often employed includes nebulized bronchodilators, magnesium, corticosteroids, and mechanical ventilation. Additional considerations, although rarely used, include sedatives, neuromuscular blockade, or inhaled anesthetics [1]. Case reports of sevoflurane use in emergency departments and the pediatric population exist for the treatment of status asthmaticus prior to extracorporeal membrane oxygenation (ECMO) [2]. However, data regarding the use during pregnancy is limited. Matters are further complicated by the potential of hepatotoxicity with use of halogenated inhaled anesthetics. With informed patient consent, we present a case of refractory status asthmaticus during pregnancy with resultant hepatotoxicity.

2. Case

A 31-year-old, gravida 2 para 1001, patient was transferred to our medical ICU at 23 2/7 weeks of gestation with status asthmaticus complicated by acute hypercarbic respiratory failure. She was intubated and paralyzed with a pH < 7.0 and pCO2 > 130. The picture was further complicated by marked bronchoconstriction with elevated PEEP and increased airway resistance nonresponsive to nebulized beta agonists, glucocorticoid, magnesium, and epinephrine treatments. She was initially stabilized on continuous nebulizers, magnesium, propofol, ketamine, and inhaled helium-oxygen (heliox) mixture. Due to persistent difficulty with oxygenation and limited ventilation over a 24-hour period, ECMO was considered: during this time, the patient's oxygen saturation was 85–94% with arterial pH 6.8–7.2. However, due to the potential complications associated with ECMO use during

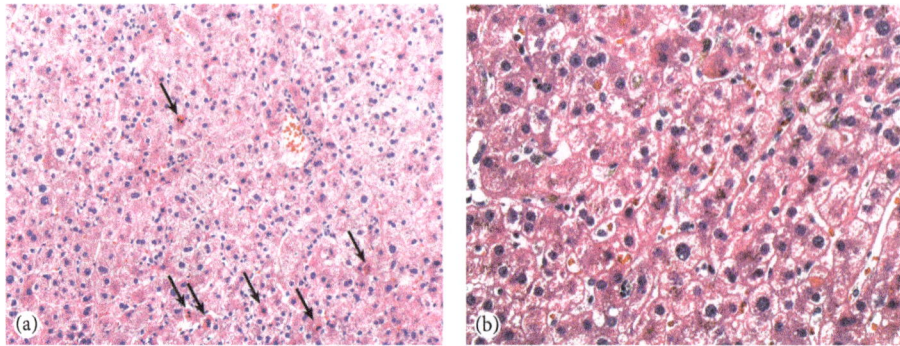

FIGURE 1: Liver biopsy. (a) Hematoxylin and eosin ×20: liver biopsy specimen showing lobular disarray with numerous apoptotic hepatocytes (arrows) and increased sinusoidal inflammatory cells. No steatosis or frank necrosis is present. (b) Hematoxylin and eosin ×40: liver biopsy specimen showing lobular disarray, prominent apoptotic hepatocytes, and biliary stasis, compatible with recent drug induced liver injury.

pregnancy, a decision was made to add an inhaled anesthetic for its bronchodilator effects. The patient was transitioned to an anesthesia ventilator system that could provide heliox with inhaled anesthetic. Sevoflurane was initiated, allowing us to lower our peak pressures and maintain oxygen saturations >95%. During this time, the patient was noted to have elevated blood pressure (137–166/70–82 mmHg) requiring intravenous treatment. A 24-hour urine protein was found to be elevated at 739 mg. On review of the patient's previous records, it was determined that the patient was likely a chronic hypertensive with history of antihypertensive medication use and no further workup was undertaken.

Over the next 24 hours, the patient was noted to have improved oxygenation and the sevoflurane was discontinued. She was transitioned back to a traditional ventilator. She remained hypercapnic but maintained a normal pH while on heliox, steroids, propofol, and ketamine. The following day, the patient was noted to have an acute rise in her liver enzymes with an AST of 91 U/L and ALT of 32 U/L; platelets at that time were 243 K/UL. The liver enzymes were noted to progressively rise over the next 10 days while the platelet count remained normal (196–316 K/UL).

The patient's respiratory status continued to slowly improve during this time as she was weaned off of the paralytic, corticosteroids, and ketamine. We were able to decrease her peak pressures and elevated PEEP. She was ultimately extubated on hospital day 10. Due to altered mental status, she was reintubated. CT head was negative. Her laboratory evaluation at that time showed AST 161 U/L, ALT 329 U/L, Cr 0.28 mg/dL, Hgb 9.4 g/dL, Plt 261 K/UL, LDH 1029 U/L, and 24-hour urine protein 1245 mg. Diagnosis of atypical hemolysis, elevated liver enzymes, and low platelet count syndrome (HELLP syndrome) was considered a possibility. However, due to her periviable gestational age, hematology and hepatology were consulted to rule out other potential etiologies. An extensive autoimmune and infectious workup was done that included antinuclear antibody, anti-mitochondrial antibody, anti-smooth muscle antibody, ADAMTS-13, acute and chronic hepatitis panels, Epstein-Barr virus, cytomegalovirus, herpes simplex virus, and human herpes virus 6, all of which were unremarkable. Of

note, the maternal Rhesus status was negative. Given that maternal blood transfusion did not occur, Rh incompatibility was unlikely to explain the maternal findings. Abdominal ultrasound was performed and noted to be within normal limits. The patient was reextubated 2 days later.

On hospital day 15, the patient's AST peaked at 1146 U/L and ALT peaked at 3168 U/L. Alkaline phosphatase and total bilirubin remained within normal limits. A liver biopsy showed acute hepatitis with prominent apoptotic hepatocytes, cholestasis, and increased sinusoidal inflammatory cells (Figure 1). Immunostains for herpes simplex virus I and II and in situ hybridization for Epstein-Barr virus were negative. There was no significant steatosis or fibrosis, frank necrosis, or fibrin deposition. Given the absence of features of an underlying chronic liver disease and a negative viral and autoimmune hepatitis workup, the findings were consistent with acute drug induced liver injury, most likely due to sevoflurane exposure. Her respiratory status continued to improve and she was discharged from the hospital. No additional episodes of hypertension were noted. Liver enzymes returned to normal over a two-month period (AST 16 U/L and ALT 7 U/L) and repeat 24-hour urine protein was 188 mg two months after the episode. With prolonged periods of maternal hypoxia during the initial 24 hours of hospitalization, there was concern for fetal hypoxic encephalopathy. However, a fetal MRI performed four weeks after the inciting maternal event failed to demonstrate evidence of hypoxic insult. The patient was induced at term due to new-onset oligohydramnios. A healthy term neonate was delivered via spontaneous vaginal delivery without short-term complications despite prolonged maternal hypoxia, acidemia, and permissive hypercarbia.

3. Discussion

Severe, acute asthma generally leads to significant air trapping, hyperinflation, decreased venous return, and potentially detrimental hemodynamic consequences. The mainstay of treatment revolves around the administration of inhaled bronchodilators and systemic glucocorticoids. The decision to intubate a patient with a severe asthma exacerbation is based upon clinical judgment in conjunction with arterial blood gas measurement. As a general rule, if the patient demonstrates progressive fatigue, continued work of breathing, or alterations in consciousness, intubation is indicated [3]. These patients often will also require deep sedation and paralysis to prevent further complications. In life-threatening exacerbations, such as the patient presented here, nontraditional therapies may be utilized. This can include a helium-oxygen mixture to decrease airflow resistance, magnesium sulfate for bronchodilatory effects, ketamine for potential bronchodilatory effects, or inhalational anesthetics [3]. The mechanism of action for inhaled anesthetics is unclear, but it is thought that these agents have direct bronchodilatory effects on the airways and an increase in cholinergic tone. Halothane, isoflurane, and sevoflurane have been shown to be effective in case reports [2]. Hypotension is usually the limiting factor with use of these agents and bronchoconstriction can be seen after discontinuation of the medications. Additionally, when maternal ventilation is suboptimal, a concern for fetal hypoxemia exists. In our case, particularly due to gestational age, our focus was improving maternal ventilation as opposed to delivery of a periviable neonate. While cordocentesis is an option to assess fetal oxygen saturation, we felt the clinical benefit would be minimal in this situation. Additionally, in the presence of maternal academia, the fetal oxygen disassociation curve would experience a left-ward shift allowing for increased amounts of oxygen delivery to the neonate despite fetal acidosis.

HELLP syndrome, a disorder marked by hemolysis, elevated liver enzymes, and low platelets, has a typical onset in the third trimester. It can be difficult to differentiate HELLP syndrome from other disease processes due to multiorgan involvement. The differential diagnoses include acute fatty liver of pregnancy, thrombotic thrombocytopenic purpura, hemolytic uremic syndrome, systemic lupus erythematosus, and antiphospholipid syndrome [4]. At this gestational age, maternal mortality is reported at ~1% with perinatal mortality rate of 7–22% [5]. Rare case reports of HELLP syndrome occurring at periviable gestational age have been reported in the literature [6–9], all associated with triploidy, molar pregnancy, or antiphospholipid syndrome. It is important to ensure that the diagnosis of HELLP syndrome is accurate during the periviable period as it has significant implications on pregnancy outcome. Continuing the pregnancy may result in significant maternal morbidity/mortality with severe end organ damage but treatment requires delivery of a fetus who will require a prolonged NICU admission and will face high rates of morbidity and mortality. As such, when a patient presents with hepatic dysfunction at an early gestational age, a thorough assessment of hepatotoxicity should include consideration of disorders beyond the spectrum of hypertensive disorders of pregnancy. Furthermore, evaluation via liver biopsy may assist with making an accurate diagnosis and guiding appropriate treatment.

In our case, a thorough evaluation by hepatology and hematology was performed, including a negative viral and autoimmune workup. Eventually a liver biopsy was performed, and the histologic features were consistent with drug induced livery injury. The typical findings of HELLP syndrome including frank necrosis, periportal hemorrhage, and fibrin deposition were not observed [5]. Sevoflurane, the halogenated inhaled anesthetic used to treat the patient's status asthmaticus, was the presumed inciting agent. Review of the literature has rare reports of sevoflurane-associated hepatotoxicity, primarily in Japanese literature [10]. The patient's overall state of persistent acidosis likely made her more susceptible to hepatotoxicity. Older halogenated anesthetics cause hepatotoxicity via production of trifluoroacetic acid (TFA) that subsequently produce trifluoroacetylated components and cause an immunogenic response in the patient, resulting in hepatitis. Compared to these older halogenated anesthetics, sevoflurane has low hepatotoxic potential as it is metabolized into hexafluoroisopropanol (HFIP) rather than TFA. HFIP has less protein binding capacity, does not accumulate, and is rapidly converted into a stable nontoxic compound that is excreted in the urine. Ultimately, its low hepatotoxic potential makes it the preferred inhaled anesthetic for patients with hepatic disease or at risk for postoperative hepatic injury; however, the risk of hepatotoxicity from TFA still exists [11].

The use of sevoflurane for the treatment of persistent status asthmaticus is an option during pregnancy. Should failure of traditional therapy occur, the addition of sevoflurane has the potential to improve the patient's clinical course. Practitioners should remain aware of the potential of hepatotoxicity, particularly in the presence of acidosis.

References

[1] D. Elsayegh and J. M. Shapiro, "Management of the obstetric patient with status asthmaticus," *Journal of Intensive Care Medicine*, vol. 23, no. 6, pp. 396–402, 2008.

[2] D. Schutte, A. M. Zwitserloot, R. Houmes, M. De Hoog, J. M. Draaisma, and J. Lemson, "Sevoflurane therapy for life-threatening asthma in children," *British Journal of Anaesthesia*, vol. 111, no. 6, pp. 967–970, 2013.

[3] M. Oddo, F. Feihl, M.-D. Schaller, and C. Perret, "Management of mechanical ventilation in acute severe asthma: practical aspects," *Intensive Care Medicine*, vol. 32, no. 4, pp. 501–510, 2006.

[4] O. Pourrat, R. Coudroy, and F. Pierre, "Differentiation between severe HELLP syndrome and thrombotic microangiopathy, thrombotic thrombocytopenic purpura and other imitators," *European Journal of Obstetrics & Gynecology and Reproductive Biology*, vol. 189, pp. 68–72, 2015.

[5] N. M. Lee and C. W. Brady, "Liver disease in pregnancy," *World Journal of Gastroenterology*, vol. 15, no. 8, pp. 897–906, 2009.

[6] E. Myer and J. Hill, "First trimester hemolysis, elevated liver enzymes, low platelets syndrome in a surrogate pregnancy," *American Journal of Perinatology Reports*, vol. 5, pp. e212–e214, 2015.

[7]   E. Bornstein, Y. Barnhard, R. Atkin, and M. Y. Divon, "HELLP syndrome: a rare, early presentation at 17 weeks of gestation," *Obstetrics and Gynecology*, vol. 110, no. 2, pp. 525–527, 2007.

[8]   T. Stefos, N. Plachouras, G. Mari, E. Cosmi, and D. Lolis, "A case of partial mole and atypical type I triploidy associated with severe HELLP syndrome at 18 weeks' gestation," *Ultrasound in Obstetrics and Gynecology*, vol. 20, no. 4, pp. 403–404, 2002.

[9]   K. Haram, J. Trovik, P. M. Sandset, and K. Hordnes, "Severe syndrome of hemolysis, elevated liver enzymes and low platelets (HELLP) in the 18th week of pregnancy associated with the antiphospholipid-antibody syndrome," *Acta Obstetricia et Gynecologica Scandinavica*, vol. 82, no. 7, pp. 679–680, 2003.

[10] Y. Jang and I. Kim, "Severe hepatotoxicity after sevoflurane anesthesia in a child with mild renal dysfunction," *Paediatric Anaesthesia*, vol. 15, pp. 1140–1144, 2005.

[11] S. Safari, M. Motavaf, S. A. S. Siamdoust, and S. M. Alavian, "Hepatotoxicity of halogenated inhalational anesthetics," *Iranian Red Crescent Medical Journal*, vol. 16, no. 9, Article ID e20153, 2014.

5

The Cytoreductive Effect of Radiotherapy for Small Cell Ovarian Carcinoma of the Pulmonary Type

Shuhei Terada (ⓘ), **Takashi Suzuki, Akihiro Hasegawa,
Satoru Nakayama, and Hiroshi Adachi**

Department of Gynecology, Seirei Hamamatsu General Hospital, 2-12-12 Sumiyoshi, Naka-ku, Hamamatsu, Shizuoka 430-8558, Japan

Correspondence should be addressed to Shuhei Terada; shuheiterada@gmail.com

Academic Editor: Maria Grazia Porpora

Small cell ovarian carcinoma of the pulmonary type is a rare and highly aggressive tumor for which a suitable treatment strategy has not been established. A 45-year-old woman presented with abdominal swelling, and primary ovarian carcinoma was suspected. The postoperative pathological diagnosis was small cell ovarian carcinoma of the pulmonary type. She also had complicated grade 1 endometrioid carcinoma of the uterine corpus. Three courses of cisplatin and etoposide therapy were administered as adjuvant chemotherapy. Because the tumor was chemotherapy resistant, she underwent palliative abdominal irradiation at a dose of 26 Gy in 13 fractions, which induced cytoreduction and provided symptomatic relief. She died 4 months after surgery. Lactate dehydrogenase was a useful tumor marker during treatment. Here, we present an extremely rare case of a patient with small cell ovarian carcinoma of the pulmonary type treated with radiotherapy after surgery and chemotherapy.

1. Introduction

Small cell ovarian carcinoma pulmonary type (SCOCPT) is defined as a small cell carcinoma that resembles a neuroendocrine type of pulmonary small cell carcinoma. Most patients with SCOCPT are postmenopausal and present with symptoms such as a pelvic or abdominal mass. SCOCPTs are highly aggressive neoplasms, which usually present at an advanced stage, and the overall prognosis is poor. Only 26 cases of SCOCPT have been reported in the literature, and most patients have typically been treated with surgery followed by chemotherapy. Palliative brain irradiation was administered to control seizures in the previous report [1], but the cytoreductive effect of radiotherapy on the primary lesions is unknown. Here we present a case in which a patient with chemotherapy-resistant SCOCPT underwent abdominal radiotherapy. We describe the outcomes of the radiotherapy and also present evidence on lactate dehydrogenase (LDH) potentially acting as a good tumor marker during the course of treatment.

2. Case Presentation

A 45-year-old woman (gravida 1, para 1) presented at our hospital with abdominal swelling. She had undergone laser ablation of cervical intraepithelial neoplasia 3 (CIN3) 12 years previously. She had a family history of paternal prostate cancer. Physical examination showed a large solid tumor in her pelvic region. Abdominal magnetic resonance imaging (MRI) identified a unilateral ovarian mass and small ascites. The tumor, approximately 12 cm in diameter, revealed a mixed pattern of multicystic and solid parts. Uterine endometrial thickening was also observed, and endometrial biopsy revealed grade 1 endometrioid carcinoma. Computed tomography (CT) revealed no lymph node metastasis or extrapelvic tumors. The laboratory data showed an elevated level of LDH (1246 U/L, normal < 210 U/L). Isozyme analysis results were as follows: LD1 15%, LD2 30%, LD3 27%, LD4 18%, and LD5 10%. The serum level of cancer antigen 125 (CA125) was 156.7 U/mL (normal < 35 U/mL). The serum calcium level was normal. Double cancer of the ovary and endometrium was suspected, and a staging laparotomy was

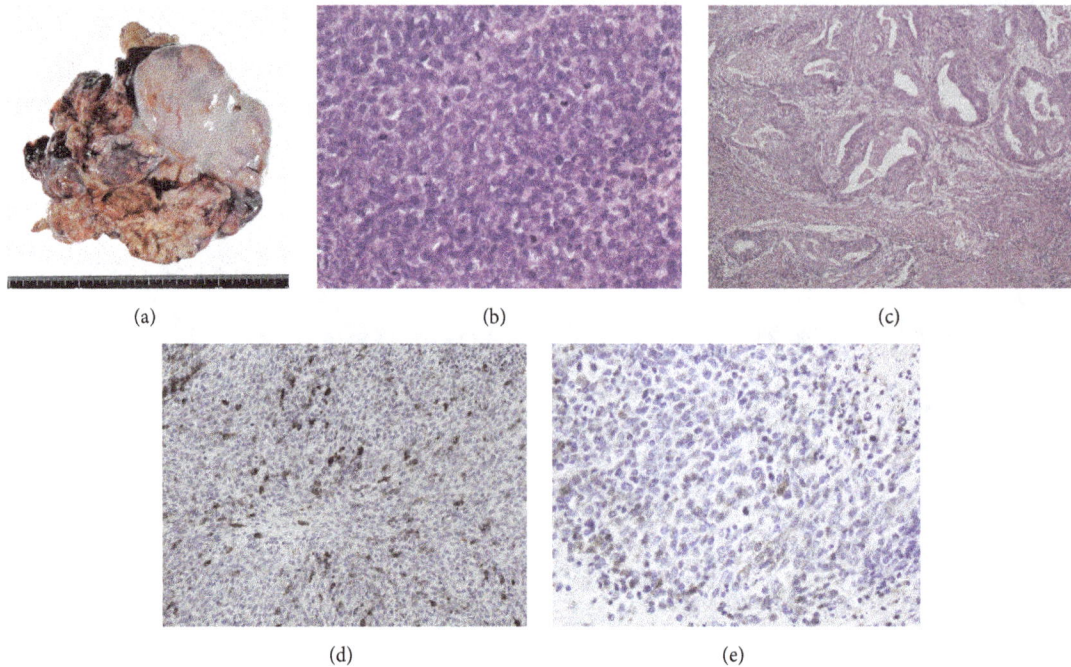

FIGURE 1: (a) Macroscopic findings: an irregular, white, and solid tumor of the right ovary. ((b)–(d)) Microscopic findings. (b) Tumor cells are round to ovoid with hyperchromatic nuclei, scant cytoplasm, abundant mitosis, and apoptosis with conspicuous necrosis (hematoxylin-eosin stain (HE), ×300). (c) Endometrial carcinoma grade 1 in uterine corpus (HE, ×30) with less than half myometrial invasion and no vascular invasion. ((d), (e)) Tumor cells are positive for synaptophysin and neuron-specific enolase (immunostaining, ×300).

scheduled. Eighteen days after first consultation, the patient complained of severe abdominal pain, and ultrasonography revealed that the tumor had enlarged to 16 cm in diameter, with an accumulation of ascitic fluid and newly diagnosed peritoneal dissemination. The tumor was rapidly progressing, and tumor rupture was also suspected. She underwent an urgent laparotomy, which revealed that a white and solid tumor of the right ovary had spontaneously ruptured in the intra-abdominal cavity (Figure 1(a)). There was massive bloody ascites of approximately 2700 mL in volume. The tumor was strongly adherent to the bladder and sigmoid colon and was difficult to decorticate. Multiple, but small, peritoneal disseminations were observed in the pelvic cavity. Total abdominal hysterectomy, bilateral salpingo-oophorectomy, and partial omentectomy were performed, and a 5 × 4 cm tumor remained behind the bladder due to the strong adhesion. The pathological diagnosis was SCOCPT (Figure 1(b)) and grade 1 endometrioid carcinoma of the uterine corpus (Figure 1(c)). Immunostaining of the ovarian tumor was positive for epithelial membrane antigen, synaptophysin (Figure 1(d)), neuron-specific enolase (NSE) (Figure 1(e)), p16, and cluster of differentiation (CD) 56 and negative for cytokeratin 20, Wilms Tumor 1, thyroid transcription factor 1, and anti-cytokeratin (CK) antibodies CK18, CK19, and CD99. Thus, we diagnosed primary ovarian cancer stage IIIC (pT3cNxM0) and endometrial cancer stage IA (pT1aNxM0) according to the International Federation of Gynecology and Obstetrics classification system. The serum level of NSE after surgery was 28.1 ng/mL (normal < 16.3 ng/mL).

Twenty days after surgery, a CT scan revealed that the remaining tumor in the pelvic cavity had enlarged to 14.8 cm. At 21 days after surgery, the patient received adjuvant chemotherapy combining cisplatin (60 mg/m^2 on day 1) and etoposide (100 mg/m^2 on days 1 to 3) administered every 3 weeks by intravenous infusion. After each course, CT scanning revealed slight shrinkage of the residual tumor, but it enlarged during the drug holidays. After 3 courses of this regimen, the tumor was observed to have enlarged to 20.3 cm on CT. The patient's performance status, as measured using the Eastern Cooperative Oncology Group (ECOG) grading scale, was grade 3, and she complained of abdominal swelling. Therefore, irradiation of the abdominal tumor was initiated. A total dose of 26 Gy was given in 13 fractions, and the tumor size decreased to 15.3 cm with improved symptoms (Figure 2). However, several hypointensity lesions suggestive of intratumor gas were observed in the pelvic tumor. The patient gradually felt severely fatigued and refused any treatment. She was transferred to a hospice and died 135 days after the surgery. An autopsy was not performed. During the course of treatment, serum LDH levels repeatedly decreased soon after the chemotherapy but increased during drug holidays (Figure 3).

3. Discussion

We identified two important clinical issues. Palliative radiotherapy for SCOCPT can be considered in patients with abdominal swelling, and LDH is a useful tumor marker.

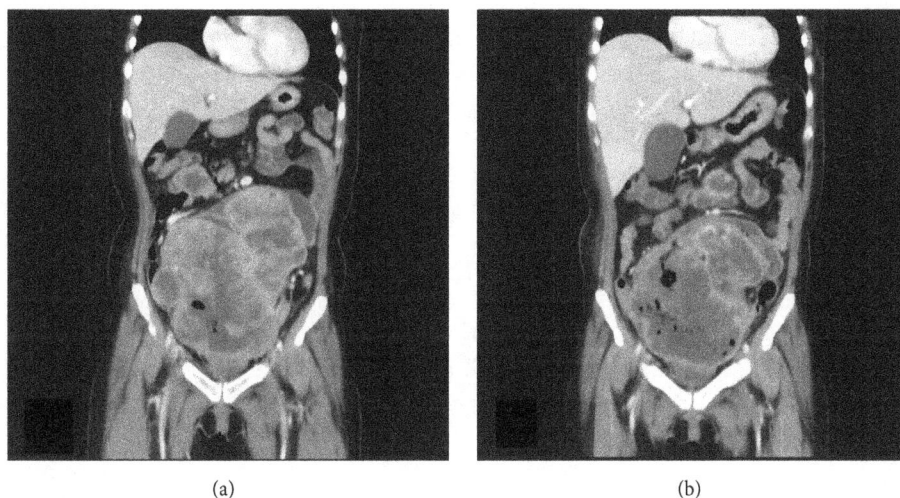

(a)   (b)

FIGURE 2: (a) Enhanced abdominal computed tomography (coronal section) reveals the remaining tumor is approximately 20.3 cm in diameter before irradiation. (b) After radiation therapy, the tumor size decreased to 15.3 cm.

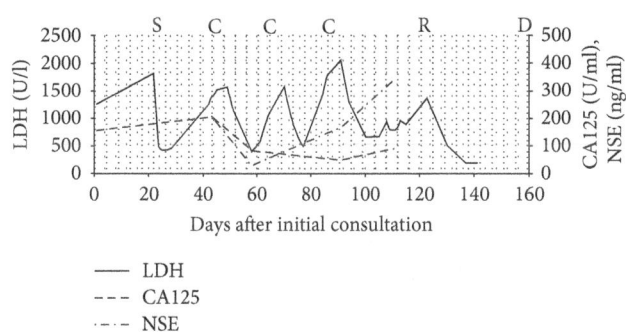

FIGURE 3: The graph shows the time course of the levels of serum lactate dehydrogenase (LDH), cancer antigen 125 (CA125), and neuron-specific enolase (NSE). The patient underwent surgery (S) on day 21; chemotherapy (C) on days 43, 65, and 86; and abdominal irradiation (R) from day 120 to day 140. She died on day 157 (D). The solid line shows levels of LDH, the dashed-line shows levels of CA125, and the dashed-dotted line shows levels of NSE.

First, with regard to palliative radiotherapy as a cytoreductive effect for SCOCPT, a total of 26 cases of SCOCPT have been reported in the literature, and 18 of these were treated with chemotherapy postoperatively (Table 1) [1–15]. To our knowledge, this is the first report of SCOCPT treated with radiotherapy except for brain irradiation to control seizures with brain metastasis. Palliative radiotherapy at a dose of 26 Gy for the residual abdominal tumor contributed to tumor shrinkage by approximately 25%. Intratumor gas was observed, but it was not ascertained that the fistula between the tumor and the intestines was attributable to radiotherapy. It is not clear if radiotherapy improved the prognosis. However, we believe that radiotherapy was at least effective for improving the symptoms associated with tumor enlargement.

There are many reports regarding the effectiveness of radiotherapy in small cell carcinoma in other organs. Radiotherapy plays a vital role in the management of the full spectrum of small cell lung cancer, from its ability to palliate symptoms to improvements in survival [16]. Thoracic radiotherapy combined with chemotherapy improves survival in patients with limited-stage small cell lung cancer [17, 18]. According to the National Comprehensive Cancer Network guideline, concurrent chemoradiotherapy (CCRT) is recommended for limited-stage small cell lung cancer in excess of T1-2 N0 [19]. According to reports on small cell carcinoma in other sex organs, including the uterine cervix, endometrium, and vagina, multimodality therapy is likely the treatment of choice [20]. Patients with SCOCPT never received pelvic or abdominal radiation in previous reports. It is reasonable to follow treatment trends for small cell carcinoma of the lung, since tumors are histologically indistinguishable and exhibit a similar aggressive behavior.

Second, with regard to LDH as a useful tumor marker of SCOCPT, CA125 (positive rate 82.4%), NSE (85.7%), and CA19-9 (37.5%) have been reported as tumor markers for SCOCPT [21], but LDH has not been reported. Increased LDH is a prognostic tumor marker in many other solid tumors, including non-small cell lung cancer [22], breast cancer [23], and prostate cancer [24]. It has long been known that many human cancers have higher LDH levels than normal tissues [25]. The serum level of LDH is thought to be correlated with the tumor burden and to reflect the tumor's growth and invasive potential [26]. In this case, chemotherapy and radiotherapy transiently inhibited the growth of both tumor cells and LDH production, which led to an acute decrease in the serum LDH level. Because of the highly proliferative capacity of SCOCPT, serum LDH levels increased during the drug holidays. Although LDH has five isoforms with different distributions, it was not necessary to detect these isoforms separately because no specific isoform was characteristically increased. This is useful, because total serum LDH assessment is convenient and inexpensive [27]. Serum LDH can be a useful tumor marker to evaluate the effectiveness of the treatment and to assess the prognosis.

TABLE 1: A review of the literature: the characteristics, the treatment, and the outcome of small cell ovarian carcinoma, pulmonary type.

Author	Year	Age	Stage	Operation	Postoperative treatment	Outcome
		62	1a	RSO	None	DOD, 4 Mo
		59	1a	TAH, RSO	Unknown	Unknown
		55	1a	TAH, BSO	Unknown	Unknown
		28	1c	TAH, BSO, OMT, appendectomy, peritoneal biopsies	Unknown	AWD, 6 Mo
		85	2b	BSO	None	DOD, 1 Mo
Eichhorn et al. [1]	1992	76	3b	BSO (subtotal resection)	Unknown	DOD, 12 Mo
		50	3b	LSO	Unknown	Unknown
		72	3b	TAH, BSO, OMT	CDDP, CPM	DOD, 12 Mo
		64	3b	TAH, BSO, OMT, LND, colectomy, appendectomy	CDDP, CPM, ADR	AWD, 8 Mo
		49	3b	LSO, ileocolectomy, right para-aortic LND	CDDP, CPM, ADR, MTX, 5-FU	DOD, 13 Mo
		46	3c	TAH, BSO, retroperitoneal LND	CDDP, CPM, ADR, VP-16, VCR	ANED, 7.5 years
Chang et al. [2]	1992	22	1a	LSO, enucleation of the right ovarian tumor	CDDP, CPM, ADR	ANED, 84 Mo
Fukunaga et al. [3]	1997	64	1a	TAH, BSO, OMT, pelvic and para-aortic LND	CDDP, CPM	DOD, 10 Mo
Lim et al. [4]	1998	28	4b	TAH, BSO	CDDP, VP-16, BLM	ANED, 34 Mo
Mebis et al. [5]	2004	54	3c	TAH, BSO, OMT	CDDP, IFM, VP-16	DOD, 14 Mo
Rund and Fischer [6]	2006	56	3c	TAH, BSO, OMT, pelvic LND, splenectomy, segmental resection of ileum and sigmoid colon	CDDP, VP-16	AWD, 7 Mo
	2006	39	3a	TAH, BSO, OMT	CDDP, VP-16, PTX	DOD, 16 Mo
Grandjean et al. [7]	2007	32	1a	BSO, OMT, left pelvic LND	CDDP, VP-16	ANED
Saitoh-Sekiguchi et al. [8]	2007	55	3c	TAH, BSO, OMT, cytoreductive surgery of dissemination	CDDP, CPT-11	ANED, 12 Mo
Suzuki et al. [9]	2007	49	1c(a)	TAH, BSO, pelvic and para-aortic LND, OMT	CBDCA, PTX	ANED, 36 Mo
Reckova et al. [10]	2010	67	4b	TAH, BSO, OMT, appendectomy	CBDCA, VP-16	DOD, 24 Mo
Ikota et al. [11]	2012	68	1a	TAH, BSO, OMT	None	ANED, 10 Mo
Kira et al. [12]	2012	33	3c	TAH, BSO, OMT, pelvic and para-aortic LND	CDDP, CPT-11	DOD, 6 Mo
Tsolakidis et al. [13]	2012	55	3c	TAH, BSO, OMT, sigmoidectomy, pelvic and para-aortic LND	CBDCA, VP-16	AEND, 21 Mo
Kurasaki et al. [14]	2013	54	3a	TAH, BSO, OMT	CBDCA, PTX	ANED, 22 Mo
Rubio et al. [15]	2015	37	3b	TAH, BSO, OMT, pelvic LND	CDDP, VP-16	DOD, 4 Mo

TAH, total abdominal hysterectomy; BSO, bilateral salpingo-oophorectomy; LND, lymph node dissection; OMT, omentectomy; CDDP, cisplatin; CBDCA, carboplatin; PTX, paclitaxel; ADR, doxorubicin; CPM, cyclophosphamide; VP-16, etoposide; CPT-11, irinotecan; IFM, ifosfamide; BLM, bleomycin; VCR, vincristine; MTX, methotrexate; 5-FU, 5-fluorouracil; DOD, dead of disease; ANED, alive with no evidence of disease; AWD, alive with recurrent or residual disease; Mo, months.

4. Conclusion

Palliative radiotherapy for SCOCPT can be considered in patients with abdominal swelling, and LDH might be a useful tumor marker. Radiotherapy might be considered as an option if the tumor is resistant to chemotherapy after a staging laparotomy. Furthermore, multimodality therapy might be appropriate in patients thought to be candidates for aggressive, potentially curative treatments, but further research is required to establish the treatment strategy for SCOCPT.

Consent

Written informed consent was obtained from the patient for publication of this case report.

Acknowledgments

The authors thank Dr. Yoshiro Otsuki (Department of Pathology, Seirei Hamamatsu General Hospital) and Dr. Ayse Ayhan (Department of Pathology, Seirei Mikatahara General Hospital) for their helpful comments.

References

[1] J. H. Eichhorn, R. H. Young, and R. E. Scully, "Primary ovarian small cell carcinoma of pulmonary type: A clinicopathologic, immunohistologic, and flow cytometric analysis of 11 cases," *The American Journal of Surgical Pathology*, vol. 16, no. 10, pp. 926–938, 1992.

[2] D. H.-C. Chang, S. Hsueh, and Y.-K. Soong, "Small cell carcinoma with neurosecretory granules arising in an ovarian dermoid cyst," *Gynecologic Oncology*, vol. 46, no. 2, pp. 246–250, 1992.

[3] M. Fukunaga, Y. Endo, Y. Miyazawa, and S. Ushigome, "Small cell neuroendocrine carcinoma of the ovary," *Virchows Archiv*, vol. 430, no. 4, pp. 343–348, 1997.

[4] S.-C. Lim, S. J. Choi, and C. H. Suh, "A case of small cell carcinoma arising in a mature cystic teratoma of the ovary," *Pathology International*, vol. 48, no. 10, pp. 834–839, 1998.

[5] J. Mebis, H. De Raeve, M. Baekelandt, W. A. A. Tjalma, and J. B. Vermorken, "Primary ovarian small cell carcinoma of the pulmonary type: A case report and review of the literature," *European Journal of Gynaecological Oncology*, vol. 25, no. 2, pp. 239–241, 2004.

[6] C. R. Rund and E. G. Fischer, "Perinuclear dot-like cytokeratin 20 staining in small cell neuroendocrine carcinoma of the ovary (pulmonary-type)," *Applied Immunohistochemistry & Molecular Morphology*, vol. 14, no. 2, pp. 244–248, 2006.

[7] M. Grandjean, L. Legrand, M. Waterkeyn et al., "Small cell carcinoma of pulmonary type inside a microinvasive mucinous cystadenocarcinoma of the ovary: A case report," *International Journal of Gynecological Pathology*, vol. 26, no. 4, pp. 426–431, 2007.

[8] M. Saitoh-Sekiguchi, K. Nakahara, T. Kojimahara et al., "Complete remission of ovarian small cell carcinoma treated with irinotecan and cisplatin: A case report," *Anticancer Reseach*, vol. 27, no. 4 C, pp. 2685–2687, 2007.

[9] N. Suzuki, K. Kameyama, T. Hirao, N. Susumu, M. Mukai, and D. Aoki, "A case of pulmonary type of ovarian small cell carcinoma," *Journal of Obstetrics and Gynaecology Research*, vol. 33, no. 2, pp. 203–206, 2007.

[10] M. Reckova, M. Mego, K. Rejlekova, Z. Sycova-Mila, Z. Obertova, and J. Mardiak, "Small-cell carcinoma of the ovary with breast metastases: A case report," *Klinicka Onkologie*, vol. 23, no. 1, pp. 43–45, 2010.

[11] H. Ikota, K. Kaneko, S. Takahashi et al., "Malignant transformation of ovarian mature cystic teratoma with a predominant pulmonary type small cell carcinoma component," *Pathology International*, vol. 62, no. 4, pp. 276–280, 2012.

[12] N. Kira, N. Takai, T. Ishii et al., "Ovarian small cell carcinoma complicated by carcinomatous meningitis," *Rare Tumors*, vol. 4, no. 2, p. e26, 2012.

[13] D. Tsolakidis, A. Papanikolaou, K. Ktenidis, and S. Pervana, "Primary ovarian small cell carcinoma of pulmonary type with enlarged paraaortic lymph node masses: A case report and review of the literature," *European Journal of Gynaecological Oncology*, vol. 33, no. 3, pp. 312–315, 2012.

[14] A. Kurasaki, N. Sakurai, Y. Yamamoto, H. Taoka, K. Takahashi, and K. Kubushiro, "Ovarian pulmonary-type small cell carcinoma: Case report and review of the literature," *International Journal of Gynecological Pathology*, vol. 32, no. 5, pp. 464–470, 2013.

[15] A. Rubio, M. Schuldt, C. Chamorro, V. Crespo-Lora, and F. F. Nogales, "Ovarian small cell carcinoma of pulmonary type arising in mature cystic teratomas with metastases to the contralateral ovary," *International Journal of Surgical Pathology*, vol. 23, no. 5, pp. 388–392, 2015.

[16] D. K. Woolf, B. J. Slotman, and C. Faivre-Finn, "The Current Role of Radiotherapy in the Treatment of Small Cell Lung Cancer," *Clinical Oncology*, vol. 28, no. 11, pp. 712–719, 2016.

[17] J.-P. Pignon, R. Arriagada, D. C. Ihde et al., "A meta-analysis of thoracic radiotherapy for small-cell lung cancer," *The New England Journal of Medicine*, vol. 327, no. 23, pp. 1618–1624, 1992.

[18] P. Warde and D. Payne, "Does thoracic irradiation improve survival and local control in limited-stage small-cell carcinoma of the lung? A meta-analysis," *Journal of Clinical Oncology*, vol. 10, no. 6, pp. 890–895, 1992.

[19] National Comprehensive Cancer Network. NCCN Clinical Practice Guidlines in Oncology: Small Cell Lung Cancer, In: P. Gregory, M. Kalemkerian (ed.), 2016.

[20] S. Crowder and E. Tuller, "Small Cell Carcinoma of the Female Genital Tract," *Seminars in Oncology*, vol. 34, no. 1, pp. 57–63, 2007.

[21] K. Münstedt, R. Estel, T. Dreyer, A. Kurata, and A. Benz, "Small cell ovarian carcinomas - Characterisation of two rare tumor entities," *Geburtshilfe und Frauenheilkunde*, vol. 73, no. 7, pp. 698–704, 2013.

[22] K. S. Albain, J. J. Crowley, M. LeBlanc, and R. B. Livingston, "Survival determinants in extensive-stage non-small-cell lung cancer: the southwest oncology group experience," *Journal of Clinical Oncology*, vol. 9, no. 9, pp. 1618–1626, 1991.

[23] J. E. Brown, R. J. Cook, A. Lipton, and R. E. Coleman, "Serum lactate dehydrogenase is prognostic for survival in patients with bone metastases from breast cancer: A retrospective analysis in

bisphosphonate-treated patients," *Clinical Cancer Research*, vol. 18, no. 22, pp. 6348–6355, 2012.

[24] S. Halabi, E. J. Small, P. W. Kantoff et al., "Prognostic model for predicting survival in men with hormone-refractory metastatic prostate cancer," *Journal of Clinical Oncology*, vol. 21, no. 7, pp. 1232–1237, 2003.

[25] R. D. Goldman, N. O. Kaplan, and T. C. Hall, "Lactic Dehydrogenase in Human Neoplastic Tissues," *Cancer Research*, vol. 24, pp. 389–399, 1964.

[26] S.-Y. Suh and H.-Y. Ahn, "Lactate dehydrogenase as a prognostic factor for survival time of terminally ill cancer patients: A preliminary study," *European Journal of Cancer*, vol. 43, no. 6, pp. 1051–1059, 2007.

[27] R. Liu, J. Cao, X. Gao et al., "Overall survival of cancer patients with serum lactate dehydrogenase greater than 1000 IU/L," *Tumor Biology*, vol. 37, no. 10, pp. 14083–14088, 2016.

Epidural Anesthesia for Cesarean Section in a Pregnant Woman with Marfan Syndrome and Dural Ectasia

Franco Pepe,[1] Mariagrazia Stracquadanio,[2] Francesco De Luca,[3] Agata Privitera,[3] Elisabetta Sanalitro,[4] and Puccio Scarpinati[4]

[1]U.O.C. Ostetricia e Ginecologia e PS, Ospedale Santo Bambino, Catania, Italy
[2]Istituto di Patologia Ostetrica e Ginecologica, Ospedale Santo Bambino, Catania, Italy
[3]U.O. Cardiologia Pediatrica, Ospedale Santo Bambino, Catania, Italy
[4]Modulo Dipartimentale Anestesia Ostetrica, Ospedale Santo Bambino, Catania, Italy

Correspondence should be addressed to Mariagrazia Stracquadanio; mariagrazia.stracquadanio@gmail.com

Academic Editor: Michael Geary

Marfan syndrome (MFS) is a genetic disorder of connective tissue, characterized by variable clinical features and multisystem complications. The anesthetic management during delivery is debated. Regional anesthesia has been used with success during cesarean delivery, but in some MFS patients there is a probability of erratic and inadequate spread of intrathecal local anesthetics as a result of dural ectasia. In these cases, epidural anesthesia may be a particularly useful technique during cesarean delivery because it allows an adequate spread and action of local anesthetic with a controlled onset of anesthesia, analgesia, and sympathetic block and a low risk of perioperative complications. We report the perioperative management of a patient with MFS and dural ectasia who successfully underwent cesarean section using epidural technique anesthesia. The previous pregnancy of this woman ended with cesarean section with a failed spinal anesthesia that was converted to general anesthesia due to unknown dural ectasia at that time.

1. Introduction

Marfan syndrome (MFS) is an autosomal dominant hereditary disorder of connective tissue; its incidence is estimated to be around 1 : 5.000, with no differences in gender or ethnic background. In 90% of cases, it is associated with mutations in the FBN1 gene that encodes fibrillin [1]. The clinical manifestations of the gene may involve multiple organs with various severity, particularly affecting the cardiovascular, skeletal, and ocular systems. The clinical and instrumental diagnosis is based on observation of the Ghent criteria, proposed in 1996 by De Paepe et al. [2], ranging from the familiarity to multiorgan involvement and they were recently revised by Loeys et al. in 2010 [3]. Some manifestations are evident since childhood (such as ectopia lentis), while others were at a later date, such as the lumbosacral dural ectasia; the main cause of morbidity and mortality is related to aortic dilation and acute aortic dissection. Cardiovascular manifestations, such as aortic dilatation and dissection, are

responsible for 90% of deaths attributed to MFS [4, 5]. The disease is not associated with a reduction in fertility; in fact it is common to find a pregnant woman with the syndrome. In such a case, it would be appropriate to have an accurate clinical evaluation before pregnancy, particularly an echocardiography, to assess the size of the aortic root: a diameter greater than 40 mm puts the patient at risk of its rupture.

As reported in literature, the obstetric management of women with MFS seems now well coded, with favorable outcome if the aortic root diameter is less than 40 mm. The increase in aortic size during pregnancy is not unique in women with MFS but is known to occur during normal healthy pregnancies and with increased severity in women with preeclampsia [6].

Some recent guidelines advise women with MFS to avoid pregnancy or, alternatively, undergo surgical ascending aortic replacement prior to conception, if the aorta measures > 4 cm [7].

Literature suggests a 1% risk of aortic dissection or significant cardiac event in women with an aortic root diameter of <40 mm [8]. The risk is increased when the aortic root diameter is >40 mm, if there is a rapid increase in aortic dimensions or in the context of a family history of dissection [9].

However, the presence of ectasia of the dural sac has been considered the major cause of failure of locoregional anesthesia during cesarean section. The purpose of this study is to present the case of a MFS pregnant woman at term with an extensive dural ectasia who had a successful cesarean section with epidural anesthesia during her second pregnancy.

2. Case Report

F. S. is a 35-year-old, 180 cm tall, 85 Kg patient, suffering from MSF with a lumbosacral dural ectasia, who was subjected to a cesarean section at 37 weeks and 3 days of gestation. She reports that the mother was very high and died suddenly before the age of 50; her maternal grandfather was particularly high too, and her brother was myopic and had severe scoliosis. Medical history was positive for ectopia lentis (diagnosed when she was 6 years old), dorsal scoliosis (treated with corset from 10 to 14 years of age), and mild ectasia of the aortic arch. Previously she underwent right saphenectomy and right breast fibroadenoma enucleation. Physical examination showed skeletal abnormalities such as high arched palate, opening of the arms greater than height, pectus carinatum internalized to the right, flat feet, bilateral valgus, and arachnodactyly. Striae were evident on the skin of her chest, shoulders, back, and abdomen. On cardiovascular examination, a metallic click and systolic murmur were auscultated with a stethoscope. Heart sounded valid and rhythmic, with good hemodynamic compensation, and ECG had a normal sinus rhythm and normal track with a medium pulse of 65 beats per minute. The patient was normotensive (BP 120/70 mmHg). Echocardiogram showed a mild dilatation of the aortic root (42 mm), normal ventricular function, and a mild mitral valve prolapse without regurgitation.

The obstetric history showed an uneventful previous C-section delivery in 2004. She had a spinal block anesthesia after spinal anesthesia, which was converted into a general one. In the postoperative period, she had a hemorrhage due to uterine atony treated with oxytocin and prostaglandins and recovery in intensive care. After five days, the patient was discharged in good medical condition and she was followed up every 6 months and had a prophylactic therapy with beta-blockers. In 2007, because of a lumbar pain, she performed a lumbosacral MRI that showed ectasia of the distal dural sac with cystic dilatation of some nerve roots. This finding is one of the major diagnostic criteria of MFS. In 2009, she started a second pregnancy and she was under the care of the outpatient obstetric clinic of the Santo Bambino Hospital in Catania (Sicily). During her first trimester of pregnancy, the patient was asymptomatic with good cardiovascular compensation and she did not take any medication. She has been monthly subjected to obstetric visits; she also had three ultrasound scans (one for each trimester of pregnancy),

two cardiological examinations (at the beginning and near term), and two maternal echocardiographies (at 22 weeks and near term) in order to monitor the aortic root. The fetal growth was regular. At 37 weeks + 3 days, because of the occurrence of uterine contractions, the patient was admitted to the hospital for cesarean section. Considering the previous bad experience during spinal anesthesia (lack of efficacy with use of general anesthesia), being aware of the presence of the ectasia of the dural sac during the preoperative evaluation of the patient, epidural anesthesia was proposed to perform her second cesarean section. This type of anesthesia allows a better circulation and distribution of the anesthetic, overcoming the problems related to spinal anesthesia in the presence of dural ectasia. The drugs administered epidurally require dosages from 5 to 10 times higher and volumes greater than those calculated for the subarachnoid space. The advantages of an epidural block include a lower incidence and severity of maternal hypotension, thanks to the reduced rate of sympathetic block, a lower risk of headache due to accidental dural puncture, and the possibility of an accurate control of level and duration of anesthesia. The patient was informed about the type of regional anesthesia chosen and monitored. She was continuously under noninvasive monitoring (ECG, arterial blood pressure, and oxygen saturation) and she was premedicated with ranitidine 50 mg and metoclopramide 10 mg in saline solution. She was placed in a sitting position and then the locoregional block in epidural anesthesia was performed by a midline approach with the placement of an epidural catheter, through a 17-gauge Tuohy needle, positioned between L2 and L3. She was given lidocaine 400 mg (20 ml of 2%) with 1 mEq of sodium bicarbonate and 50 mcg of fentanyl. The anesthetic block was manifested within three minutes without side effects. After 15 minutes, the cesarean section started, because the sensory block was sufficiently high (T4) for cesarean section. The systolic blood pressure remained stable (110–125/70 mmHg) for the entire duration of surgery and the postoperative period. There was no evidence of intraoperative and postoperative complications and the patient did not report any pain symptoms. Short-term prophylaxis for infection was administered (3 g ampicillin/sulbactam) after the delivery of the baby as well as 20 IU of oxytocin. After 30 minutes from the anesthetic block, 1 mg of morphine + 75 mcg of clonidine and 12 mg of naropine were injected in the epidural space through the catheter. After an hour from the beginning of the anesthetic block, an ongoing anesthesia with 0,1% naropine, 250 mg at 10 ml/h, was placed in the infusion pump for epidural. At the end of the surgery, for further analgesia, a 75 mg of diclofenac i.m and 0.2 mg of methylergometrine i.m. were administered. The patient was kept under observation for 2 hours and then transferred to the ward. The male newborn was 3.250 g, and he was extracted after 30 minutes since the moment epidural catheter was placed and 1 minute after the skin incision. The Apgar score in the first minute was 9, and it was 10 after five minutes. The epidural catheter was removed 12 hours after cesarean section. The postoperative course was regular, with her discharge on the fourth day after C-section. A 12-day heparin prophylaxis was performed for venous thromboembolism prevention. After a follow-up of five years, we can assert that the patient is in good health and the aortic root diameter is always 42 mm.

3. Discussion

MFS is an autosomal dominant disorder of the connective tissue related to mutation of the gene for fibrillin, a glycoprotein that is the major component of extracellular microfibrils, whose gene maps to chromosome 15. MFS involves different organs and systems with varying severity: for this reason, its diagnosis is mainly clinical and instrumental and, then, molecular. It is based on the observation of the Ghent criteria and revised criteria [10].

In literature, there are many experiences on the management of pregnant women with MS [9–13]. Pregnancy can be considered at low risk in the absence of significant aortic dilatation and mitral insufficiency. In women with low cardiac involvement, the risk of aortic dissection, endocarditis, and congestive heart failure in pregnancy is estimated to be only 1%. The risk is higher during the third trimester of pregnancy due to the increase of the hemodynamic stress. During pregnancy and postpartum period, echocardiography should be frequently performed, depending on the extent of the initial dilatation of the aortic root, in order to monitor the cardiovascular system and the possible progressive aortic dilatation.

Beta-blockers reduce the risk of aortic dilatation and cardiac complications, but they seem to increase the tone and uterine contractility, and they might reduce the flow in the umbilical artery causing low birth weight infants. They were not used in our pregnant woman.

The dural ectasia is one of the major criteria for diagnosis of MFS and it is present in over 2/3 of adults affected [14–16] and the prevalence of severe (degrees 2 and 3) involvement of dura mater was higher in patients harboring premature termination codon mutations compared to those carrying missense mutations [17]. It is hypothesized that, in Marfan's syndrome, the dura mater is weaker and, as a result, cerebrospinal fluid pulsation eventually leads to dural ectasia with gradual bone erosion. The dural ectasia is characterized by a swelling of the dural sac and of the spinal canal and, sometimes, of the nerve sheaths. Although it can occur along the entire channel, the most frequent site is the lumbosacral spine. The most common clinical symptoms, which can be intensified by the supine position, are low back pain, headache, asthenia, decreased sensitivity below and around the affected section, and, occasionally, rectal pain and/or discomfort in the genital area [16, 18]. The extension of the dural expansion is variable; sometimes the lesion is confined to focal dilation of the dural coating of the nerve roots, near their exit from the spinal column: they are called "radicular cysts." The chronic dilatation of the dural sac can also exert an erosive effect against adjacent bone structures of the spine. The indirect signs of bone damage can be observed with radiographic test (Rx) and by examination of Computed Tomography (CT). However, the gold standard for the evaluation of dural ectasia is RM, for the quality of anatomical detail and for its multiplanarity. The prevalence of dural ectasia in patients with MS is variable from 63%

to 92%, probably in relation to the imaging modality used in the various studies [19–21]. In a study published in 1999, out of 83 MFS patients examined by MRI, the dural ectasia was detected in 92% of cases and in none of the patients in the control group. However, high prevalence of dural ectasia (41%) exits even in patients with MFS without back pain [16]. No correlation was found with the presence of aortic dilatation; therefore, dural ectasia has no predictive value on cardiovascular prognosis in these patients. Regarding the clinical expression, dural ectasia is often clinically silent or can be occasionally associated with low back pain or lumbosciatica. However, a clear correlation between low back pain and dural ectasia has not been demonstrated.

For the best management of labor and delivery of MFS patients, it is clear that the primary goal is the reduction of cardiovascular stress, and cesarean section is often performed for the prevention of cardiovascular complications. Patients with an aortic root < 4 cm in diameter at the time of delivery have a similar outcome for vaginal and cesarean section delivery, but cesarean section is preferred in patients with an aortic root > 4 cm because the risk for cardiac decompensation is extremely high [22]. However, aortic dissection has been reported even in the absence of preexisting aortic root dilatation [22].

Fluctuation in hemodynamic parameters secondary to pain and anxiety of labor may have negative effects on the cardiovascular system; high blood pressure tends to develop aortic aneurysms due to weakened vascular media in patients with MFS, and myocardial ischemia and heart failure can also be caused by an increased myocardial oxygen demand resulting in high blood pressure; thus, the main goal is to prevent high blood pressure [23]. For all these reasons, cesarean section is frequently planned.

The type of anesthesia has been discussed too. General anesthesia causes blood pressure variations during intubation; therefore peripheral anesthesia seems preferable because of slow onset and gradual progression of epidural block. Since the spontaneous birth determines increase in blood pressure during contractions, the use of epidural analgesia reduces pain, blood pressure, and heart rate. Cesarean section was performed in our patient because she already had a cesarean section.

In some studies, regional anesthesia has been practiced successfully in MFS patients, both during labor analgesia and during cesarean section. Combined spinal-epidural anesthesia is preferred over general anesthesia for cesarean section in patents with MFS because combined spinal-epidural anesthesia provides excellent hemodynamic stability, and adequate postoperative pain control may be obtained via epidural analgesia. However, many cases of spinal anesthesia failure have been reported in Marfan patients, possibly due to dural ectasia [24, 25]. Few cases of incorrect or inadequate spread of intrathecal local anesthetic in patients with this syndrome have been described. Lacassie et al. [26] performed continuous spinal anesthesia in two patients with an incrementally increased dose of bupivacaine, but they stopped further administration of bupivacaine after 21 ml for the fear of potential neurological damage. They also reported an irregular distribution of spinal anesthesia due to unpredictable and inadequate spread of intrathecal local anesthetics in patients with MFS. One of the most important factors influencing the height of the block in patients receiving spinal anesthesia is the volume of CSF in the lumbosacral space, which contributes to the variability in the spread of spinal block. Kim et al. [27] reported a successful perioperative management of a patient with MFS and dural ectasia for cesarean section using epidural anesthesia. The surgically adequate level of anesthesia was achieved 30 min after the epidural injection of 27 ml of 2% lidocaine with epinephrine (1 : 200) and fentanyl (100 mcg).

In summary, the evaluation of pregnant women with MFS requires multidisciplinary management with a close cooperation between gynecologist, cardiologist, anesthesiologist, and neonatologist. Pregnancy should be programmed after complete evaluation of the patient and the definition of specific risks. Relevant is the echocardiographic assessment of aortic root dilation. During pregnancy, the obstetric management is not significantly different, but it is burdened with a higher frequency of premature rupture of membranes, the side effects of the drugs used, where indicated, for the prevention of aortic rupture, and the risk of aortic dissection. The anesthetic management during delivery is debated. Regional anesthesia has been successfully used during cesarean section, but there is a significant probability of erratic and inadequate intrathecal spread of local anesthetics, most likely as a result of dural ectasia. In these patients, epidural anesthesia may be a particularly useful technique during cesarean delivery because it allows adequate spread and action of local anesthetic and controlled onset of anesthesia, analgesia, and sympathetic block with low risk of complications. We report the perioperative management of a patient with MFS and lumbosacral dural ectasia who underwent successful cesarean delivery using epidural technique anesthesia. In her previous pregnancy, the failed spinal anesthesia during cesarean section was converted to general anesthesia due to the unknown presence of dural ectasia at that time.

References

[1] R. E. Pyeritz and V. A. McKusick, "The Marfan syndrome: diagnosis and management," *The New England Journal of Medicine*, vol. 300, no. 14, pp. 772–777, 1979.

[2] A. De Paepe, R. B. Devereux, H. C. Dietz, R. C. M. Hennekam, and R. E. Pyeritz, "Revised diagnostic criteria for the Marfan syndrome," *American Journal of Medical Genetics*, vol. 62, no. 4, pp. 417–426, 1996.

[3] B. L. Loeys, H. C. Dietz, A. C. Braverman et al., "The revised Ghent nosology for the Marfan syndrome," *Journal of Medical Genetics*, vol. 47, no. 7, pp. 476–485, 2010.

[4] D. M. Paternoster, C. Santarossa, N. Vettore et al., "Obstetric complications in Marfan's syndrome pregnancy," *Minerva Ginecologica*, vol. 50, pp. 441–443, 1999.

[5] P. Beigthon, A. De Paepe, D. Danks et al., "International nosology of heritable disorders of connective tissue, Berlin,

1986," *American Journal of Medical Genetics*, vol. 29, pp. 581–589, 1988.

[6] T. R. Easterling, T. J. Benedetti, B. C. Schumaker et al., "Maternal hemodynamics and aortic diameter in normal and hypertensive pregnancies," *Obstetrics & Gynecology*, vol. 78, pp. 1073–1077, 1991.

[7] L. F. Hiratzka, G. L. Bakris, J. A. Beckman et al., "ACCF/AHA/AATS/ACR/ASA/SCA/SCAI/SIR/STS/SVM guidelines for the diagnosis and management of patients with thoracic aortic disease," *Journal of the American College of Cardiology*, vol. 55, pp. e27-129, 2010.

[8] V. Regitz-Zagrosek, C. B. Lundqvist, C. Borghi et al., "ESC guidelines on the management of cardiovascular diseases during pregnancy: the taskforce on the management of cardiovascular disease during pregnancy of the European Society of Cardiology (ESC)," *European Heart Journal*, vol. 32, pp. 3147–3197, 2011.

[9] L. J. Meijboom, F. E. Vos, J. Timmermans, G. H. Boers, A. H. Zwinderman, and B. J. M. Mulder, "Pregnancy and aortic root growth in the Marfan syndrome: A prospective study," *European Heart Journal*, vol. 26, no. 9, pp. 914–920, 2005.

[10] S. Lalchandani and M. Wingfield, "Pregnancy in women with Marfan's Syndrome," *European Journal of Obstetrics Gynecology and Reproductive Biology*, vol. 110, no. 2, pp. 125–130, 2003.

[11] U. Elkayam, E. Ostrzega, A. Shotan, and A. Mehra, "Cardiovascular problems in pregnant women with the Marfan syndrome," *Annals of Internal Medicine*, vol. 123, no. 2, pp. 117–122, 1995.

[12] R. T. Buser, M. M. Mordecai, and S. J. Brull, "Combined spinal-epidural analgesia for labor in a patient with Marfan's syndrome," *International Journal of Obstetric Anesthesia*, vol. 16, no. 3, pp. 274–276, 2007.

[13] K. J. Lipscomb, J. C. Smith, B. Clarke, P. Donnai, and R. Harris, "Outcome of pregnancy in women with Marfan's syndrome," *An International Journal of Obstetrics and Gynaecology*, vol. 104, no. 2, pp. 201–206, 1997.

[14] R. E. Pyeritz, E. K. Fishman, B. A. Bernhardt, and S. S. Siegelman, "Dural ectasia is a common feature of the Marfan syndrome," *American Journal of Human Genetics*, vol. 43, no. 5, pp. 726–732, 1988.

[15] R. Fattori, C. A. Nienaber, B. Descovich et al., "Importance of dural ectasia in phenotypic assessment of Marfan's syndrome," *The Lancet*, vol. 354, no. 9182, pp. 910–913, 1999.

[16] N. U. Ahn, P. D. Sponseller, U. M. Ahn, L. Nallamshetty, B. S. Kuszyk, and S. J. Zinreich, "Dural ectasia is associated with back pain in marfan syndrome," *Spine*, vol. 25, no. 12, pp. 1562–1568, 2000.

[17] M. Attanasio, E. Pratelli, M. C. Porciani et al., "Dural ectasia and FBN1 mutation screening of 40 patients with Marfan syndrome and related disorders: role of dural ectasia for the diagnosis," *European Journal of Medical Genetics*, vol. 56, no. 7, pp. 356–360, 2013.

[18] A. A. Sánchez, C. D. Iglesias, C. D. López et al., "Rectothecal fistula secondary to an anterior sacral meningocele: Case report," *Journal of Neurosurgery: Spine*, vol. 8, no. 5, pp. 487–489, 2008.

[19] R. Lundby, S. Rand-Hendriksen, J. K. Hald et al., "Dural ectasia in Marfan syndrome: A case control study," *American Journal of Neuroradiology*, vol. 30, no. 8, pp. 1534–1540, 2009.

[20] G. M. Villeirs, A. J. Van Tongerloo, K. L. Verstraete, M. F. Kunnen, and A. M. De Paepe, "Widening of the spinal canal and dural ectasia in Marfan's syndrome: assessment by CT," *Neuroradiology*, vol. 41, no. 11, pp. 850–854, 1999.

[21] N. C. Ho, D. W. Hadley, P. K. Jain, and C. A. Francomano, "Case 47: dural ectasia associated with Marfan syndrome," *Radiology*, vol. 223, no. 3, pp. 767–771, 2002.

[22] J. Rahman, F. Z. Rahman, W. Rahman, S. A. Al-Suleiman, and M. S. Rahman, "Obstetric and ginecologic complications in women under general anesthesia," *The Journal of Reproductive Medicine*, vol. 48, pp. 723–728, 2003.

[23] D. W. Kim and Y. G. Lim, "A case report of marfan syndrome under general anesthesia," *Korean Journal of Anesthesiology*, vol. 26, no. 5, pp. 1055–1058, 1993.

[24] V. A. McKusik, Marfan syndrome, MFS. Online Mendelian Inheritance in Man. OMIM, MIM no 154700, Baltimore (MD): John Hopkins University, 2003.

[25] P. D. W. Fettes, J.-R. Jansson, and J. A. W. Wildsmith, "Failed spinal anaesthesia: mechanisms, management, and prevention," *British Journal of Anaesthesia*, vol. 102, no. 6, pp. 739–748, 2009.

[26] H. J. Lacassie, S. Millar, L. G. Leithe et al., "Dural ectasia: a likely cause of inadequate spinal anaesthesia in two parturients with Marfan's syndrome," *British Journal of Anaesthesia*, vol. 94, no. 4, pp. 500–504, 2005.

[27] G. Kim, J. S. Ko, and D. H. Choi, "Epidural anesthesia for cesarean section in a patient with Marfan syndrome and dural ectasia," *Korean Journal of Anesthesiology*, vol. 60, no. 3, pp. 214–216, 2011.

7

Uterine Tumor Resembling Ovarian Sex-Cord Tumors Initially Diagnosed as a Prolapsed Fibroid

Fernando Augusto Rozário Garcia (iD),[1] **Vanessa Pereira Gaigher,**[1]
Rodrigo Neves Ferreira,[2] **and Antônio Chambô Filho**[3,4]

[1]*Medical Resident, Department of Obstetrics and Gynecology, Hospital Santa Casa de Misericórdia de Vitória, Vitória, ES, Brazil*
[2]*Pathologist, Hospital Santa Casa de Misericórdia de Vitória, Vitória, ES, Brazil*
[3]*MD, PhD, Full Professor, Department of Obstetrics and Gynecology, Escola Superior de Ciências,*
Santa Casa de Misericórdia de Vitória, ES, Brazil
[4]*Head of the Department of Obstetrics and Gynecology, Hospital Santa Casa de Misericórdia de Vitória, Vitória, ES, Brazil*

Correspondence should be addressed to Fernando Augusto Rozário Garcia; fernando_241@hotmail.com

Academic Editor: Yoshio Yoshida

Background. First described in 1945 by Morehead and Bowman, uterine tumors resembling ovarian sex-cord tumors (UTROSCT) are rare tumors of the uterine body that tend to occur in menopausal women presenting with abnormal vaginal bleeding, abdominal pain, and increased uterine volume. UTROSCT are usually diagnosed from incidental histological findings following hysterectomy performed due to a suspected endometrial polyp or uterine fibroids. *Objective.* To report on a 46-year-old patient with abnormal vaginal bleeding. At physical examination, a pediculated nodular lesion was found protruding from the external cervical os. Histopathology of the resected lesion led to a diagnosis of UTROSCT. Total abdominal hysterectomy with bilateral adnexectomy was then performed. The patient is currently undergoing regular outpatient follow-up, with no evidence of disease after one year. *Methods.* Data were retrieved from the patient's records, and macroscopic and microscopic images of the tumor were obtained. *Discussion.* Reports of metastasis or recurrence are rare. UTROSCT are considered of uncertain malignant potential and no particular form of treatment is formally recommended, with hysterectomy currently being the treatment of choice. This patient will be followed up for five years during which clinical examination and tomography of the chest, abdomen, and pelvis will be performed annually.

1. Introduction

Uterine tumors resembling ovarian sex-cord tumors (UTROSCT) represent a rare form of tumors that affect the uterine body [1]. Up to the present moment, fewer than 100 cases have been reported in the literature [2].

Morehead and Bowman published the first descriptions of UTROSCT in 1945 [3]. In 1976, Clemente and Scully studied these tumors and classified them into two groups: Group 1: endometrial stromal tumors with sex-cord-like elements (ESTSCLE) and Group 2: UTROSCT [4]. Diagnosis is reached following histopathology, with immunohistochemistry playing a crucial role, particularly with respect to the differential diagnosis [5].

Clinically, these tumor types generally occur in menopausal women, who may present with symptoms of abnormal vaginal bleeding, abdominal pain, and increased uterine volume [6]. Treatment options include hysterectomy with bilateral salpingo-oophorectomy or even hysteroscopic resection of the tumor; however, the management, prognosis, morbidity, and mortality associated with this pathology remain the subject of debate due to the scarcity of such cases in current literature [7].

This paper describes the case of a 46-year old patient with abnormal vaginal bleeding. She presented with a pelvic mass, identified at histopathology as a UTROSCT. Her follow-up and treatment after diagnosis are discussed.

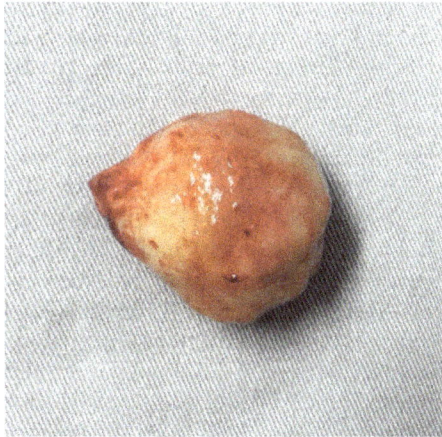

FIGURE 1: UTROSCT removed from the patient's uterus.

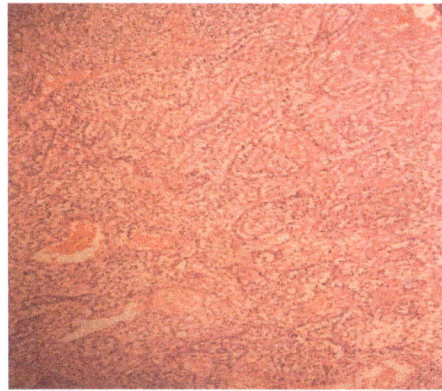

FIGURE 2: Hematoxylin-eosin (HE) staining, magnification 400x, clear cell cords resembling Sertoli cells.

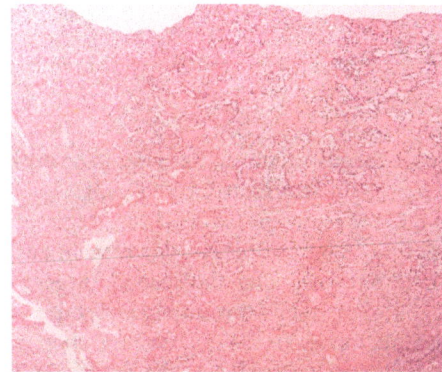

FIGURE 3: Hematoxylin-eosin, magnification 200x, clear cell cords resembling ovarian sex cord.

2. Case Presentation

A 46-year-old, brown-skinned woman with regular menstrual cycles and one child presented at the gynecology department of a philanthropic hospital in Vitória, Espírito Santo, Brazil, reporting a 6-month history of intense vaginal bleeding associated with abdominal pain. She had suffered vaginal discomfort over the previous week. She had no prior history of allergy, comorbidities, use of medication, or surgery. There was no family history of gynecological cancer. At physical examination, she was found to be in good general health, alert, pale, with a flaccid abdomen, and no signs of peritoneal irritation. A hypogastric mass was detected. There were no vulvar lesions. Speculum examination showed no lesions in the vagina but revealed the presence of a bleeding mass extruding from the external cervical os and associated with intense bleeding at manipulation. At bimanual pelvic examination, it was possible to palpate the pedicle of the lesion through the cervical os.

In view of the initial diagnostic hypothesis of a prolapsed fibroid, vaginal myomectomy was performed. There were no complications following surgery and the patient was discharged from hospital the following day in good clinical conditions.

Macroscopically, the pinkish-colored nodule measured 3.5 x 3 x 4 cm (Figure 1). Microscopically, it consisted of a proliferative spindle cell nodule with gland-like, epithelioid, trabecular, and glomeruloid elements, without atypia. In some parts, the cells formed clear cell cords resembling ovarian sex cords. The core was rounded and normochromatic, and the cytoplasm was clear, resembling Sertoli cells. The stroma was partially hyalinized, resembling smooth muscle strips. There was no sign of necrosis and the mitotic index was low (2 mitoses/20 high-power fields) (Figures 2 and 3).

Immunohistochemistry confirmed the diagnostic hypothesis of a UTROSCT, with positive expression for CD56, smooth muscle actin, CD10, desmin, and pan-cytokeratin. The immunohistochemical markers for calretinin and inhibin were negative (Table 1).

The patient was readmitted to the department and metastatic screening was performed using computed tomography (CT) of the abdomen and chest. No abnormalities were found in the chest CT results. However, abdominal imaging showed the uterus to be greatly increased in size, with heterogeneous enhancement, an image resembling a cyst, probably of ovarian origin, in the left parauterine region, and a small amount of free fluid in the pelvis. No other abnormalities were found.

Serum levels of carcinoembryonic antigen (CEA) and CA 125 were <50 ng/ml and 15.50 U/ml, respectively.

Once the possibility of implantation metastasis had been ruled out, it was decided to submit the patient to a total abdominal hysterectomy with bilateral salpingooophorectomy. When accessing the abdominal cavity, a small amount of ascites was found and the left ovary was increased in volume, with a cystic appearance. The cecal appendix was normal. There were no complications following surgery and the patient was discharged from hospital the following day.

Histopathology performed on the surgical specimen obtained during the latest surgical procedure revealed uterine fibroids and focal adenomyosis, an endometrium with simple hyperplasia and no atypia, and a cervix with chronic cervicitis and squamous metaplasia. The right ovary was normal, while

TABLE 1: Immunohistochemical analysis revealing a uterine tumor resembling ovarian sex-cord tumors (UTROSCT), Hospital Santa Casa de Misericórdia de Vitória, Vitória, ES, Brazil.

Markers	Tumor expression
CD56 – N-CAM (clone 123C3)	Positive
Smooth muscle actin (clone 1A4)	Positive
Pan-cytokeratin (clone AE1/ AE3)	Positive (multifocal)
Calretinin (clone CRT01)	Negative
Inhibin (clone R1)	Negative
CD10 (CALLA) (clone SS2/ 36)	Positive
Desmin (clone DE-R-11)	Positive (multifocal)

a hemorrhagic corpus luteum cyst was found on the left ovary. There was no sign of any residual UTROSCT.

The patient has been followed up regularly at the gynecological oncology outpatient department and remains asymptomatic one year after the second surgery. She will continue to be followed up as an outpatient for five years, with clinical examination and tomography of the chest, abdomen, and pelvis performed annually. At the end of the follow-up period, she will continue to undergo annual gynecological and clinical examination.

3. Discussion

A 46-year-old patient with abnormal vaginal bleeding underwent a surgical procedure to remove a pediculated nodular lesion protruding from the external cervical os. Histopathology led to a diagnosis of UTROSCT. Total abdominal hysterectomy with bilateral adnexectomy was then performed. Uterine fibroids and focal adenomyosis were identified in the surgical specimen, with no findings of residual UTROSCT. The patient is currently undergoing regular outpatient follow-up, with no evidence of disease after one year.

In 1976, Clemente and Scully classified these tumors into two groups: Group 1: ESTSCLE and Group II: UTROSCT. In ESTSCLE, less than 50% of the total tumor mass is composed of structural areas resembling sex cords and the tumor behavior is malignant in around 15% of cases [4, 5]. On the other hand, in UTROSCT, more than 50% of the total tumor mass resembles sex cords and in the great majority of cases its behavior is benign; however, there are cases in the literature involving metastasis and recurrence [7].

As in the case reported here, UTROSCT are more common between the fourth and sixth decades of life, with the principal symptoms being abnormal uterine bleeding and pelvic pain. Because of the rarity of this type of tumor, its incidence and mortality rates remain unknown [7].

Diagnosis can only be confirmed by histology after tumor resection, in most cases incidentally following hysterectomy performed because of a suspected endometrial polyp or uterine fibroids. Up to the present time, no noninvasive diagnostic tests such as specific serum markers or imaging findings have become available [6]. Although the potential for malignancy is low, there have been reports of UTROSCT associated with lymph node and extrauterine metastases [8].

Microscopically, these tumors are well demarcated; however, in rare cases they can be infiltrated between muscle fibers and may present with different microscopic forms such as sheets, tight nests, thin cords, trabeculae with wide interconnections, irregular islands, and hollow or solid tubules, with varying amounts of fibrous or hyalinized stroma. Cells with small amounts of clear or foam eosinophilic cytoplasm remaining from Sertoli and granulosa cells may be present. Typically, mitotic indexes are low with this type of tumor. It should also be emphasized that neoplastic endometrial stroma should not be found in the histological analysis of UTROSCT [9]. Differential histological diagnosis should be made between epithelioid and plexiform leiomyomas, uterine sarcoma, endometrial carcinoma, and metastatic sex-cord tumors of the ovary [10].

The tumor site varies and it may be submucous, intramural, or subserous. In the present report, the tumor was submucous, since pathological analysis of the uterine body showed no sign of the tumor after it had been removed [8]. Immunohistochemistry aids diagnosis, since the tumor shows positivity for the sex-cord markers calretinin, inhibin, CD99, Wilms' tumor protein 1, and melanoma antigen recognized by T cells (MART-1), for the epithelial markers pan-cytokeratin and epithelial membrane antigen (EMA), for the myeloid markers smooth muscle actin (SMA), desmin, and histone deacetylase 8, and for a range of other markers such as CD10, estrogen receptors, progesterone receptors, S100, and CD117, characterizing the varying phenotypes of this rare form of tumor [8].

There are few reports of metastasis and recurrence in the literature. In a systematic review published in 2018 that evaluated prognostic factors of recurrence in UTROSCT, recurrence rates of 6.3% were found for the 79 patients evaluated. Disease-free survival is high and is associated only with the type of surgery: 86% for patients submitted to resection of the tumor alone and 96% for those submitted to total hysterectomy, both for a five-year period [11]. The UTROSCT is considered of uncertain malignant potential, and there are no formal recommendations regarding treatment [7]. Up to the present time, hysterectomy has been the treatment of choice. Nevertheless, there are reports of some individual cases in which the patient wanted to go on to have children and the tumor was resected at hysteroscopy [7].

Although there is currently no consensus with respect to the follow-up regimen for cases of UTROSCT, the patient in the present report is undergoing annual outpatient follow-up, with no signs of metastasis or tumor recurrence twelve months after surgery. She will continue to be evaluated for five years, with clinical examination and tomography to assess for metastases in abdominal and pelvic organs.

This is the first reported case of a UTROSCT in a prolapsed fibroid protruding into the vagina through the cervix. The initial surgical procedure performed (vaginal myomectomy) would have been sufficient to completely resect the tumor in this case, since histopathology following the second procedure (total abdominal hysterectomy and bilateral adnexectomy) failed to detect any signs of residual UTROSCT, confirming the low malignant potential of this type of tumor.

References

[1] M. G. Uçar, T. T. Ilhan, A. Gül, C. Ugurluoglu, and Ç. Çelik, "Uterine tumour resembling ovarian sex cord tumour- A rare entity," *Journal of Clinical and Diagnostic Research*, vol. 10, no. 12, pp. QD05–QD07, 2016.

[2] S. M. Schraag, R. Caduff, K. J. Dedes, D. Fink, and A.-M. Schmidt, "Uterine tumors resembling ovarian sex cord tumors – treatment, recurrence, pregnancy and brief review," *Gynecologic Oncology Reports*, vol. 19, pp. 53–56, 2017.

[3] R. P. Morehead and M. C. Bowman, "Heterologous mesodermal tumors of the uterus: report of a neoplasm resembling a granulosa cell tumor," *American Journal of Pathology*, vol. 21, no. 1, pp. 53–61, 1945.

[4] P. B. Clement and R. E. Scully, "Uterine tumors resembling ovarian sex-cord tumors: a clinicopathologic analysis of fourteen cases," *American Journal of Clinical Pathology*, vol. 66, no. 3, pp. 512–525, 1976.

[5] C.-Y. Liu, Y. Shen, J.-G. Zhao, and P.-P. Qu, "Clinical experience of uterine tumors resembling ovarian sex cord tumors: A clinicopathological analysis of 6 cases," *International Journal of Clinical and Experimental Pathology*, vol. 8, no. 4, pp. 4158–4164, 2015.

[6] J. M. Byun, K. T. Kim, H. K. Yoon et al., "Uterine tumors resembling ovarian sex cord tumor in postmenopausal woman," *The Journal of Obstetrics and Gynecology of India*, vol. 65, no. 4, pp. 273–277, 2015.

[7] M. L. Kuznicki, S. E. Robertson, A. Hakam, and M. M. Shahzad, "Metastatic uterine tumor resembling ovarian sex cord tumor: A case report and review of the literature," *Gynecologic Oncology Reports*, vol. 22, pp. 64–68, 2017.

[8] N. Cetinkaya, S. Bas, Z. F. Cuylan, O. Erdem, S. Erkaya, and T. Gungor, "Uterine tumors resembling ovarian sex cord tumors: A case report and literature review," *Oncology Letters*, vol. 11, no. 2, pp. 1496–1498, 2016.

[9] E. Oliva, "Pure mesenchymal and mixed müllerian tumors of the uterus," in *Gynecologic Pathology*, R. M. Nucci and E. Oliva, Eds., pp. 261–329, Churchill Livingstone, London, UK, 2009.

[10] A. A. Hashmi, N. Faridi, M. M. Edhi, and M. Khan, "Uterine tumor resembling ovarian sex cord tumor (UTROSCT), case report with literature review," *International Archives of Medicine*, vol. 7, no. 1, p. 47, 2014.

[11] G. K. Comert, C. Kilic, D. Cavusoglu et al., "Recurrence in uterine tumors with ovarian sex-cord tumor resemblance: a case report and systematic review," *Turkish Journal of Pathology*, 2018.

8

Two Case Reports of Intravenous Leiomyomatosis with Hyaluronan Expression

Haruhisa Konishi ⓘ,[1] Iemasa Koh,[1] Noriyuki Shiroma,[2] Yukie Kidani,[1] Satoshi Urabe,[1] Norifumi Tanaka,[1] Eiji Hirata,[1] Koji Arihiro,[2] and Yoshiki Kudo[1]

[1]*Department of Obstetrics and Gynecology, Graduate School of Biomedical Science, Hiroshima University, Japan*
[2]*Department of Anatomical Pathology, Hiroshima University Hospital, Japan*

Correspondence should be addressed to Haruhisa Konishi; haru.konishi@gmail.com

Academic Editor: Maria Grazia Porpora

Intravenous leiomyomatosis (IVL) is a rare benign neoplasm. Herein, we describe two cases of IVL at different levels of progression. The tumor in Case 1 was extensive, invading the right atrium after a hysterectomy for a uterine myoma. The tumor temporarily responded to hormonal treatment; however, tumor regrowth occurred. In contrast, the tumor in Case 2 extended only to the pelvic veins and was revealed preoperatively. Hysterectomy and bilateral salpingo-oophorectomy were performed, resulting in the complete surgical resection of the tumor. In Case 2, no recurrence has been observed. Tumor samples were evaluated for hyaluronan expression using Alcian blue staining (with and without hyaluronidase digestion). The tumor in Case 1 stained strongly positive for hyaluronan while the tumor in Case 2 stained weakly positive for hyaluronan. In contrast, a large non-IVL uterine leiomyoma (control) stained negative for hyaluronan. These results suggest a relationship between tumor hyaluronan expression and IVL progression, similar to that in other cancers.

1. Introduction

Leiomyomas are the most common type of benign neoplasm in the uterus. Intravenous leiomyomatosis (IVL) is a rare variant of leiomyoma; IVL tumors grow within the uterine and extrauterine venous system. Although IVL tumors are histologically benign, IVL is potentially life-threatening, as the tumor can extend into the inferior vena cava (IVC), right cardiac chambers, and pulmonary arteries. Thus, patients with IVL can present with findings of hemodynamic compromise, such as dyspnea, syncope, congestive heart failure, or sudden death. Although IVL may be incidentally discovered early (in the uterine veins alone) when a patient undergoes a hysterectomy for reasons other than leiomyoma, most reports are of patients in the advanced stage of the disease, with right cardiac chamber or pulmonary artery involvement.

Hyaluronan is known to enhance tumor growth by promoting angiogenesis in various tumors [1, 2]. Herein, we report two cases of IVL at different levels of progression, concordant with different hyaluronan expression levels. Thus, these cases suggest a relationship between tumor hyaluronan expression and IVL progression.

2. Case Reports

2.1. Case 1. A 55-year-old woman (gravida 1, para 1) was referred to our hospital because of the progression of a lower abdominal tumor. At 45 years of age, she underwent a total abdominal hysterectomy (TAH) at another hospital for a leiomyoma, which persisted after the surgery. One year later, an attempt to reduce the progressing residual tumor was unsuccessful. Two years after the TAH, the tumor had extended into the IVC and right cardiac chamber; thus, she underwent tumor resection surgery at another hospital and was admitted to our care some years after her last surgery. Computerized tomography (CT) revealed a large tumor occupying the abdominal cavity and multiple bilateral pulmonary nodules (Figure 1(a)). The patient's course was complicated by renal failure due to ureteric stenosis,

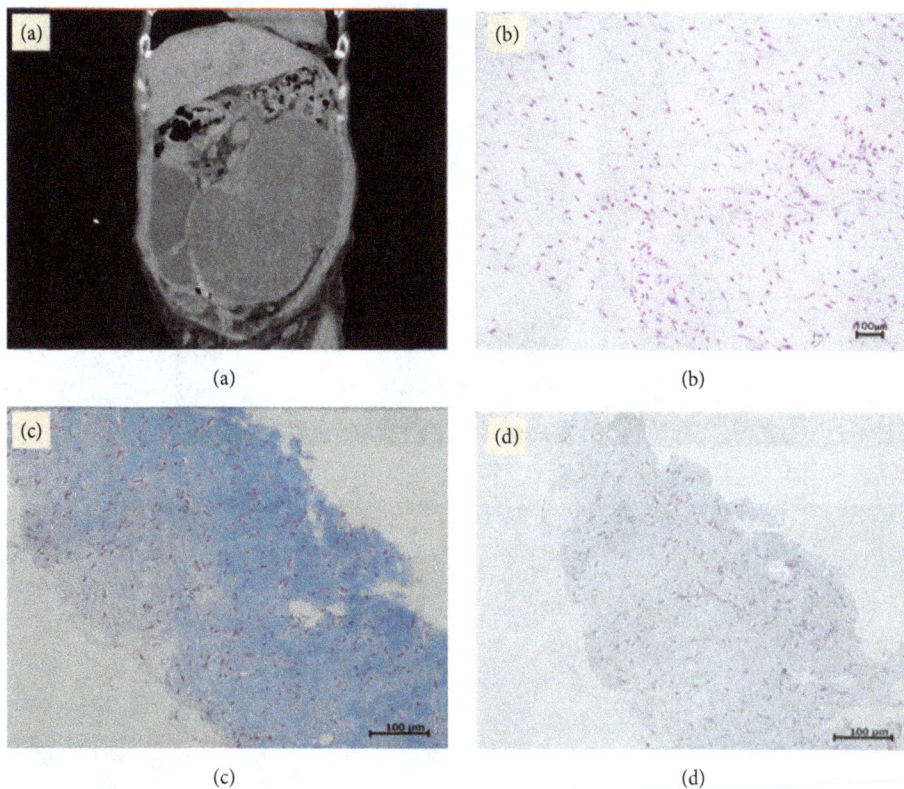

FIGURE 1: (a) Large tumor occupying the abdominal cavity on a computerized tomography scan. (b) The histopathological diagnosis is leiomyoma (H&E 200×), based on the absence of nuclear atypia and a low mitotic index. (c) Tumor cells stained strongly positive for Alcian blue at a pH of 2.5 (200×). (d) Alcian blue staining disappears after hyaluronidase digestion (200×).

secondary to the expanding tumor. Her serum estradiol level was 11 pg/ml and FSH level was 103 mIU.

A transabdominal needle biopsy was performed to exclude a malignant tumor; there was no nuclear atypia and the mitotic index was low. Thus, the final histopathological diagnosis was leiomyoma (Figure 1(b)). On immunohisto-chemistry, the tumor was positive for estrogen and proges-terone receptors. In addition, the tumor cells stained strongly positive for Alcian blue (pH = 2.5). Moreover, the staining disappeared after hyaluronidase digestion, suggesting that the tumor contained abundant hyaluronan (Figures 1(c) and 1(d)). Thus, she was diagnosed with IVL and benign metastasizing leiomyoma.

The tumor temporarily responded to hormonal treatment (letrozole, medroxyprogesterone) and became smaller. How-ever, the tumor eventually progressed. Among other condi-tions, she had a progressing lung metastasis, gastrointestinal obstruction, repeated cellulitis, and leg edema. The patient died of multiple organ failure due to tumor progression, 13 years after her initial surgery.

2.2. Case 2.

A 46-year-old woman (gravida 2, para 2) was referred to our hospital complaining of a lower abdominal mass and pain. Her medical history was unremarkable. She was initially diagnosed with a uterine leiomyoma by tran-scervical needle biopsy. CT revealed a large heterogeneous tumor occupying the pelvic cavity and an intravascular tumor

within the dilated left internal iliac and ovarian veins (Figures 2(a) and 2(b)). Her preoperative cervical cytology results were negative for intraepithelial lesions and malignancy. The endometrial cytology and needle biopsy results were also negative. Thus, the preoperative diagnosis was IVL, with extension of the tumor into the left internal iliac and ovarian veins.

Intraoperatively, multiple myomas were found within the uterine corpus and cervix, and the tumor extended to the parametrium and paracolpium. Detachment of the tumor from the left ureter and vaginal wall was very difficult. Intravenous tumors in the left internal iliac and ovarian veins could be palpated. The left internal iliac vein forming the common iliac vein was transected at the bifurcation region. In addition, TAH and bilateral salpingo-oophorectomy (BSO) were performed, resulting in the complete surgical resection of the tumor (operative time, 11 hours; blood loss, 8462 g). The resected uterus and adnexa weighed 897 g (Figures 2(c) and 2(d)). There was no residual tumor detected in the venous resection stump.

The nodule resected from the uterus and the internal iliac and ovarian veins consisted of a proliferation of spindle cells. There was no nuclear atypia and the mitotic index was low. In addition, vessel endothelium cells and a vascular smooth muscle layer covered the IVL (Figures 3(a) and 3(b)). The tumor cells stained positive for Alcian blue (pH = 2.5) and the staining disappeared after hyaluronidase digestion. However,

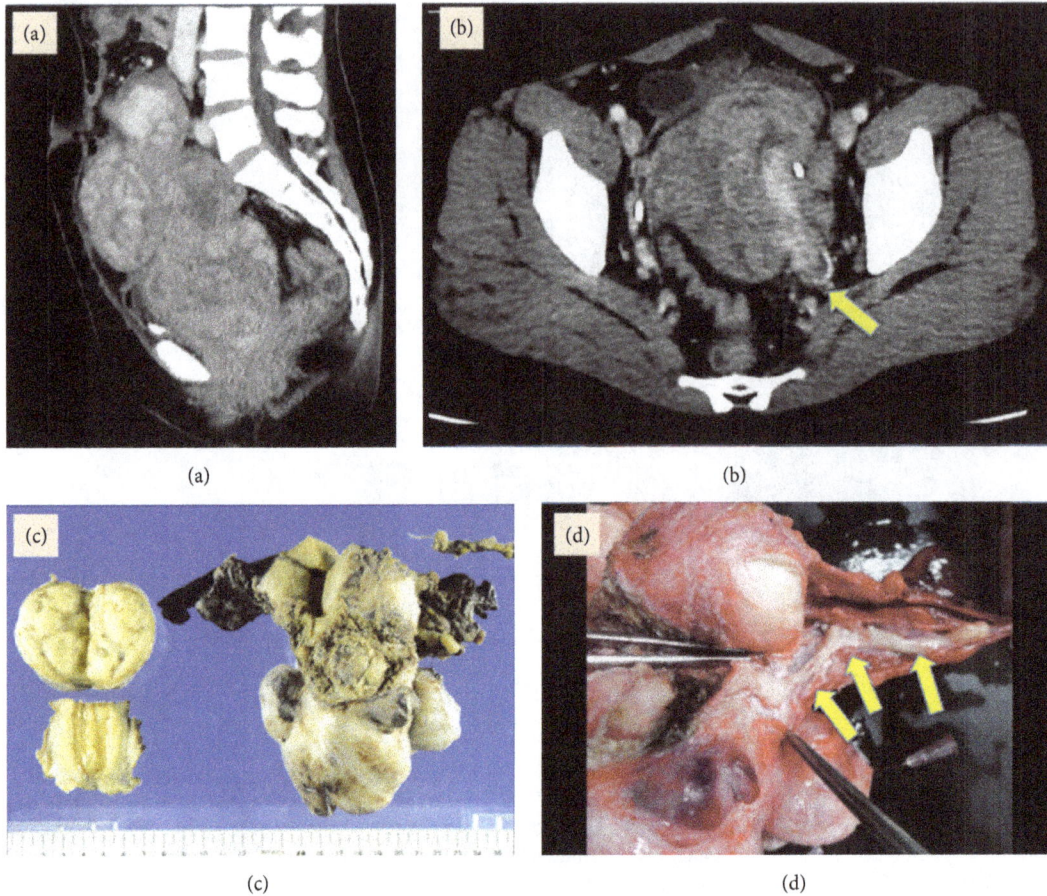

FIGURE 2: (a) Heterogeneous large tumor occupying the pelvic cavity on a computerized tomography scan. (b) Intravascular tumor within the dilated left internal iliac vein on a computerized tomography scan. (c) Multiple leiomyomas within the uterine corpus and cervix. (d) Tumor growth extending into the left ovarian vein.

compared to that in Case 1, the intensity of the staining was weaker and less diffuse (Figures 3(c) and 3(d)). Similar findings for hyaluronan expression were obtained using the sample retrieved from the preoperative needle biopsy.

The histopathological diagnosis of the uterine and intravascular tumors was IVL. There has been no evidence of IVL recurrence, with the most recent follow-up at 38 months postoperatively.

3. Discussion

IVL was first described by Hirschfield in 1896 [3] and was defined by Norris and Parmly in 1975 [4]. IVL is histologically defined as a benign smooth muscle cell tumor; however, given their potential to grow within the uterine venous system, IVL tumors can cause a fatal cardiac obstruction. The early diagnosis of this condition is rare because of its low prevalence and nonspecific initial manifestations. Not infrequently, the diagnosis is made after death due to congestive heart failure. Differential diagnoses include leiomyosarcoma, endometrial stromal sarcoma, and diffuse uterine leiomyomatosis. The true rate of recurrence of completely resected IVL is unknown, but regrowth has been

documented in up to 30% of patients. Thus, long-term follow-up imaging is recommended. CT appears to adequately detect the regrowth [5].

Although the precise pathogenesis of the intravenous invasion remains unclear, there are two theories regarding the origin of IVL tumors. The first suggests that the tumors arise from smooth muscle in the vessel wall, while the second considers IVL to be the consequence of a uterine leiomyoma invading into the surrounding vessels [6, 7]. Recently, Fukuyama et al. [8] reported that tumors advance by stretching the vascular wall (rather than by breaking the wall), progressing into the vein like a polyp, covered in endothelium cells. We are inclined to support the latter theory regarding the pathogenesis of IVL, as our pathological findings were of a tumor covered in endothelium cells (Figures 3(a) and 3(b)).

Controversy exists regarding the treatment of IVL. Given that IVL tumors are positive for estrogen and progesterone receptors, BSO is essential and exogenous estrogen must be avoided. Although hormonal treatments, such as gonadotropin releasing hormone (GnRH) analogs and antiestrogens, have been used to prevent tumor growth, evidence regarding their efficacy is inconsistent [4]. In Case 1, treatment with Letrozole (an aromatase inhibitor)

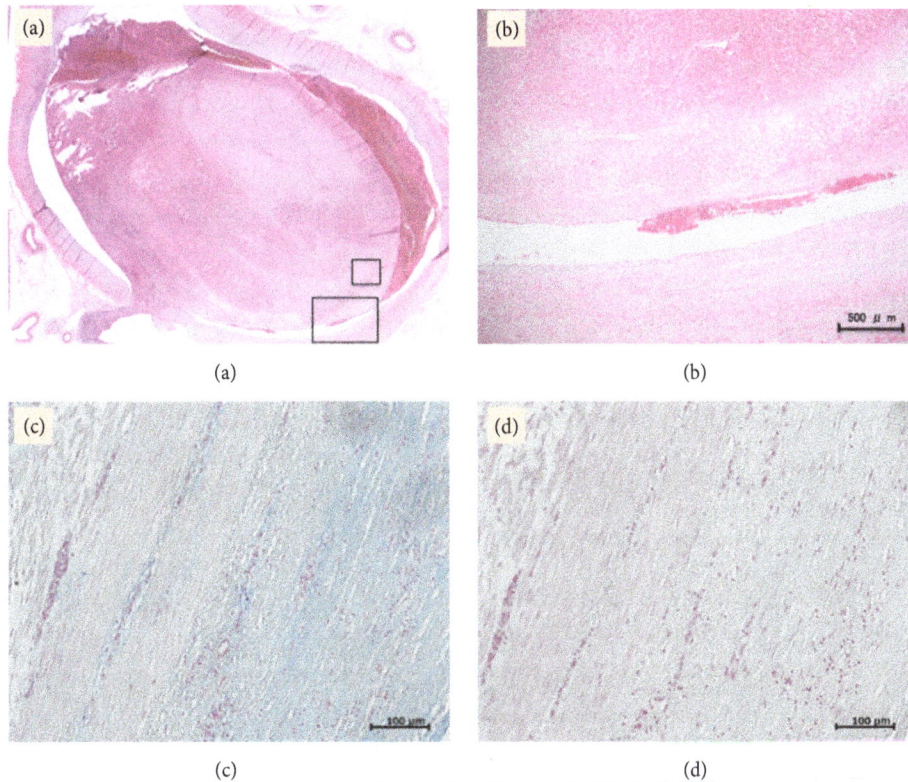

FIGURE 3: (a) The intravenous tumor (H&E magnifying lens). (b) Vessel endothelium cells and vascular smooth muscle layer covered the intravenous leiomyoma (H&E 40×); an enlarged view of the area in Figure 3(a) is surrounded by a large black box. (c) Tumor cells stained strongly for positive Alcian blue at a pH of 2.5 (200×); an enlarged view of the area in Figure 3(a) is surrounded by a small black box. (d) Alcian blue staining disappears after hyaluronidase digestion (200×); the same area as that in Figure 3(c) is shown.

and medroxyprogesterone resulted in a temporary response; however, the tumor eventually progressed. Currently, the complete resection of all existing and visible tumors is recommended, if possible [9]. However, an early-stage diagnosis is critical for a complete resection and good prognosis, which is rare, as the clinical presentation is initially nonspecific (e.g., pelvic pain and abdominal discomfort). In Case 2, we suspected IVL because of the enlarged veins and intravenous tumors on CT imaging. This preoperative diagnosis enabled the necessary preparations for a complete resection.

Hyaluronan is a component of the extracellular matrix and is involved in various aspects of mammalian tissue physiology. Hyaluronan binds to CD44 receptors, mediating many cellular events, including cellular regeneration and wound healing. However, abnormalities in hyaluronan production, resulting in Rho A and PI3K Rac cascade activation, have been implicated in many diseases, including cancer [1, 2]. In addition, high levels of hyaluronan expression have been observed in IVL tumors [10, 11]. We noted that hyaluronan was expressed in the IVL tumors in both of our cases. Furthermore, the tumor in Case 1 had a higher level of hyaluronan expression and more progressed IVL compared to that in Case 2. In contrast, hyaluronan expression in a large leiomyoma was negative (data not shown). Thus, increased hyaluronan expression in IVL tumors may indicate that the tumors are highly angiogenic and have a potential for

invasion. Consistent with this, a close relationship between tumor hyaluronan expression and the progression of breast and colorectal cancers has been demonstrated [12, 13].

Alcian blue staining was used to evaluate the hyaluronan expression level in IVL tumors. Alcian blue staining is a common and well-validated staining technique that is used to detect acid mucopolysaccharides, including chondroitin sulfate and hyaluronan. Hyaluronan can be distinguished from other materials by the disappearance of the stain after hyaluronidase digestion. Myxoid leiomyomas and myxoid leiomyosarcoma have also been reported to stain positive with Alcian blue [14].

In this report, we described two cases of IVL with different outcomes. The accumulation of additional cases is needed to further evaluate a relationship between hyaluronan expression, assessed with Alcian blue staining, and IVL progression.

References

[1] T. Chanmee, P. Ontong, and N. Itano, "Hyaluronan: A modulator of the tumor microenvironment," *Cancer Letters*, vol. 375, no. 1, pp. 20–30, 2016.

[2] Y. Gouëffic, C. Guilluy, P. Guérin, P. Patra, P. Pacaud, and G. Loirand, "Hyaluronan induces vascular smooth muscle cell migration through RHAMM-mediated PI3K-dependent Rac activation," *Cardiovascular Research*, vol. 72, no. 2, pp. 339–348, 2006.

[3] B. Hirschfeld, *DMW - Deutsche Medizinische Wochenschrift*, FCW Vogel, Leipzig, Germany, 5th edition, 1896.

[4] H. J. Norris and T. Parmley, "Mesenchymal tumors of the uterus. V. Intravenous leiomyomatosis. A clinical and pathologic study of 14 cases," *Cancer*, vol. 36, no. 6, pp. 2164–2178, 1975.

[5] V. Valdés Devesa, C. R. Conley, W. M. Stone, J. M. Collins, and J. F. Magrina, "Update on intravenous leiomyomatosis: Report of five patients and literature review," *European Journal of Obstetrics & Gynecology and Reproductive Biology*, vol. 171, no. 2, pp. 209–213, 2013.

[6] L. Grella, T. E. Arnold, K. H. V. Kvilekval, and F. Giron, "Intravenous leiomyomatosis," *Journal of Vascular Surgery*, vol. 20, no. 6, pp. 987–994, 1994.

[7] G. Kir, M. Kir, A. Gurbuz, A. Karateke, and F. Aker, "Estrogen and progesterone expression of vessel walls with intravascular leiomyomatosis; Discussion of histogenesis," *European Journal of Gynaecological Oncology*, vol. 25, no. 3, pp. 362–366, 2004.

[8] A. Fukuyama, Y. Yokoyama, M. Futagami, T. Shigeto, R. Wada, and H. Mizunuma, "A case of uterine leiomyoma with intravenous leiomyomatosis -histological investigation of the pathological condition," *Pathology & Oncology Research*, vol. 17, no. 1, pp. 171–174, 2011.

[9] C. Mizoguchi, H. Matsumoto, K. Nasu, M. Arakane, K. Kai, and H. Narahara, "Intravenous leiomyomatosis treated with radical hysterectomy and adjuvant aromatase inhibitor therapy," *Journal of Obstetrics and Gynaecology Research*, vol. 42, no. 10, pp. 1405–1408, 2016.

[10] C. Yaguchi, H. Oi, H. Kobayashi, K. Miura, and N. Kanayama, "A case of intravenous leiomyomatosis with high levels of hyaluronan," *Journal of Obstetrics and Gynaecology Research*, vol. 36, no. 2, pp. 454–458, 2010.

[11] M.-J. Chen, Y. Peng, Y.-S. Yang, S.-C. Huang, S.-N. Chow, and P.-L. Torng, "Increased hyaluronan and CD44 expressions in intravenous leiomyomatosis," *Acta Obstetricia et Gynecologica Scandinavica*, vol. 84, no. 4, pp. 322–328, 2005.

[12] P. Auvinen, R. Tammi, J. Parkkinen et al., "Hyaluronan in peritumoral stroma and malignant cells associates with breast cancer spreading and predicts survival," *The American Journal of Pathology*, vol. 156, no. 2, pp. 529–536, 2000.

[13] K. Ropponen, M. Tammi, J. Parkkinen et al., "Tumor cell-associated hyaluronan as an unfavorable prognostic factor in colorectal cancer," *Cancer Research*, vol. 58, no. 2, pp. 342–347, 1998.

[14] G. Toledo and E. Oliva, "Smooth muscle tumors of the uterus: a practical approach," *Archives of Pathology & Laboratory Medicine*, vol. 132, no. 4, pp. 595–605, 2008.

9

Gestational Tubal Choriocarcinoma Presenting as a Pregnancy of Unknown Location following Ovarian Induction

Lawrence Hsu Lin ⓘ,[1] Koji Fushida,[1] Eliane Azeka Hase,[1] Regina Schultz ⓘ,[2] Laysa Manatta Tenorio,[1] Fabricia Andrea Rosa Madia,[3] Evelin Aline Zanardo,[3] Leslie Domenici Kulikowski,[3] and Rossana Pulcineli Vieira Francisco ⓘ[1]

[1]University of Sao Paulo Trophoblastic Disease Center, University of Sao Paulo Medical School, Sao Paulo, SP, Brazil
[2]Department of Pathology, University of Sao Paulo Medical School, Sao Paulo, SP, Brazil
[3]Cytogenomic Laboratory, Department of Pathology, University of Sao Paulo Medical School, Sao Paulo, SP, Brazil

Correspondence should be addressed to Lawrence Hsu Lin; l.lin@hc.fm.usp.br

Academic Editor: Erich Cosmi

The management of pregnancy of unknown location (PUL) can be a challenging situation, since it can present as several different conditions. Here we describe a rare case of gestational choriocarcinoma arising in the fallopian tube after ovarian induction in an infertile patient. The patient received clomiphene for ovarian induction and had rising levels of human chorionic gonadotropin (hCG) over nine months without sign of pregnancy. After referral to our center, the patient was diagnosed with a paraovarian tumor, which revealed a gestational choriocarcinoma arising in the fallopian tube; the final diagnosis was supported by pathological and cytogenomic analysis. Malignancies, such as gestational trophoblastic disease, should be in the differential diagnosis of PUL; the early recognition of these conditions is key for the proper treatment and favorable outcome.

1. Introduction

Pregnancy of unknown location (PUL) is a condition that can be particularly challenging for clinicians due to the variety of diagnoses that PUL can represent [1]. PUL can occur via either spontaneous conception or assisted reproduction treatment (ART). In certain cases, the use of ART should raise concerns, since ART is an important risk factor for ectopic pregnancies, which are associated with high rates of life-threatening complications [2]. However, PUL can also be the initial presentation of a variety of human chorionic gonadotropin- (hCG-) secreting malignancies [3].

Here, we report a case of tubal choriocarcinoma that initially presented as PUL in an infertile patient after ovarian induction. The gestational origin of the tumor was confirmed via short tandem repeat (STR) analysis of samples from the tumor and serum samples from the patient and her partner.

2. Case Report

A 38-year-old nulliparous woman was referred to the University of Sao Paulo Trophoblastic Disease Center due to PUL with increasing hCG levels, amenorrhea for 9 months, and no sign of an hCG-producing site. She had a prior history of primary infertility for years and had received clomiphene for ovarian induction. Her hCG rose from an initial level of 2,845 mIU/mL to 3,917 mIU/mL after 2 days, 5,533 mIU/mL after two weeks, and 381,808 mIU/mL after 9 months, with serial normal ultrasound scans performed during follow-up at another institution.

When the patient was referred to our institution, her hCG level was 267,836 mIU/mL, and ultrasound showed a normal uterus, a normal left ovary, a large cystic structure on the right ovary that measured 7.5 cm × 5.5 cm, and an irregular left paraovarian mass that measured 4.6 cm × 3.7 cm and exhibited intense low-resistance peripheral vascularization on Doppler examinations (Figures 1(a) and

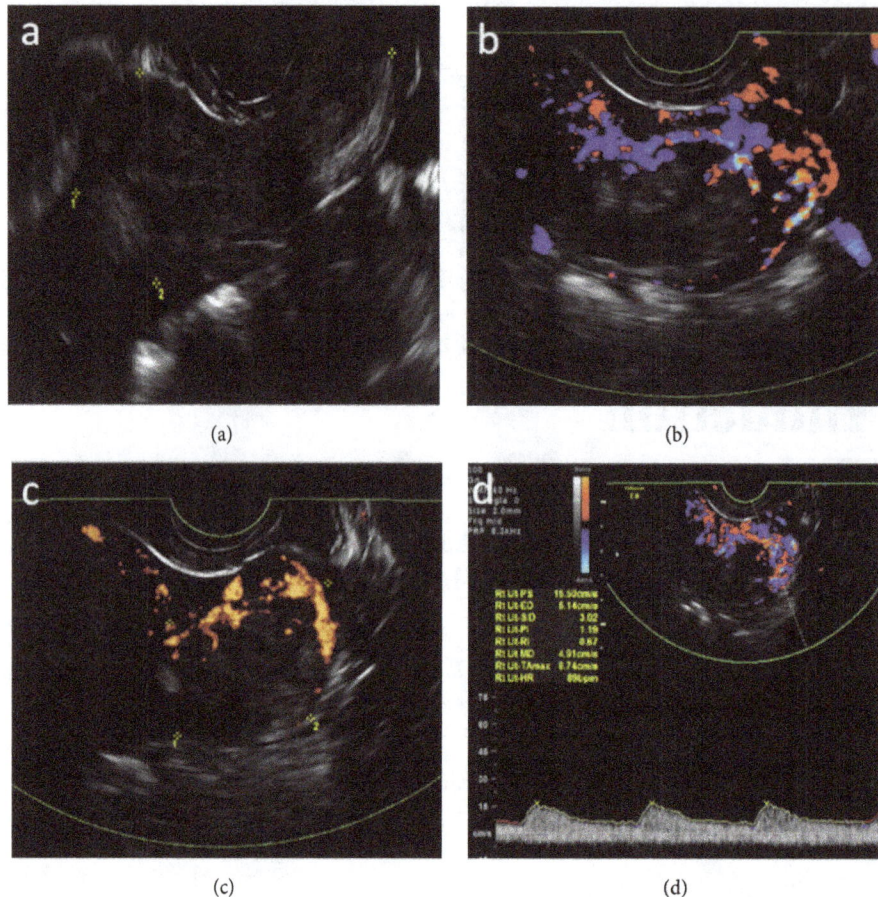

(a)

(b)

(c)

(d)

FIGURE 1: (a) Transvaginal sonographic sagittal section of the uterus revealing no signs of intrauterine pregnancy. (b) Color Doppler and (c) power Doppler transvaginal sonographic transverse sections of the left paraovarian tumor with strong peripheral vascularization. (d) Pulsed Doppler analysis of tumor vascularization, showing a pattern of low resistance.

1(b)). Pelvic magnetic resonance imaging was performed to further evaluate the origin of these findings; this imaging confirmed the presence of a solid-cystic lesion measuring 4.5 cm × 3.2 cm with a clear cleavage interface to the left ovary and postcontrast enhancement (Figures 2(a) and 2(b)). Brain, chest, and upper abdomen CT scans showed normal results.

An exploratory laparotomy was performed, resulting in visualization of a 5 cm vascularized left tubal mass, an 8 cm serous right ovarian cyst, and no other evidence of abdominal disease. Excision of the right ovarian cyst and the left uterine tube was performed. Pathological and immunohistochemical analyses revealed a choriocarcinoma infiltrating the tubal wall up to the serosa, the presence of vascular infiltration in tubal vessels, and a corpus luteum as the right ovarian cyst (Figure 3).

Also, in order to clarify the origin of the tumor we performed the differential diagnosis by genotyping seven autosomal STR loci (D13S317, D7S820, D2S1338, D21S11, D16S539, D18S51, CSF1PO, and FGA) and the sex-determining marker using AmpFLSTR® MiniFiler™ PCR Amplification Kit (Life Technologies™, California, USA) according to manufacturer's instructions.

Cytogenomic analysis showed the presence of paternal alleles in choriocarcinoma tissue, confirming the gestational origin of the tumor (Figure 4).

The patient received 8 cycles of methotrexate, and her hCG levels normalized 4 months after surgery. The patient remains healthy 2 years after the completion of chemotherapy, with no signs of recurrence.

3. Discussion

PUL can be a challenging dilemma in medical practice, since several clinical entities can present with increased hCG levels and no visible sign of pregnancy [1, 2]. Early or failing intrauterine pregnancies, ectopic pregnancies, heterophile antibodies, and hCG-secreting tumors are examples of medical conditions that could initially present as PUL [2, 3]. Most guidelines suggest a diagnostic flow diagram based on levels and trends of hCG [17]. Increasing levels of hCG are more commonly associated with viable pregnancies than with other medical conditions; however, extremely high hCG values typically indicate a neoplastic process, particularly if no pregnancy is readily detectable.

Gestational trophoblastic disease (GTD) is a spectrum of disorders that arise from the placental trophoblast [18, 19].

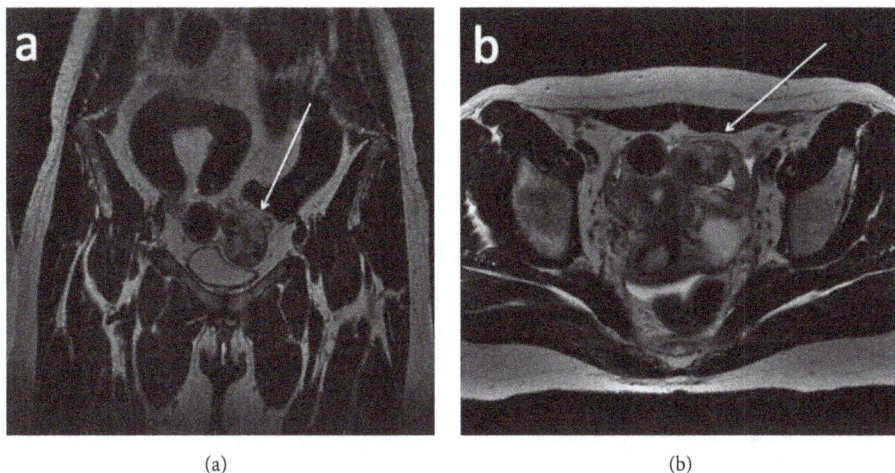

(a) (b)

FIGURE 2: (a) T1-weighted coronal and (b) axial pelvic magnetic resonance imaging showing a cystic-solid lesion originating from the left fallopian tube (white arrow).

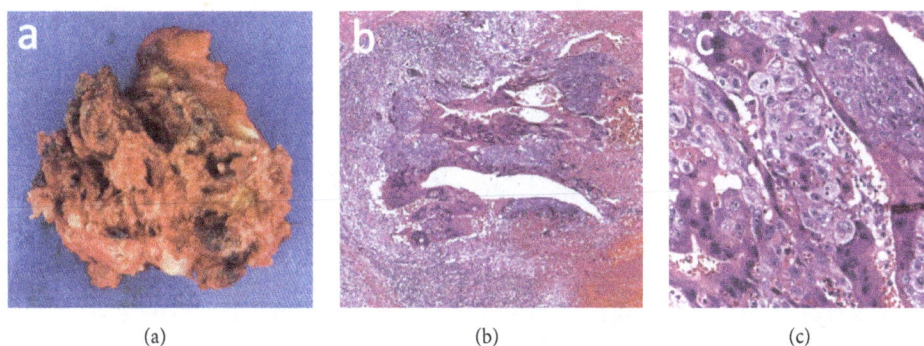

(a) (b) (c)

FIGURE 3: (a) Macroscopic appearance of the tumor. ((b) and (c)) Histological section of the tumor displaying clusters of abnormal syncytiotrophoblast and cytotrophoblast cells (hematoxylin-eosin staining, (b) ×50 magnification and (c) ×200 magnification).

One of the most aggressive types of GTD is gestational choriocarcinoma, which typically arises in the uterus. The presence of choriocarcinoma in the fallopian tube is extremely rare, with only four cases involving this phenomenon reported among 6,708 patients with GTD at Weston Park Hospital and six such cases among 2,100 cases of GTD at the New England Trophoblastic Disease Center [20, 21]. A tubal choriocarcinoma can be mistaken for an ectopic pregnancy due to the presence of an adnexal mass with raised hCG levels and can even present with tubal rupture and hemoperitoneum; therefore, pathological evaluation of tubal specimens is critical for appropriate differential diagnosis [11, 20]. In the case described here, besides presenting with very high hCG levels, the adnexal tumor showed peripheral low-resistance vascularization with an avascular central region (Figures 1(b), 1(c), and 1(d)), which resembles the compact pattern described by Hsieh et al. (1994), commonly associated with choriocarcinoma [22]. Table 1 summarizes the data from recently published cases of tubal choriocarcinoma in the literature, showing that most patients presented with symptoms that resemble ectopic pregnancies and higher hCG levels (median serum hCG: 15,000 mIU/mL; range: 3160–326,100 mIU/mL).

Since GTD is a rare condition, the relationship between ART and development of GTD has been debated in the literature. A retrospective report from United States of America disclosed a higher frequency of hydatidiform moles following ART (1 : 659 pregnancies) as compared to spontaneous pregnancies (estimated incidence 1 : 1000 pregnancies), even though it represents a rare complication [23, 24]. There seems to be a high percentage of multiple pregnancies with complete mole and coexisting fetus following ART, reaching 13% in a large retrospective cohort [24, 25]. However, a retrospective study in the United Kingdom found no statistical difference in the frequency of infertility treatment in patients with normal pregnancies and the ones with GTD [26].

ART is a risk factor for developing extrauterine pregnancies; therefore, ART may potentially increase the risk for gestational choriocarcinoma arising in unusual locations [10]. Other reports have described cases of tubal choriocarcinoma following ovarian induction with intrauterine insemination [10] and with in vitro fertilization [27]. However, data from the literature indicate that ART does not seem to influence the development of gestational trophoblastic neoplasia after hydatidiform moles [24, 26].

TABLE 1: Well-documented tubal choriocarcinoma case reports published in the literature in the last 10 years.

Study	Age	Last menstrual period	hCG levels (mIU/mL)	Clinical presentation	Tumor size (cm)	Surgical management	Chemotherapy	Genetic analysis
Bacalbasa et al., 2018 [4]	19	NA	NA	Abdominal pain and vaginal bleeding at presentation. Sigmoid colon invasion at recurrence	5	Unilateral salpingectomy at presentation. Recurrence managed with total hysterectomy, contralateral adnexectomy and sigmoid colon resection	MTX and ActD	No
Boynukalin et al., 2011 [5]	38	7 weeks	>15,000	Abdominal pain and vaginal bleeding	3.4	Unilateral salpingectomy	NA	NA
Butler et al., 2010 [6]	24	6 weeks	15,000	Abdominal pain and vaginal bleeding	3	Unilateral salpingectomy	MTX	No
Cianci et al., 2014 [7]	30	20 weeks	24,474	Coexisting intrauterine pregnancy and abdominal pain. Pulmonary metastasis	8	Unilateral adnexectomy at 20 weeks (delivery at 31 weeks)	EMA-CO after delivery	No
Davies et al., 2010 [8]	24	6 weeks	15,000	Abdominal pain and vaginal bleeding	3	Unilateral salpingectomy	MTX	No
Jia et al., 2017 [9]	39	6 weeks	7,158	Vaginal bleeding and palpable abdominal mass. Pulmonary metastasis	14	Total abdominal hysterectomy and bilateral adnexectomy	Yes (type not reported)	No
Jwa et al., 2017 [10]	34	6 weeks	7,054	Asymptomatic	2	Unilateral salpingectomy	EMA-CO	No
Karaman et al., 2015 [11]	31	7 weeks	29,251	Abdominal pain, fatigue, hypotension and tachycardia	4	Unilateral salpingectomy	MTX	No
Lin et al., 2017	38	9 months	267,836	Asymptomatic	4.6	Unilateral salpingectomy	MTX	Yes
Mehrotra et al., 2012 [12]	30	3.5 months	326,100	Abdominal pain, fever, fatigue, tachycardia, palpable mass 1 month after first trimester abortion	16	Unilateral adnexectomy	EMA-CO	No
Nakayama et al., 2011 [13]	26	5 months	9,903	Vaginal bleeding	6.4	Unilateral salpingectomy	None	Yes
Rettenmaier et al., 2013 [14]	32	NA	4,759	Abdominal pain	NA	Unilateral salpingectomy	Patient refused	No
Ubayasiri et al., 2010 [15]	36	6 weeks	3,160	Vaginal bleeding	3	Unilateral salpingectomy	MTX	No
Wan et al., 2014 [16]	54	3 months	291,116	Vaginal bleeding	4	Total abdominal hysterectomy and bilateral adnexectomy	5-Fu and KSM	No

NA: not available; hCG: human chorionic gonadotropin; cm: centimeter; MTX: methotrexate; ActD: actinomycin D; EMA-CO: etoposide, methotrexate, actinomycin D, cyclophosphamide, vincristine; 5-FU: 5-fluorouracil; KSM: kengshengmycin.

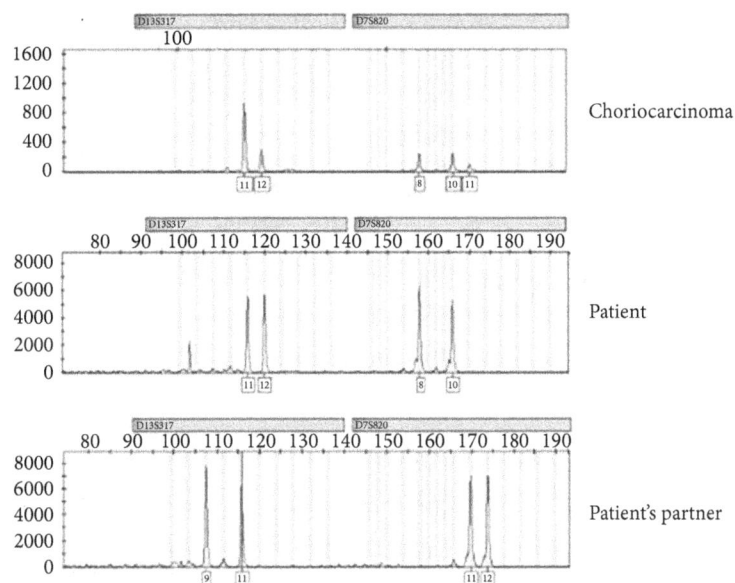

FIGURE 4: Results of genotyping of two autosomal STR loci (D13S317, D7S820) obtained from choriocarcinoma, patient, and patient's partner. The choriocarcinoma's electropherogram shows the presence of three allele for each STR loci. In the D13S317 presents the alleles 11 and 12, patient origin, and allele 11, patient's partner origin. The D7S820 presents the alleles 8 and 10, patient origin, and allele 11, patient's partner origin.

hCG is a key tumor marker in the management of patients with GTD because its levels are correlated with disease burden [18, 19]. In the presented case, the ectopic hCG-producing site was not initially detected using standard diagnostic methods, possibly because it was insufficiently large at first presentation. Since hCG is highly produced by choriocarcinoma cells, the same hCG level in a choriocarcinoma would reflect a much smaller mass of trophoblastic cells than of nonneoplastic trophoblasts, which are present in ectopic pregnancies [17, 18]. Most cases recently reported in the literature showed larger pelvic tumors, with a median size of 4 cm, ranging from 2 cm to 16 cm (Table 1).

Choriocarcinoma, particularly when presenting in unusual locations, can be of gestational or nongestational origin. STR analysis is a useful tool for determining tumor origin, which can impact treatment modalities and outcomes for patients with this tumor [28–30]. Gestational choriocarcinoma is highly sensitive to chemotherapy, as was observed for the patient described in this case report; in contrast, nongestational tumors are less sensitive to chemotherapy and demand more aggressive therapy because of worse outcomes [28, 29]. Since most centers do not have genetic analysis readily available (Table 1 shows that only 1 of 13 recently published cases of tubal choriocarcinoma reported genetic analysis of the tumor), differentiation between gestational and nongestation origin is based on clinical data, which is not always accurate, especially in trophoblastic tumors with unusual presentations [29].

In conclusion, differential diagnosis for PUL includes a variety of medical conditions. Early recognition of the hCG-producing source is key for the appropriate management of patients, particularly patients with neoplastic processes, which might be suspected based on extremely high and increasing levels of hCG combined with no signs of pregnancy.

Consent

Written consent has been obtained from the patient for the publication of this case report.

References

[1] K. Barnhart, N. M. Van Mello, T. Bourne et al., "Pregnancy of unknown location: A consensus statement of nomenclature, definitions, and outcome," *Fertility and Sterility*, vol. 95, no. 3, pp. 857–866, 2011.

[2] E. Kirk, C. Bottomley, and T. Bourne, "Diagnosing ectopic pregnancy and current concepts in the management of pregnancy of unknown location," *Human Reproduction Update*, vol. 20, no. 2, pp. 250–261, 2014.

[3] A. Larish, A. Kumar, S. Kerr, and C. Langstraat, "Primary gastric choriocarcinoma presenting as a pregnancy of unknown location," *Obstetrics & Gynecology*, vol. 129, no. 2, pp. 281–284, 2017.

[4] N. Bacalbasa, I. Balescu, V. Brasoveanu, and A. F. Anca, "Debulking surgery for pelvic recurrence after surgically-treated tubal gestational choriocarcinoma - A case report and literature review," *Anticancer Reseach*, vol. 38, no. 1, pp. 423–426, 2018.

[5] F. Boynukalin, Z. Erol, A. Aral, and I. Boyar, "Gestational choriocarcinoma arising in a tubal ectopic pregnancy: case report," *European Journal of Gynaecological Oncology*, vol. 32, no. 5, pp. 592-593, 2011.

[6] R. Butler, Y. Chadha, J. Davies, and M. Singh, "A case of primary tubal gestational choriocarcinoma: Case Reports," *Australian and New Zealand Journal of Obstetrics and Gynaecology*, vol. 50, no. 2, pp. 200-201, 2010.

[7] S. Cianci, SG. Vitale, R. Tozzi, P. Cignini, F. Padula, and L. D'Emidio, "Tubal primary metastatic choriocarcinoma coexistent with a viable early pregnancy?: a case report," *Journal of Prenatal Medicine*, vol. 8, no. 3-4, pp. 47–49, 2014.

[8] J. Davies, R. Butler, Y. Chadha, and M. Singh, "Primary tubal choriocarcinoma," *Journal of Clinical Pathology*, vol. 63, no. 12, pp. 1130–1132, 2010.

[9] H.-R. Jia, J. Zhang, and Y.-M. Guo, "MRI characteristics of primary fallopian tube choriocarcinoma: a case report," *Radiology Case Reports*, vol. 12, no. 2, pp. 300–303, 2017.

[10] S. C. Jwa, S. Kamiyama, H. Takayama, Y. Tokunaga, T. Sakumoto, and M. Higashi, "Extrauterine Choriocarcinoma in the Fallopian Tube Following Infertility Treatment: Implications for the Management of Early-Detected Ectopic Pregnancies," *Journal of Minimally Invasive Gynecology*, vol. 24, no. 5, pp. 855–858, 2017.

[11] E. Karaman, O. Çetin, A. Kolusarı, and I. Bayram, "Primary tubal choriocarcinoma presented as ruptured ectopic pregnancy," *Journal of Clinical and Diagnostic Research*, vol. 9, no. 9, pp. QD17–QD18, 2015.

[12] S. Mehrotra, U. Singh, M. Goel, and S. Chauhan, "Ectopic tubal choriocarcinoma: a rarity.," *BMJ Case Reports*, vol. 2012, 2012.

[13] M. Nakayama, A. Namba, M. Yasuda, M. Hara, O. Ishihara, and A. Itakura, "Gestational choriocarcinoma of Fallopian tube diagnosed with a combination of p57KIP2 immunostaining and short tandem repeat analysis: case report.," *Journal of Obstetrics and Gynaecology Research*, vol. 37, no. 10, pp. 1493–1496, 2011.

[14] M. A. Rettenmaier, H. J. Khan, H. D. Epstein, D. Nguyen, L. N. Abaid, and B. H. Goldstein, "Gestational choriocarcinoma in the fallopian tube," *Journal of Obstetrics & Gynaecology*, vol. 33, no. 8, pp. 912–914, 2013.

[15] K. Ubayasiri, B. Hancock, and T. Duncan, "A case of primary choriocarcinoma of the fallopian tube," *Journal of Obstetrics & Gynaecology*, vol. 30, no. 8, pp. 881–883, 2010.

[16] J. Wan, X. Li, and J. Gu, "Primary choriocarcinoma of the fallopian tube: a case report and literature review," *European Journal of Gynaecological Oncology*, vol. 35, no. 5, pp. 604–607, 2014.

[17] N. M. van Mello, F. Mol, B. C. Opmeer et al., "Diagnostic value of serum hCG on the outcome of pregnancy of unknown location: A systematic review and meta-analysis," *Human Reproduction Update*, vol. 18, no. 6, Article ID dms035, pp. 603–617, 2012.

[18] H. Y. Ngan, E. I. Kohorn, L. A. Cole et al., "Trophoblastic disease," *International Journal of Gynecology & Obstetrics*, vol. 125, no. 1, pp. 93-93, 2014.

[19] M. J. Seckl, N. J. Sebire, and R. S. Berkowitz, "Gestational trophoblastic disease," *The Lancet*, vol. 376, no. 9742, pp. 717–729, 2010.

[20] A. Hassadia, F. M. Kew, J. A. Tidy, M. Wells, and B. W. Hancock, "Ectopic gestational trophoblastic disease: a case series review.," *The Journal of Reproductive Medicine*, vol. 57, no. 7-8, pp. 297–300, 2012.

[21] M. G. Muto, J. M. Lage, R. S. Berkowitz, D. P. Goldstein, and M. R. Bernstein, "Gestational trophoblastic disease of the fallopian tube," *The Journal of Reproductive Medicine*, vol. 36, no. 1, pp. 57–60, 1991.

[22] F. Hsieh, C. Wu, C. Lee et al., "Vascular patterns of gestational trophoblastic tumors by color doppler ultrasound," *Cancer*, vol. 74, no. 8, pp. 2361–2365, 1994.

[23] C. I. Schneiderman and B. Waxman, "Clomid therapy and subsequent hydatidiform mole formation: A case report," *Obstetrics & Gynecology*, vol. 39, no. 5, pp. 787-788, 1972.

[24] P. Petignat, P. Vassilakos, and A. Campana, "Are fertility drugs a risk factor for persistent trophoblastic tumour?" *Human Reproduction*, vol. 17, no. 6, pp. 1610–1615, 2002.

[25] L. H. Lin, I. Maestá, A. Braga et al., "Multiple pregnancies with complete mole and coexisting normal fetus in North and South America: A retrospective multicenter cohort and literature review," *Gynecologic Oncology*, vol. 145, no. 1, pp. 88–95, 2017.

[26] M. Bates, J. Everard, L. Wall, J. M. Horsman, and B. W. Hancock, "Is there a relationship between treatment for infertility and gestational trophoblastic disease?" *Human Reproduction*, vol. 19, no. 2, pp. 365–367, 2004.

[27] F. Flam, V. Lundstrom, J. Lindstedt, and C. Silfversward, "Choriocarcinoma of the fallopian tube associated with induced superovulation in an IVF program; a case report," *European Journal of Obstetrics & Gynecology and Reproductive Biology*, vol. 33, no. 2, pp. 183–186, 1989.

[28] R. A. Fisher, P. M. Savage, C. MacDermott et al., "The impact of molecular genetic diagnosis on the management of women with hCG-producing malignancies," *Gynecologic Oncology*, vol. 107, no. 3, pp. 413–419, 2007.

[29] J. Aranake-Chrisinger, P. C. Huettner, A. R. Hagemann, and J. D. Pfeifer, "Use of short tandem repeat analysis in unusual presentations of trophoblastic tumors and their mimics," *Human Pathology*, vol. 52, pp. 92–100, 2016.

[30] J. Savage, E. Adams, E. Veras, K. M. Murphy, and B. M. Ronnett, "Choriocarcinoma in Women: Analysis of a Case Series with Genotyping," *The American Journal of Surgical Pathology*, vol. 41, no. 12, pp. 1593–1606, 2017.

10

Severe Postpartum Hemorrhage Complicated with Liver Infarction Resulting in Hepatic Failure Necessitating Liver Transplantation

I-Ting Peng ⓘ,[1] Ming-Ting Chung ⓘ,[1,2] and Ching-Chung Lin[1]

[1]*Department of Obstetrics and Gynecology, Chi Mei Medical Center, Taiwan*
[2]*Chia Nan University of Pharmacy & Science, Taiwan*

Correspondence should be addressed to Ming-Ting Chung; mtasrm@gmail.com

Academic Editor: Kyousuke Takeuchi

Postpartum hemorrhage remains a major threat to maternal health. Intervention after critical blood loss or development of disseminated intravascular coagulation may lead to disastrous organ failure and poor outcomes. A 30-year-old woman was transferred to our emergency department due to massive postpartum hemorrhage. Shock and disseminated intravascular coagulation ensued, and the patient's condition quickly deteriorated. We performed an emergency hysterectomy, but blood loss had been massive. Moreover, there was another episode of internal bleeding that led to further blood loss. Ischemic injury to the liver was tremendous, with resulting progressive jaundice and hepatic encephalopathy. The patient required liver transplantation. Imaging studies and operative findings showed a large area of hepatic infarction. Unfortunately, the patient died of intractable sepsis shortly after liver transplantation. Disseminated intravascular coagulation and resultant hepatic infarction combined with ischemic hepatitis were the direct cause of death in our case.

1. Introduction

Hemorrhage is the leading cause of maternal mortality in developing and developed countries [1]. Although several risk factors are associated with postpartum hemorrhage (PPH), it is still impossible to predict it. As a result, early recognition of PPH and prompt action to curtail it are crucial to a good outcome. If we do not stop the bleeding at an early stage, severe consequences including disseminated intravascular coagulation (DIC) and organ failure can develop. We present a case of severe PPH complicated by DIC and hepatic infarction resulting in acute hepatic failure. The patient did not survive even after liver transplantation and died on the 36th day after the primary PPH episode.

2. Case Presentation

A 30-year-old woman was transferred to our emergency department five hours after delivering her baby at a clinic. She was a primipara at 41 weeks of gestation. She delivered a baby with vertex presentation vaginally, without dystocia. Massive vaginal bleeding started 2 hours after delivery. After excluding birth canal laceration and retaining placental tissue, the obstetrician began IV fluid and uterotonic treatment, but the bleeding continued. She was then transferred to our hospital due to PPH. However, when she arrived, she had severe tachycardia (heart rate, 160 bpm) and hypotension (BP, 44/34 mmHg). Her consciousness was clear, but she was agitated. We immediately began transfusion of packed red blood cells (6 units), fresh frozen plasma (4 units), apheresis platelets (2 units), and whole blood (2 units) as we simultaneously examined the patient. Signs of DIC developed with continuous blood loss (Figure 1), and her consciousness deteriorated within 30 minutes after arriving at the emergency department.

Uterine atony and an ischemic uterus were found during emergency laparotomy. A subtotal hysterectomy was completed. Intraoperative blood loss was 800 mL. The patient was transferred to the ICU after surgery. Her postoperative fibrinogen level was 54.6 mg/dL (normal: 200–400 mg/dL).

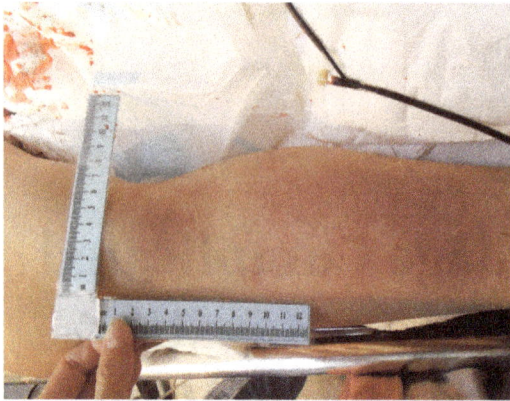

FIGURE 1: Ecchymosis on calves developed as one of the signs of DIC after uncontrollable PPH.

We transfused fresh frozen plasma and cryoprecipitate to achieve a fibrinogen level greater than 100 mg/dL. However, unstable blood pressure and progressive abdominal distension were found 4 hours after the primary surgery. We rushed the patient back into surgery due to suspicion of internal bleeding. Hemoperitoneum of 2000 mL and active bleeding from ruptured pararectal vessels were identified. After the secondary surgery for ligation of the bleeding vessels, the patient had acute kidney injury with anuria, intractable hyperkalemia, and metabolic acidosis. Thus she underwent continuous venovenous hemofiltration (CVVH).

The patient's hemodynamic status and ventilation function gradually improved after hemostasis. CVVH was shifted to intermittent hemodialysis on postoperative day 10. She was extubated on the same day.

Unfortunately, hyperbilirubinemia progressed and became the main problem (Figure 2). Liver enzyme levels peaked on postoperative day 3 and then settled to about 100–200 IU/L (Figure 3). Thrombocytopenia continued, along with prolonged prothrombin time (INR, 1.2–1.5) and activated partial thromboplastin time (1.5–2.5 times of normal control) (Figure 4). Abdominal ultrasonography revealed no biliary tract obstruction but an ill-defined hypoechoic lesion in the right lobe of the liver, about 6.5 × 6.5 cm, probably due to an inflammatory process or tumor growth. Abdominal CT was indicated to confirm the characteristic of the lesion but was postponed due to the patient's poor renal function. After consultation with a gastrointestinal expert, the lesion was thought to be a liver abscess or focal necrosis due to ischemic change. Her consciousness had been deteriorating since post-PPH day 20 in combination with intractable fever. Brain CT showed no intracranial lesion. Worsening cognition was likely due to metabolic encephalopathy of hepatic or infectious origin.

A liver transplantation was indicated, and a pretransplantation CT scan showed poor enhancement of the right hepatic lobe on the periphery covering about 50% of the total area, which was suggestive of liver infarction (Figure 5). Living donor liver transplantation was performed 28 days after PPH. The donor was her younger brother, and the graft liver weight was 840 gm. The graft-to-recipient weight ratio was 1.24%.

Intraoperatively, there were multiple micronodular lesions on the liver surface with marked swelling of the liver parenchyma and diffuse devitalized liver tissue in the right lobe of liver with necrosis and in the left lobe peripheral zone accounting for about 70%–80 % of the total liver volume (Figures 6 and 7).

The patient's bilirubin level improved on the first three days but increased again on the 4th day after transplantation. The coagulation parameters did not change significantly after liver transplantation. Serial liver ultrasonography showed acceptable vascular status of the transplanted liver, without thrombosis or biliary obstruction. Fever, tachycardia, and hypotension occurred on the 6th day after transplantation as well as vaginal and anal stool leakage. An emergency colostomy and perianal debridement were done under the suspicion of a perianal abscess and rectovaginal fistula. Unfortunately, the patient died of an intractable infection the next day.

3. Discussion

Maternal mortality rate (MMR) is an important index of fetomaternal health. WHO announced in 2016 that 99% of all maternal deaths occur in developing countries. MMR in developing countries in 2015 was 239 per 100 000 live births versus 12 per 100 000 live births in developed countries. The MMR in Taiwan in 2015 was 11.7 per 100 000 live births. There were 25 maternal deaths reported in 2015. This is a relatively low MMR compared to other areas worldwide. However, this number could be underestimated [2]. Up to two-thirds of all maternal deaths would be missed if we relied on the death registration only [3]. In addition, the true incidence of other obstetric complications is even harder to calculate accurately. For example, severe preeclampsia complicated with aortic dissection or peripartum cardiomyopathy might be erroneously linked to hypertensive cardiovascular disease but not gestation-related. Likewise, PPH may cause multiple organ failure, including acute renal failure, stroke, and ischemic liver failure, but the incidence of these complications is unknown.

In a previous report, a patient with severe PPH experienced an acute myocardial infarction on the 7th postpartum day [4]. She also had ischemic hepatitis, and her AST and ALT levels peaked on the 3rd day after PPH (her liver enzyme trend was similar to that of our patient). Her liver function then recovered spontaneously after correction of hypoperfusion and left no obvious sequela. In contrast, our patient experienced serious complications, including intractable hepatic failure. What is the difference between the two cases? We hypothesize that the large area of hepatic infarction might have played a pivotal role in our patient.

Ischemic hepatitis and hepatic infarction are two different mechanisms of vascular injury to liver tissue. Ischemic hepatitis involves the whole liver. It is caused by systemic hypoperfusion, or it may be caused by decreased perfusion from the hepatic artery and/or portal vein. For example, it can occur in patients who undergo liver transplantation and have hepatic artery thrombosis. It is mostly a self-limiting disease,

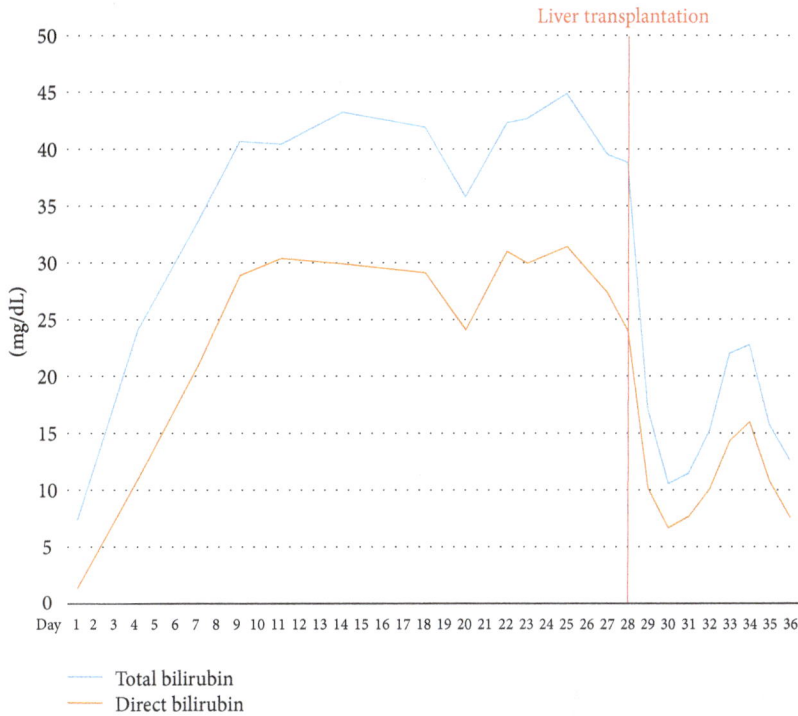

FIGURE 2: Trend of bilirubin levels.

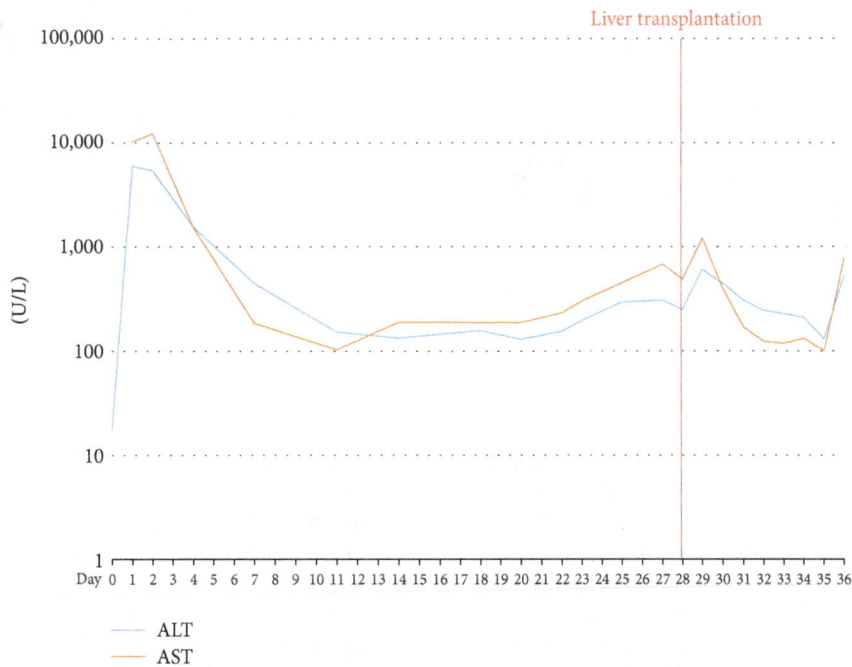

FIGURE 3: Trend of AST/ALT levels.

and the only effective treatment is to remove the insult that caused the liver hypoperfusion. In contrast, hepatic infarction represents focal ischemic injury to the liver. Most of the time this infarction is caused by occlusion of an intrahepatic branch of the hepatic artery. It may occur accidentally during ligation of the hepatic artery during surgery, after hepatic artery chemoembolization, or in a hypercoagulable state,

with related thrombosis formation [5]. In our patient, we presumed that thrombosis formation due to DIC was the cause of the hepatic infarction. Pathologic examination of the resected liver showed small artery thrombosis. This finding supports our hypothesis. Severe ischemic hepatitis combined with a large area of hepatic infarction explains why the hepatic function of our patient remained poor even

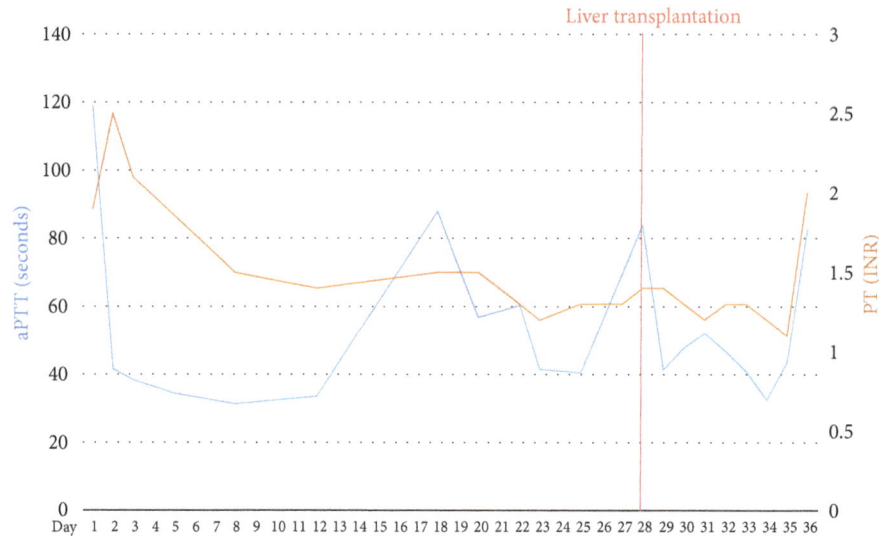

FIGURE 4: Trend of PT/aPTT.

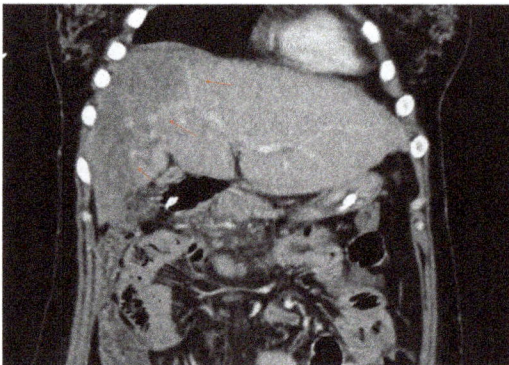

FIGURE 5: Pretransplantation CT scan showed a large area of infarction in the right lobe of the liver (arrows).

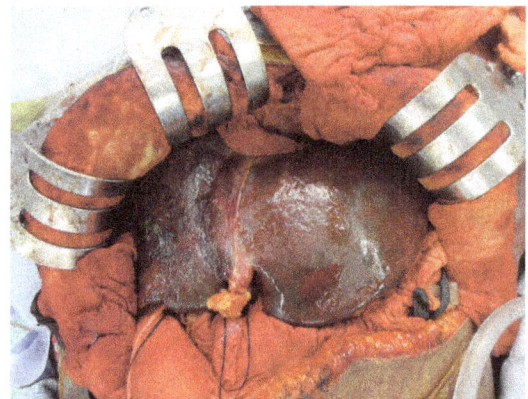

FIGURE 6: Gross appearance of the patient's liver during liver transplantation

though her hemodynamic compromise had been corrected. It was difficult to predict whether or when the liver function will spontaneously recover in a patient with acute liver failure [6]. Hepatic encephalopathy, prolonged jaundice, and concomitant renal failure suggested a poor prognosis [7]. In such circumstances, the short-term mortality rate is high, even though we intervened with liver transplantation.

The timing of effective hemostasis plays a substantial role in determining a woman's prognosis after PPH. Intervening earlier when the estimated blood loss is less seems to improve outcome [8]. The PPH episode we reported occurred in an urban clinic at a distance that takes about 30 minutes by car to the nearest tertiary center. The patient had experienced significant hypotension before arrival at our center, and DIC developed shortly afterwards. The blood loss before her transfer could have been of large amount. She underwent a hysterectomy for hemostasis, yet overwhelming DIC led to the second episode of internal bleeding and hepatic infarction.

Pregnancy is a hypercoagulable status. Obstetric complications including PPH (defined as hemorrhage above 500 mL after vaginal delivery or above 1000 mL after a cesarean section), preeclampsia, hemolysis, elevated liver function tests, and low platelets (HELLP) syndrome, amniotic fluid embolism, and acute fatty liver are all conditions linked to high risk of developing DIC. A woman at 31 weeks' gestation with HELLP syndrome complicated with large area of hepatic infarction was presented in a case report [9]. This reminds us that although DIC or hepatic infarction is rare in an uncomplicated pregnant woman, we have to monitor a woman with gestational complications closely and be well prepared to detect and cope with these serious complications.

Due to the common concept of keeping the body "complete" after a person is dead among East Asian cultures, countries in this area have the lowest deceased organ donation rate in the world. In present, living donor liver transplantation (LDLT) is far more prevalent than deceased donor liver

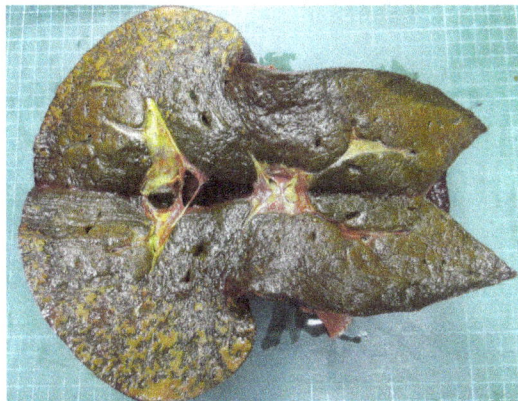

FIGURE 7: Transection of the resected native liver (1850 g).

transplantation (DDLT) in Taiwan [10]. According to the data from Taiwan Organ Registry and Sharing Center, there were 406 cases of LDLT but only 108 cases of DDLT in 2017. Furthermore, there had been 1218 candidates on the waiting list for liver donation, counted until April 2018. The decision of executing liver transplantation was quick in our case, due to her worsening hepatic encephalopathy. It was hard to get a suitable cadaver donor in time. Under these circumstances, LDLT was adopted by our transplantation team. In a meta-analysis, LDLT recipients have higher short-term complication rates including biliary complications, vascular complications, and retransplantation rate compared to DDLT recipients, with a comparable perioperative mortality rate [11]. And as the transplantation team gets more experience, the outcome will be better.

One of the concerns about LDLT in our case was the following: have we got adequate graft liver transplanted? Our donor was a healthy young man, with normal BMI. A graft-to-recipient weight ratio of 0.8-1 percent is generally adequate, which in our case was 1.24 percent. The elevation of bilirubin level on posttransplantation day 4 could not be explained with inadequate size of the graft liver but rather was a presentation of early allograft dysfunction (EAD) [12]. The underlying causes of EAD include ischemia/reperfusion injury to the graft liver and acute rejection, after excluding vascular occlusion or biliary obstruction.

In conclusion, clinicians must beware of ischemic hepatitis and hepatic infarction as possible complications in victims of severe PPH. Management of these patients needs cooperation of multiple specialties and liver transplantation is the salvage treatment.

Authors' Contributions

I-Ting Peng gathered relevant data and drafted the manuscript. Ming-Ting Chung and Ching-Chung Lin

managed the case during admission and reviewed the manuscript.

References

[1] M. S. Kramer, C. Berg, H. Abenhaim et al., "Incidence, risk factors, and temporal trends in severe postpartum hemorrhage," *American Journal of Obstetrics & Gynecology*, vol. 209, no. 5, pp. 449.e441–449.e447, 2013.

[2] S. Kao, L.-M. Chen, L. Shi, and M. C. Weinrich, "Underreporting and misclassification of maternal mortality in Taiwan," *Acta Obstetricia et Gynecologica Scandinavica*, vol. 76, no. 7, pp. 629–636, 1997.

[3] T.-P. Wu, Y.-L. Huang, F.-W. Liang, and T.-H. Lu, "Underreporting of maternal mortality in Taiwan: A data linkage study," *Taiwanese Journal of Obstetrics and Gynecology*, vol. 54, no. 6, pp. 705–708, 2015.

[4] M.-H. Chou, Y.-C. Chen, K.-S. Hwang, M.-H. Yu, and H.-Y. Su, "Myocardial infarction and ischemic hepatitis complicated by postpartum hemorrhage," *Taiwanese Journal of Obstetrics and Gynecology*, vol. 55, no. 3, pp. 437–440, 2016.

[5] M. Yoshihara, M. Mayama, M. Ukai, S. Tano, Y. Kishigami, and H. Oguchi, "Fulminant liver failure resulting from massive hepatic infarction associated with hemolysis, elevated liver enzymes, and low platelets syndrome," *Journal of Obstetrics and Gynaecology Research*, vol. 42, no. 10, pp. 1375–1378, 2016.

[6] M. Mendizabal and M. O. Silva, "Liver transplantation in acute liver failure: A challenging scenario," *World Journal of Gastroenterology*, vol. 22, no. 4, pp. 1523–1531, 2016.

[7] S. E. Yantorno, W. K. Kremers, A. E. Ruf, J. J. Trentadue, L. G. Podestá, and F. G. Villamil, "MELD is superior to King's college and Clichy's criteria to assess prognosis in fulminant hepatic failure," *Liver Transplantation*, vol. 13, no. 6, pp. 822–828, 2007.

[8] T. F. Howard and W. A. Grobman, "The relationship between timing of postpartum hemorrhage interventions and adverse outcomes," *American Journal of Obstetrics & Gynecology*, vol. 213, no. 2, pp. 239–239.e3, 2015.

[9] A. E. Mikolajczyk, J. Renz, G. Diaz, L. Alpert, J. Hart, and H. S. Te, "Massive hepatic infarction caused by HELLP syndrome," *ACG Case Reports Journal*, vol. 4, article e81, 2017.

[10] C.-L. Chen, C. S. Kabiling, and A. M. Concejero, "Why does living donor liver transplantation flourish in Asia?" *Nature Reviews Gastroenterology & Hepatology*, vol. 10, no. 12, pp. 746–751, 2013.

[11] P. Wan, X. Yu, and Q. Xia, "Operative outcomes of adult living donor liver transplantation and deceased donor liver transplantation: A systematic review and meta-analysis," *Liver Transplantation*, vol. 20, no. 4, pp. 425–436, 2014.

[12] M. Deschenes, "Early allograft dysfunction: causes, recognition, and management," *Liver Transplantation*, vol. 19, no. 2, pp. S6–S8, 2013.

11

Peritoneal Keratin Granulomatosis Associated with Endometrioid Adenocarcinoma of the Uterine Corpus in a Woman with Polycystic Ovaries: A Potential Pitfall—A Case Report and Review of the Literature

Helen J. Trihia,[1] Maria Papazian,[1] Natasa Novkovic,[1] John Provatas,[2] Sotiria Tsangouri,[3] and Dimitrios C. Papatheodorou[3]

[1]Department of Pathology, "Metaxas" Cancer Hospital, 18537 Piraeus, Greece
[2]Department of Cytology, "Metaxas" Cancer Hospital, 18537 Piraeus, Greece
[3]Department of Gynaecology, "Metaxas" Cancer Hospital, 18537 Piraeus, Greece

Correspondence should be addressed to Helen J. Trihia; eltrix@otenet.gr

Academic Editor: Kyousuke Takeuchi

Peritoneal keratin granulomatosis is a rare condition included under granulomatous lesions of the peritoneum. It can be secondary to neoplasms of the female genital tract and can mimic carcinomatosis intraoperatively. A case of a 40-year-old woman with a history of polycystic ovaries and a chief complaint of vaginal bleeding is presented. She was diagnosed with endometrioid adenocarcinoma with squamous differentiation in endometrial curettings. Intraoperatively, many peritoneal nodules were found, interpreted as peritoneal carcinomatosis. The woman underwent a total abdominal hysterectomy with bilateral salpingo-oophorectomy, omentectomy, bilateral pelvic lymphadenectomy, and appendicectomy. Multiple biopsies were taken, as well as peritoneal washings. Microscopic examination revealed multiple keratin granulomas on the serosal surface of the ovaries, fallopian tubes, appendix, and omentum. Lymph node metastasis was not found. Peritoneal keratin granulomas (PKGs) have been reported in cases of endometrioid adenocarcinoma with squamous differentiation of the uterine corpus, ovary, and atypical adenomyoma. It should be noted that the prognosis of cases of peritoneal keratin granulomas without viable tumor cells is favourable and that the histologic examination is essential for its diagnosis. We report a case of PKG in a patient with endometrial carcinoma with squamous differentiation, being the first in a woman with polycystic ovaries.

1. Introduction

Peritoneal keratin granuloma is a rare lesion included among reactive tumor-like lesions of the peritoneum. It can be secondary to endometrioid adenocarcinoma with squamous differentiation of the endometrium and ovary and atypical polypoid adenomyoma of the endometrium and in association with ruptured dermoid cysts. The prognostic significance of these lesions is unknown and it seems to have no interference with prognosis, when no viable tumor cells are detected. Here we describe a case of an endometrioid adenocarcinoma of the endometrium, in a woman with polycystic ovaries in which diffuse peritoneal keratin granulomas were found with no viable tumor implants which intraoperatively were misinterpreted as diffuse carcinomatosis.

2. Case Presentation

A 40-year-old woman with a body mass index (BMI) of 37 and a past medical history of polycystic ovary syndrome, presented to her gynaecologist complaining of irregular vaginal bleeding. Her menarche was at the age of 16 and her menstrual cycle was infrequent and irregular. Endometrial biopsies (D&C) have been examined at the age of 33 and 38 years. At the age of 38, she was diagnosed with atypical adenomatous hyperplasia of the endometrium and she was

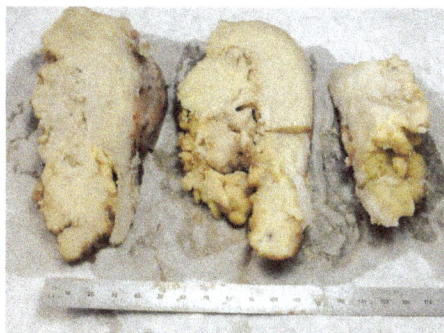

FIGURE 1: Macroscopic appearance of a cross-sectioned uterus filled with a polypoid papillary mass, extending into the uterine cervix.

put on progestagen therapy. A few months later, she experienced a new episode of irregular vaginal bleeding and after an additional D&C she was diagnosed with endometrioid adenocarcinoma of the endometrium. As a routine pre-op check, tumor markers were requested. Her serum CA125 and serum CA19.9 were elevated to 69.00 U/ml (normal < 35.00 U/ml) and 91.60 U/ml (normal < 35.00 U/ml), respectively. The magnetic resonance imaging (MRI) of the lower abdomen revealed invasion of more than 50% of the myometrium and of the uppermost uterine cervical stroma. Blurring of the sigmoid fat and prominent inguinal, para-aortic and mesenteric lymph nodes were also described with a maximum lymph node diameter of 1.5 cm. Total abdominal hysterectomy, bilateral salpingo-oophorectomy, bilateral pelvic lymph node dissection, omentectomy, and appendicectomy were performed. Intraoperative peritoneal washings were also carried out. Multiple peritoneal nodules, <0.5 cm in diameter, suspicious of disseminated carcinomatosis, were found during surgery in the pouch of Douglas, over loops of small bowel, and in the mesentery of the small bowel. Multiple biopsies were taken. Due to increased BMI, para-aortic lymphadenectomy was not performed. No frozen section was requested because it was appreciated that a positive result would not affect the overall surgical management.

Grossly, the uterine corpus, including both cornua, was filled with a polypoid papillary mass, measuring 11, 5 × 5, 5 cm, extending into the uterine cervix (Figure 1). Both ovaries were enlarged with multiple peripherally located follicular cysts and dense peripheral stroma, consistent with the clinical history of polycystic ovaries.

Histologically, the tumor of the uterine corpus was a superficially invasive, moderately differentiated, tubulopapillary adenocarcinoma of the endometrium, of endometrioid type with multiple foci of squamous differentiation (Figures 2(a)–2(c)). Immunohistochemically, there was positive expression of hormone receptors and p53 (Figure 3). The tumor was extending superficially to the uterine cervix (Figure 4). All 18 pelvic lymph nodes were unremarkable. In addition, on the serosal surface of bilateral ovaries, fallopian tubes, and the appendix, multiple microscopic granulomas were found, composed of amorphous irregularly laminated eosinophilic deposits of keratin, associated with ghost squamous cells and surrounded by foreign body giant

cells (Figures 5(a)–5(c)). There were also reactive mesothelial cells close to keratin granulomas. In retrospect, similar degenerate squamous cells were found in extensive, mainly superficial areas of the uterine tumor (Figure 6) as well as filling and distending the lumen of the fallopian tubes, bilaterally (Figures 7(a)–7(c)).

Intraoperative peritoneal washings showed scattered mesothelial cells, occasional clusters of atypical cells of mesothelial origin, rare anucleate squames, and an occasional keratin granuloma. Overall, the endometrial carcinoma was of UICC/FIGO stage II.

3. Discussion

Peritoneal keratin granuloma is a rare lesion included under granulomatous lesions of the peritoneum [1]. Such peritoneal reaction can be infectious or noninfectious in aetiology [1]. The noninfectious type can be secondary to neoplasms of the female genital tract, like endometrioid adenocarcinoma with squamous differentiation of the endometrium and ovary and atypical polypoid adenomyoma of the endometrium or seen in association with ruptured dermoid cysts. They are also found in ruptured ovarian teratoma and nonneoplastic conditions, such as spilled amniotic fluid, or in intraperitoneal renal dialysis-associated peritoneal squamous metaplasia [1].

Peritoneal keratin granulomas refer to the finding of nests of keratinized anucleate squamous cells surrounded by a foreign body type giant cell reaction, either on the peritoneal surface or within subperitoneal connective tissue. These so-called keratin granulomas do not contain any glandular epithelium. The typical histological appearances in previously reported cases were similar to ours.

Spontaneous reflux of exfoliated necrotic squamous metaplastic cells or keratin from the squamous element of the endometrial tumor to the peritoneum or its retropulsion through the tubal lumina due to endometrial sampling has been postulated as the pathogenetic mechanism of the 27 cases [2–7] of PKG associated with an endometrial adenocarcinoma with squamous differentiation [2–5]. The above induce a foreign body granulomatous reaction [3] and include frequent association with cervical stenosis, corneal location of the primary tumor, presence of keratin clumps within the lumen of the tube, and superficial location of squamous necrotic cells in the endometrial carcinoma [4]. In our case, all the above-mentioned requirements were met. The uterine cavity was filled with a tumor which was causing distention of the corneal part of the fallopian tubes and there was extensive squamous differentiation of the endometrioid adenocarcinoma, in about 1/20 of the tumor, which was more pronounced in superficial areas, where extensive degeneration and necrosis of the endometrial carcinoma were present (Figure 8). The tubes were massively distended and filled with numerous anucleate squames, which obviously spread to the peritoneum, leading to a florid granulomatous peritoneal reaction to keratin.

The commonly reported process of keratinization in endometrial carcinomas could be influenced by irradiation,

(a)

(b)

(c)

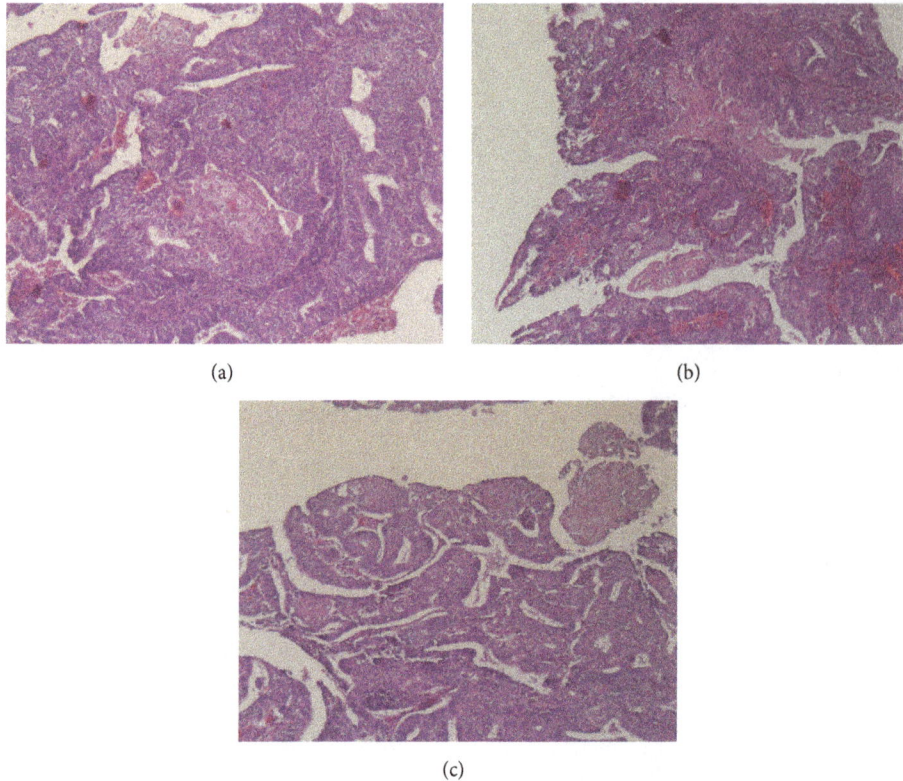

FIGURE 2: Microscopic appearance of endometrioid carcinoma with foci of squamous differentiation.

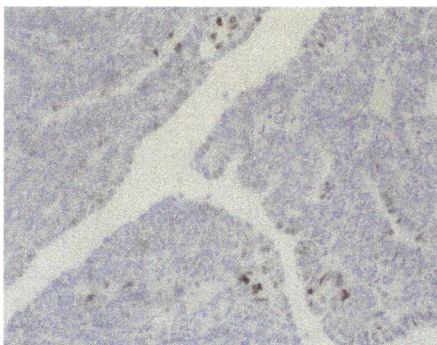

FIGURE 3: Immunostain: positive expression of p53 in endometrial carcinoma.

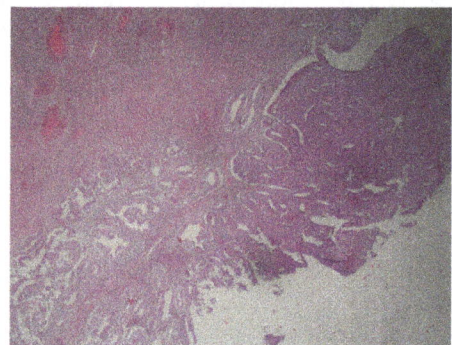

FIGURE 4: H&E stain: superficial invasion of the uterine cervix by the endometrial carcinoma.

surgical trauma, partial removal of the tumoral mass, hormonal factors, infection, or transfusion, but the aetiology is usually unknown [4]. Sometimes the tumor cells may undergo keratinization after entering into the peritoneal cavity [4]. These may be visible to the surgeon and mimic peritoneal carcinomatosis macroscopically, as it was the case with our surgeons. As long as no glandular component is identified histologically, keratin granulomas should not be considered tumor spread and should not result in upstaging. In such cases, the areas should be thoroughly sampled by the gynaecologist and carefully examined microscopically by the pathologist to exclude the presence of viable tumor cells. Furthermore, reactive mesothelial hyperplasia near the

keratin granulomas may occur. Peritoneal washings no longer contribute to endometrial cancer staging; nevertheless, they continue to be performed by the clinicians, even though a positive report may carry a risk of overdiagnosis, as it may be difficult to distinguish between reactive mesothelial and tumor cells. There is only one report on the cytohistological correlation of PKGs [8]. In our case, atypical cells in the peritoneal washings were immunoreactive for calretinin (Figure 8), indicative of mesothelial origin. There were also scattered anucleate orangeophilic squames (Figure 9), which could not have been of cutaneous origin, as the cytological sampling technique was not transcutaneous (paracentesis) and an occasional keratin granuloma, positive

(a)

(b)

(c)

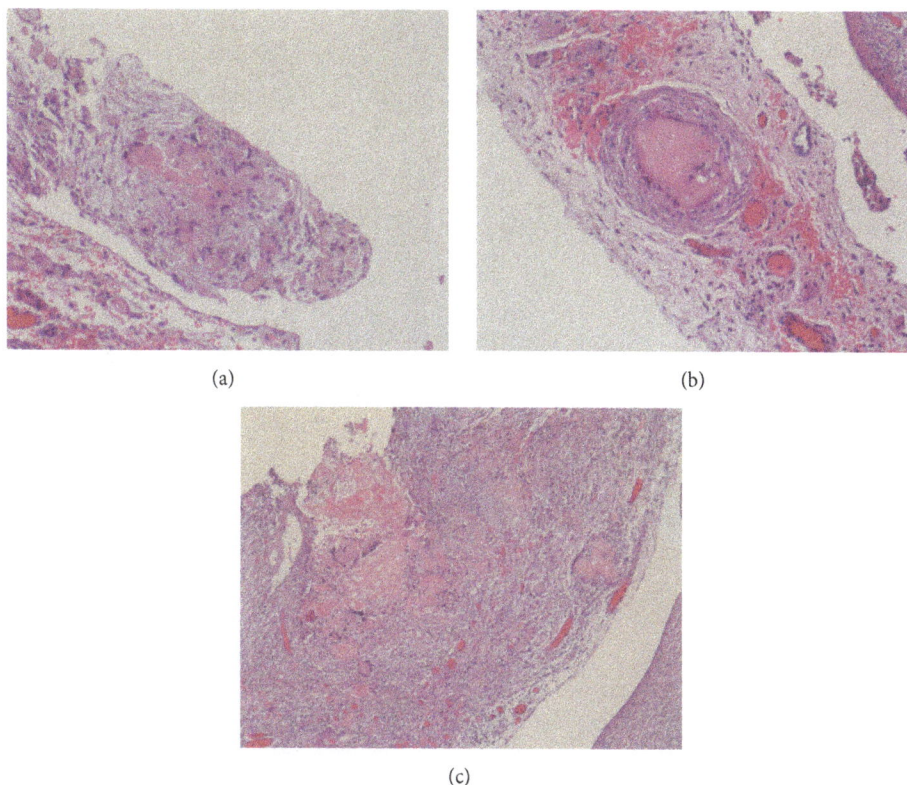

FIGURE 5: H&E stain: microscopic appearances of multiple keratin granulomas, composed of ghost squamous cells surrounded by foreign body giant cells, found on the serosal surface of bilateral ovaries, fallopian tubes, the appendix, and omentum.

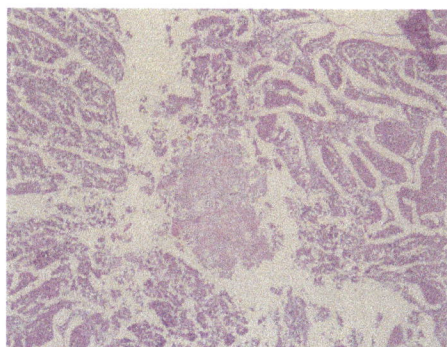

FIGURE 6: H&E stain: degenerate squamous cells found in superficial areas of the uterine tumor.

for ker5/6 (Figure 10). Cytological evidence of keratin in peritoneal washings does not infer a diagnosis of metastatic carcinoma, but careful scrutiny has to be done, to exclude the presence of malignant cells.

After revision of the literature, only 33 similar cases had been reported till 2012.

Tripathy et al. (2010) [7] and Montes et al. (1961) [9] were the first to describe a case of well-differentiated adenocarcinoma of the uterine corpus in which so-called "pigmented nodules" composed of foreign body keratin granulomas were identified on and below the serosal surface of the uterus and the proximal end of the fallopian tube. These authors suggested that squamous metaplasia and keratinization of endometriotic epithelium might lead to the formation of granulomas.

Chen (1978) [2] described five cases of uterine "adenoacanthoma" with peritoneal foreign body granulomatous reaction to keratin. These authors postulated that the pathway of entrance of keratin into the peritoneal cavity to be spontaneous reflux from the endometrial tumor, including a frequent association with cervical stenosis, a corneal location of the primary tumor leading to transtubal spreading. William et al. (1984) [10] and Wotherspoon et al. (1989) [5] reported two additional cases, associated with an "adenosquamous carcinoma" and an "adenoacanthoma" of the uterus, respectively. Kim and Scully (1990) [4] reported 22 cases of peritoneal keratin granulomas with carcinomas of endometrium and ovary and atypical polypoid adenomyoma of the endometrium, constituting the largest review of cases published in the literature. It was the first time that such peritoneal lesions were described to be related to endometrioid adenocarcinoma of the ovary (five cases). Wu et al. (2006) [11] described the other case of peritoneal keratin granuloma in association with ovarian adenocarcinoma. It was suggested by Kim and Scully (1990) [4] that tearing of the capsule of the tumor or malignant cell penetrating the ovarian surface was the way of cells in entering the peritoneal cavity. The last two published cases, by Van der Horst and Evans (2008) [6], refer to carcinomas of the endometrium also. A case with twelve-year follow-up of an endometrioid adenocarcinoma

(a)

(b)

(c)

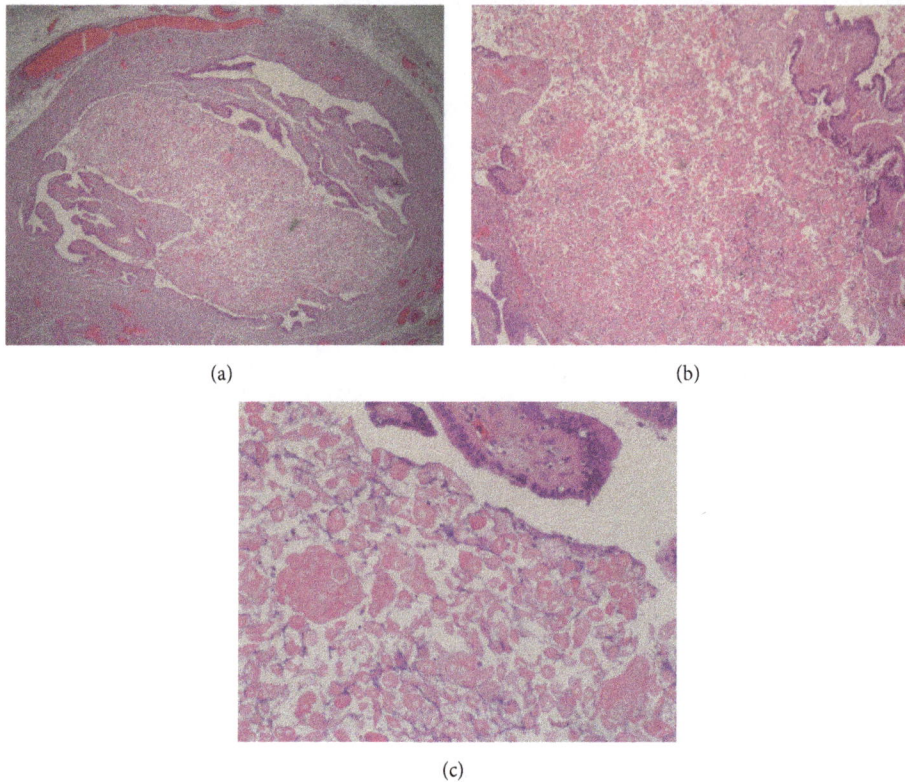

FIGURE 7: H&E stain: similar to Figure 6, degenerate squamous cells are filling and distending the lumen of the fallopian tubes (in various magnifications).

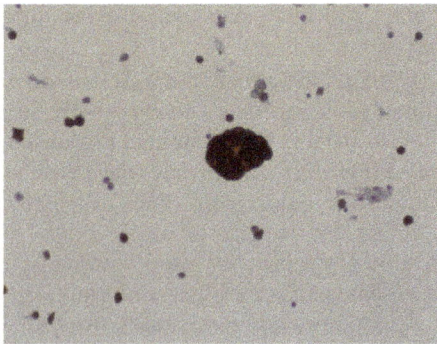

FIGURE 8: Immunostain for calretinin: atypical cell cluster in peritoneal washings of mesothelial origin.

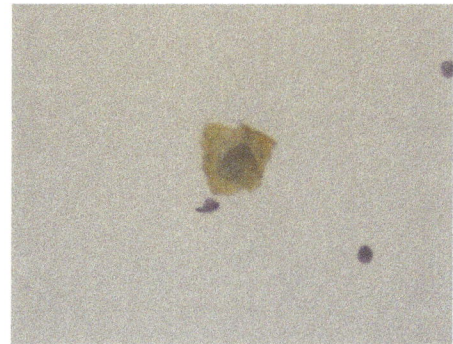

FIGURE 9: Pap stain: scattered anucleate squame in peritoneal washings.

of the endometrium with disseminated peritoneal keratin granulomas and viable tumor implants was also reported in 2012 [12]. Interpreted as disseminated disease leading to a palliative approach with only brachytherapy and hormonal therapy, the outstanding survival could suggest no adverse effect on the prognosis of such peritoneal lesions even with viable tumor implants.

The prognostic significance of keratin peritoneal granulomas with or without viable tumor implants is difficult to assess because of the small number of cases in the literature. Lack of or short follow-up in some cases and postoperative radiotherapy, chemotherapy, or both, which might have influenced the natural course of any postoperative residual peritoneal lesions, makes it more difficult to interpret the real prognostic significance of these lesions. Some authors suggest that they have no prognostic significance when no viable cells are found in the granulomas.

The combination of contrast-enhanced T1-weighted and diffusion-weighted magnetic resonance is mentioned to be helpful for the preoperative differential diagnosis [13].

In the current study, we document a very rare case involving a patient with polycystic ovaries syndrome, who

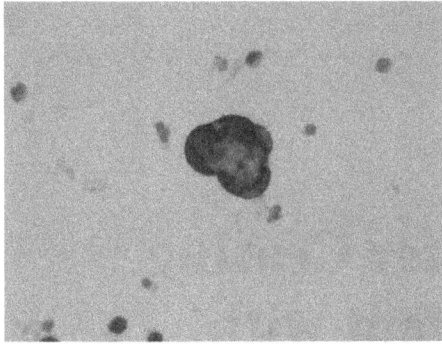

FIGURE 10: Immunostain for Ker5/6: keratin granuloma with positive expression in peritoneal washings.

presented with a huge endometrial tumor which filled the uterus and protruded through the cervical os. The tumor was an endometrioid adenocarcinoma of the endometrium which was accompanied by multiple peritoneal keratin granulomas attributed to the squamous element of the tumor, transpassing the lumen of the fallopian tubes and eliciting a giant cell reaction. Our findings are in concordance with Chen et al.'s [3] and Wotherspoon et al.'s [5] proposed pathogenetic mechanism of spontaneous reflux of keratinized squamous cells through the lumen of the fallopian tubes into the peritoneal cavity in tumors associated with cervical stenosis or a corneal location. For the first time, we confirm microscopically the proposed pathogenetic mechanism of PKG formation. The fallopian tubes in our case were distended and filled with anucleate squames originated from the squamous metaplastic element of the endometrial adenocarcinoma.

Because peritoneal granulomatosis can resemble disseminated carcinomatosis macroscopically, the knowledge of this rare entity is essential to avoid upstaging of the patient. Our patient underwent brachytherapy and whole irradiation and is well after fifteen months of follow-up.

Furthermore, the findings of scattered anucleate squames and keratin granuloma in the peritoneal washings constitute the second cytohistologic reference of PKGs [8].

Consent

Written consent has been provided from the patient.

Acknowledgments

The authors would like to express their gratitude to Nikolaos Trapezontas for his invaluable assistance with the submission process of the manuscript.

References

[1] P. B. Clement, "Reactive tumor-like lesions of the peritoneum," *American Journal of Clinical Pathology*, vol. 103, no. 6, pp. 673–676, 1995.

[2] K. T. K. Chen, "Cytology of peritoneal keratin granulomas," *Diagnostic Cytopathology*, vol. 20, no. 2, pp. 105–107, 1999.

[3] K. T. K. Chen, N. D. Kostich, and J. Rosai, "Peritoneal foreign body granulomas to keratin in uterine adenoacanthoma," *Archives of Pathology and Laboratory Medicine*, vol. 102, no. 4, pp. 174–177, 1978.

[4] K.-R. Kim and R. E. Scully, "Peritoneal keratin granulomas with carcinomas of endometrium and ovary and atypical polypoid adenomyoma of endometrium: a clinicopathological analysis of 22 cases," *American Journal of Surgical Pathology*, vol. 14, no. 10, pp. 925–932, 1990.

[5] A. C. Wotherspoon, E. Benjamin, and A. A. Boutwood, "Peritoneal keratin granulomas from transtubal spread of endometrial carcinoma with squamous metaplasia (adenoacanthoma). Case report," *British Journal of Obstetrics and Gynaecology*, vol. 96, no. 2, pp. 236–240, 1989.

[6] C. Van Der Horst and A. J. Evans, "Peritoneal keratin granulomas complicating endometrial carcinoma: a report of two cases and review of the literature," *International Journal of Gynecological Cancer*, vol. 18, no. 3, pp. 549–553, 2008.

[7] K. Tripathy, A. Misra, S. Sethi et al., "Peritoneal keratin granuloma masquerading as disseminated carcinoma," *Case Reports in Gastroenterology*, vol. 4, no. 1, pp. 31–34, 2010.

[8] F. Rivasi and A. Palicelli, "Peritoneal keratin granulomas: cytohistological correlation in a case of endometrial adenocarcinoma with squamous differentiation," *Cytopathology*, vol. 23, no. 5, pp. 342–344, 2012.

[9] M. Montes, W. Beautyman, and G. L. Haidak, "Cholesteatomatous endometriosis," *American Journal of Obstetrics and Gynecology*, vol. 82, pp. 119–123, 1961.

[10] W. D. William, K. Amazon, and A. M. Rywlin, "Peritoneal keratin globules in uterine adenosquamous carcinoma," *Southern Medical Journal*, vol. 77, no. 10, pp. 1316–1318, 1984.

[11] T. I. Wu, T. C. Chang, S. Hsueh, and C. H. Lai, "Ovarian endometrioid carcinoma with diffuse pigmented peritoneal keratin granulomas: a case report and review of the literature," *International Journal of Gynecological Cancer*, vol. 16, no. 1, pp. 426–429, 2006.

[12] D. de Freitas Pina Ferreira, D. Fernandes, T. Amaro, and A. Petiz, "Extensive peritoneal keratin granuloma in stage IV B endometrial carcinoma with an outstanding survival: a case report and review of the literature," *Gynecologic Oncology Case Reports*, vol. 2, no. 2, pp. 61–62, 2012.

[13] T. Ooyama, M. Inamine, A. Wakayama et al., "Endometrial carcinoma with peritoneal keratin granulomas mimicking peritoneal carcinomatosis: a case report and imaging diagnosis," *International Cancer Conference Journal*, vol. 1, no. 4, pp. 206–209, 2012.

12

Tumors Sharply Increased after Ceasing Pazopanib Therapy for a Patient with Advanced Uterine Leiomyosarcoma: Experience of Tumor Flare

Terumi Tanigawa, Shintaro Morisaki, Hisanobu Fukuda, Shuichiro Yoshimura, Hisayoshi Nakajima, and Kohei Kotera

Department of Obstetrics and Gynecology, Nagasaki Harbor Medical Center City Hospital, 6-39 Shinchimachi, Nagasaki-shi, Nagasaki 850-8555, Japan

Correspondence should be addressed to Terumi Tanigawa; obgytanigawa@gmail.com

Academic Editor: Yoshio Yoshida

Pazopanib has activity in patients with soft-tissue sarcoma. We report an advanced uterine leiomyosarcoma case that suddenly worsened after cessation of pazopanib therapy. A 47-year-old woman had a primary uterine leiomyosarcoma tumor and multiple lung metastases, which progressed during her initial treatment. In subsequent treatment with pazopanib for 3 months, the sum of her tumor diameters after cessation sharply increased for two weeks. Symptoms such as dyspnea suddenly worsened also. She died of the disease one month after cessation of pazopanib therapy. Given the poor prognosis of recurrent uterine leiomyosarcoma and the rapid tumor enlargement after ending pazopanib therapy, control of this disease is especially important. Therefore, the decision to discontinue pazopanib therapy requires careful consideration.

1. Introduction

Uterine leiomyosarcomas (LMS) are associated with poor prognosis, with an average five-year survival rate of around 40% [1, 2]. Moreover, median overall survival after recurrence is under 12 months [3, 4].

The treatment for unresectable advanced or recurrent uterine LMS is chemotherapy. Standard first-line chemotherapy has been doxorubicin with or without ifosfamide [5]. The response rate of this combination chemotherapy was reported as complete response in 3% to 16% of patients and partial response in 27% to 32% of patients [6, 7].

If the disease does not respond to standard chemotherapy, one agent of interest is pazopanib because of its activity in patients with soft-tissue sarcoma [8]. Pazopanib has been comprehensively defined as a synthetic indazolpyrimidine with activity as a small-molecule vascular endothelial growth factor (VEGF) inhibitor (specifically, as a multitargeted tyrosine kinase inhibitor) against VEGFs 1, 2, and 3 and platelet-derived growth factors. Pazopanib was approved as a second-line treatment after a phase III trial of this drug reported a statistically significant increase in progression-free survival [9, 10]. Pazopanib has been available in Japan for treating soft-tissue sarcoma since 2012.

Many tyrosine kinase inhibitors (TKIs) are also used in the treatment of other cancers such as non-small cell lung cancer, chronic myeloid leukemia, renal cell carcinoma, hepatocellular carcinoma, and thyroid cancer. Recently, several reports have demonstrated cases of rapid tumor size increase related to cessation of TKI treatment [11–15].

In this report, we present an advanced LMS case that suddenly worsened after cessation of pazopanib therapy.

2. Case Presentation

A 47-year-old woman (nullipara) with no past history was diagnosed with uterine LMS of FIGO stage IVB, with multiple lung, liver, and bone metastases. We retrospectively reviewed the medical records of the patient so as to assess the outcomes and adverse events of therapy. We used the

Response Evaluation Criteria in Solid Tumors (ver 1.1) to assess tumor responses and the Common Terminology Criteria for Adverse Events (ver 4.0) to assess adverse events. The growth modulation index (GMI), the ratio of time to progression (TTP) with present therapy and TTP with previous therapy, is calculated as follows: GMI = $TTP_{present\ therapy}/TTP_{previous\ therapy}$ [16]. We calculated the GMI, ratio of TTP after discontinuing pazopanib to TTP while receiving chemotherapy (docetaxel with gemcitabine, adriamycin, and pazopanib).

The patient had symptoms of genital bleeding, and a uterine tumor was identified. Findings from a tumor biopsy were suggestive of uterine LMS. The patient was treated with neoadjuvant chemotherapy (docetaxel with gemcitabine) for two courses. However, the primary tumor, peritoneal dissemination, and the lung metastases progressed. The attending physician indicated surgery in order to reduce tumor volume and to confirm diagnosis by pathology. Subsequently, she was treated with surgical resection (total abdominal hysterectomy with bilateral salpingoophorectomy and partial omentectomy). Pathological examination confirmed the uterine LMS diagnosis and the presence of metastatic tumors in both ovaries and the omentum. After resection, the patient underwent chemotherapy (adriamycin) for three courses; although lung metastases became stable, peritoneal dissemination progressed. As we judged the patient's disease to have progressed as a whole, we decided to cease the adriamycin treatment. Subsequently, we treated the patient with pazopanib therapy (800 mg) orally once daily for three months. Prior to commencing pazopanib therapy, her echocardiography findings were normal. The patient did not experience pazopanib therapy-related adverse events at severe grades but did develop grade II hypertension that responded to antihypertensive medication. A CT scan taken three months after starting pazopanib treatment showed that the tumor sizes of the liver and lung metastases and of the peritoneal dissemination were stable (Figure 2). However, pazopanib therapy was discontinued due to the new occurrence of a metastasis to the skin. At this time, we began considering a different type of chemotherapy.

After ceasing pazopanib therapy, cough symptoms sharply increased for two weeks. Her echocardiography findings were again normal. Additionally, the sum of the patient's tumor diameters increased as follows: for lung metastases, by −10% (during the 3-month-pazopanib treatment) versus by 55% (during the two weeks after ceasing treatment); for liver metastases, by 0% versus by 33%; and for peritoneal dissemination, by 12% versus by 51% (Figure 1). Particularly, the lung metastases sharply increased (Figure 2). The GMI was 0.18 (ratio of TTP after discontinuing pazopanib to TTP while receiving chemotherapy).

The patient also experienced sudden worsening of symptoms, such as severe dyspnea which was difficult to control. She had an emergency hospitalization for the severe dyspnea. Large enlargement of the right ventricle and dysfunction of the left ventricle were confirmed by echocardiography. A CT scan did not show any evidence of pulmonary infarction or pulmonary bleeding. Therefore, the patient was diagnosed with acute pulmonary heart. The dyspnea was treated with

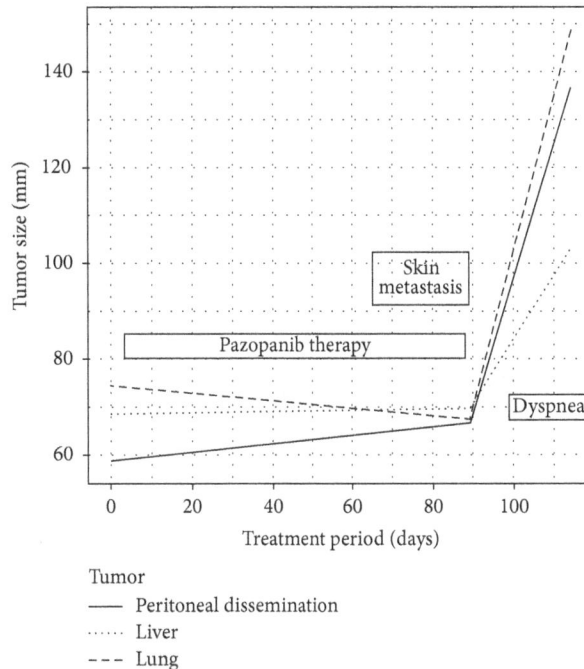

FIGURE 1: The graph shows the change of tumor size with course of treatment. The sum of the patient's tumor diameters increased after cessation of pazopanib therapy.

morphine and oxygen administration; however, the patient's symptoms did not improve. The patient died after four days under sedation. She had died one month after cessation of the pazopanib therapy.

3. Discussion

A global, double-blind, randomized, phase III trial of pazopanib for metastatic soft-tissue sarcoma compared pazopanib once daily versus placebo as second-line or later treatment for patients with advanced soft-tissue sarcoma [10]. In this trial, progression-free survival was significantly improved in the pazopanib arm (median, 4.6 versus 1.6 months; hazard ratio, 0.31; $P < .001$). On the basis of the results of the trial, pazopanib is currently recommended as one of the treatments for patients with advanced soft-tissue sarcoma after failure of standard chemotherapy.

We experienced pazopanib therapy for an advanced or recurrent uterine LMS patient whose condition suddenly worsened after cessation of pazopanib therapy. The sum of the tumor diameters after cessation sharply increased for two weeks. Furthermore, this patient's sudden tumor size increase after ceasing pazopanib therapy appeared related to uncontrolled severe dyspnea.

Some reports have claimed that the cessation of TKI therapy has been followed by the rapid progression of what is termed "flare-up" or "tumor flare" [11–15]. The mechanism for this phenomenon has not been clarified. One hypothesis is the rapid growth of TKI-sensitive clones following the

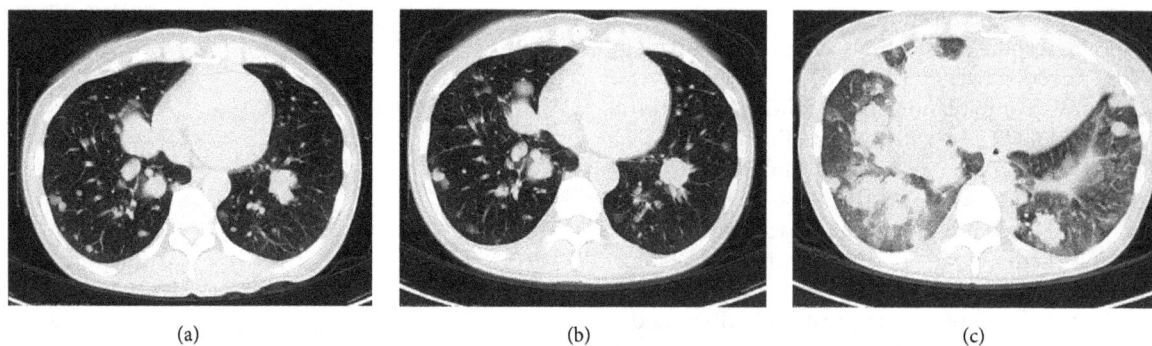

FIGURE 2: Transverse section of lung in computed tomography. (a) Start of pazopanib therapy. (b) End of pazopanib therapy. (c) After two weeks' cessation of pazopanib therapy.

discontinuation of the drug [12, 13]. Another possible explanation is that the residual inhibitory effects of the antiangiogenics disappear after cessation of therapy [14]. One such study found that some (23%) patients with EGFR-mutant lung cancer and acquired resistance to TKIs experienced disease flare after discontinuation of TKI and that the median time to flare was 8 days (range 3–21 days) [12]. Another study of tumor flare occurrence and its prognostic role after discontinuing anti-VEGF receptor TKIs investigated patients with metastatic renal cell carcinoma, similarly concluding that TKI discontinuation accelerates tumor growth rate and negatively affects prognosis [15]. Chaft et al. have reported that shorter time to progression on initial TKI treatment and the presence of pleural or central nervous system metastases are associated with tumor flares in patients with lung cancer [12].

The growth modulation index (GMI) is the ratio of time to progression (TTP) with present therapy and TTP with previous therapy. It has been suggested that GMI > 1.33 indicates a drug or drug combination is active [16]. In our patient, the GMI was 0.18 (ratio of TTP after discontinuing pazopanib to TTP while receiving pazopanib). This GMI suggests that her disease progressed suddenly after discontinuing pazopanib therapy.

A phase II study has shown that trabectedin is a useful therapeutic agent [17] and this new agent was recently approved for treatment of advanced soft-tissue sarcoma; however, we could not use it to treat our patient because it had not yet been approved.

Some studies have suggested that continuing some therapies beyond identification of progressive disease can be clinically beneficial; this is termed "beyond PD" [18, 19]. The concept of beyond PD may be relevant to avoidance of "flare-up" or "tumor flare" associated with TKI therapy.

If the patient above had continued pazopanib therapy, such symptoms might have instead been mild. Therefore, when considering this case for sudden tumor growth after ending pazopanib treatment and for absence of adverse events of severe grade, it appears that treatment could have been further continued in light of comparative risks of disease progression. The prognosis of recurrent uterine leiomyosarcomas is poor; thus, disease control is important.

4. Conclusion

In conclusion, on the basis of our experience conducting pazopanib therapy for patients with advanced LMS, we conclude that the decision to discontinue pazopanib therapy requires careful consideration.

Acknowledgments

The authors thank Charles de Kerckhove for editing as per his training through the American Medical Writers Association.

References

[1] W.-L. Wang, R. Soslow, M. Hensley et al., "Histopathologic prognostic factors in stage I leiomyosarcoma of the uterus: a detailed analysis of 27 cases," *American Journal of Surgical Pathology*, vol. 35, no. 4, pp. 522–529, 2011.

[2] D. S. Kapp, J. Y. Shin, and J. K. Chan, "Prognostic factors and survival in 1396 patients with uterine leiomyosarcomas: emphasis on impact of lymphadenectomy and oophorectomy," *Cancer*, vol. 112, no. 4, pp. 820–830, 2008.

[3] A. Gadducci, F. Landoni, E. Sartori et al., "Uterine leiomyosarcoma: analysis of treatment failures and survival," *Gynecologic Oncology*, vol. 62, no. 1, pp. 25–32, 1996.

[4] Y. Naaman, D. Shveiky, I. Ben-Shachar, A. Shushan, J. Mejia-Gomez, and A. Benshushan, "Uterine sarcoma: prognostic factors and treatment evaluation," *Israel Medical Association Journal*, vol. 13, no. 2, pp. 76–79, 2011.

[5] A. I. Spira and D. S. Ettinger, "The use of chemotherapy in soft-tissue sarcomas," *Oncologist*, vol. 7, no. 4, pp. 348–359, 2002.

[6] G. Sutton, J. A. Blessing, and J. H. Malfetano, "Ifosfamide and doxorubicin in the treatment of advanced leiomyosarcomas of the uterus: a Gynecologic Oncology Group study," *Gynecologic Oncology*, vol. 62, no. 2, pp. 226–229, 1996.

[7] S. Leyvraz, M. Zweifel, G. Jundt et al., "Swiss Group for Clinical Cancer Research. Long-term results of a multicenter SAKK trial on high-dose ifosfamide and doxorubicin in advanced or

metastatic gynecologic sarcomas," *Annals of Oncology*, vol. 17, no. 4, pp. 646–651, 2006.

[8] S. Sleijfer, I. Ray-Coquard, Z. Papai et al., "Pazopanib, a multikinase angiogenesis inhibitor, in patients with relapsed or refractory advanced soft tissue sarcoma: a phase II study from the European organisation for research and treatment of cancer-soft tissue and bone sarcoma group (EORTC Study 62043)," *Journal of Clinical Oncology*, vol. 27, no. 19, pp. 3126–3132, 2009.

[9] F. A. B. Schutz, T. K. Choueiri, and C. N. Sternberg, "Pazopanib: clinical development of a potent anti-angiogenic drug," *Critical Reviews in Oncology/Hematology*, vol. 77, no. 3, pp. 163–171, 2011.

[10] W. T. A. Van Der Graaf, J.-Y. Blay, S. P. Chawla et al., "Pazopanib for metastatic soft-tissue sarcoma (PALETTE): a randomised, double-blind, placebo-controlled phase 3 trial," *The Lancet*, vol. 379, no. 9829, pp. 1879–1886, 2012.

[11] K.-J. Yun, W. Kim, E. H. Kim et al., "Accelerated disease progression after discontinuation of sorafenib in a patient with metastatic papillary thyroid cancer," *Endocrinology and Metabolism*, vol. 29, no. 3, pp. 388–393, 2014.

[12] J. E. Chaft, G. R. Oxnard, C. S. Sima, M. G. Kris, V. A. Miller, and G. J. Riely, "Disease flare after tyrosine kinase inhibitor discontinuation in patients with EGFR-mutant lung cancer and acquired resistance to erlotinib or gefitinib: implications for clinical trial design," *Clinical Cancer Research*, vol. 17, no. 19, pp. 6298–6303, 2011.

[13] P. Wolter, B. Beuselinck, S. Pans, and P. Schffski, "Flare-up: an often unreported phenomenon nevertheless familiar to oncologists prescribing tyrosine kinase inhibitors," *Acta Oncologica*, vol. 48, no. 4, pp. 621–624, 2009.

[14] I. M. E. Desar, S. F. Mulder, A. B. Stillebroer et al., "The reverse side of the victory: flare up of symptoms after discontinuation of sunitinib or sorafenib in renal cell cancer patients. A report of three cases," *Acta Oncologica*, vol. 48, no. 6, pp. 927–931, 2009.

[15] R. Iacovelli, F. Massari, L. Albiges et al., "Evidence and clinical relevance of tumor flare in patients who discontinue tyrosine kinase inhibitors for treatment of metastatic renal cell carcinoma," *European Urology*, vol. 68, no. 1, pp. 154–160, 2015.

[16] D. D. Von Hoff, "There are no bad anticancer agents, only bad clinical trial designs- twenty-first Richard and Hinda Rosenthal foundation award lecture," *Clinical Cancer Research*, vol. 4, no. 5, pp. 1079–1086, 1998.

[17] G. D. Demetri, S. P. Chawla, M. Von Mehren et al., "Efficacy and safety of trabectedin in patients with advanced or metastatic liposarcoma or leiomyosarcoma after failure of prior anthracyclines and ifosfamide: results of a randomized phase II study of two different schedules," *Journal of Clinical Oncology*, vol. 27, no. 25, pp. 4188–4196, 2009.

[18] G. R. Oxnard, M. E. Arcila, J. Chmielecki, M. Ladanyi, V. A. Miller, and W. Pao, "New strategies in overcoming acquired resistance to epidermal growth factor receptor tyrosinekinase inhibitors in lung cancer," *Clinical Cancer Research*, vol. 17, no. 17, pp. 5530–5537, 2011.

[19] J. Bennouna, J. Sastre, D. Arnold et al., "Continuation of bevacizumab after first progression in metastatic colorectal cancer (ML18147): a randomised phase 3 trial," *The Lancet Oncology*, vol. 14, no. 1, pp. 29–37, 2013.

13

Malignant Transformation of Mature Cystic Teratoma Diagnosed after a 10-Year Interval

Mariko Jitsumori,[1] **Satoru Munakata,**[2] **and Toshiya Yamamoto**[1]

[1]Department of Obstetrics and Gynecology, Sakai City Medical Center, Sakai, Japan
[2]Department of Pathology, Sakai City Medical Center, Sakai, Japan

Correspondence should be addressed to Toshiya Yamamoto; yamamoto-to@sakai-hospital.jp

Academic Editor: Hans Rudolf Tinneberg

A 67-year-old uniparous woman had undergone surgery for acute perforated gastric ulcer 10 years prior to the current presentation. Although abdominal computed tomography (CT) performed at that point had revealed a mature cystic teratoma measuring 6 cm in diameter in the right ovary, it was left untreated. She visited the department of surgery at our hospital with chief complaints of appetite loss, nausea, and vomiting that had persisted for the prior two weeks. She was admitted with a diagnosis of ileus attributed to an abdominal incisional hernia. CT performed on admission revealed a tumor measuring 21 cm in diameter with mural nodules in the right ovary. Thus, surgery was performed under suspicion of malignant transformation of the previously detected ovarian mature cystic teratoma. While neither lymphadenopathy nor distant metastasis was detected by imaging studies, bilateral adnexectomy and repair of the abdominal incisional hernia were performed. Cytology of ascites was negative. The postoperative pathological diagnosis was squamous cell carcinoma arising from teratoma, and the postoperative clinical diagnosis was stage IA ovarian cancer. It was assumed that the mature cystic teratoma which had been detected in the right ovary 10 years earlier had undergone malignant transformation.

1. Introduction

Mature cystic teratoma, which is the most common benign ovarian tumor type, is known to occasionally undergo malignant transformation. Malignant transformation of mature cystic teratoma is extremely difficult either to predict or to detect early. Moreover, the mechanism of malignant transformation has not as yet been elucidated. We experienced a case with a mature cystic teratoma that had undergone malignant transformation over a period of 10 years. We herein present this case with a literature review.

2. Case

Our patient was a 67-year-old woman, gravida 4, para 1. Her past medical history included epilepsy diagnosed at 56 years of age, unspecified cardiopulmonary arrest at age 57 years, peritonitis due to acute perforated gastric ulcer, venous thrombosis of the lower limb, and pulmonary arterial embolism. She was also allergic to numerous drugs and diagnostic agents (e.g., contrast media, nonsteroidal anti-inflammatory drugs, and sodium valproate). She visited the department of surgery at our hospital with chief complaints of appetite loss, nausea, and vomiting that had persisted for the prior two weeks. Because abdominal plain computed tomography (CT) revealed ileus and an abdominal incisional hernia, she was immediately admitted with a diagnosis of ileus caused by the incisional hernia. Moreover, a tumor measuring 21 cm in longest diameter was detected in the pelvis (Figure 1(a)). She was thus referred to our department for detailed examination and treatment. At the initial examination, the abdomen was soft without tenderness, rebound tenderness, or muscular defense. An easily movable mass extending from the right lower abdomen to the level of the umbilicus was palpated. The patient had undergone omental implantation for acute perforated gastric ulcer 10 years earlier. Preoperative abdominal plain CT had revealed

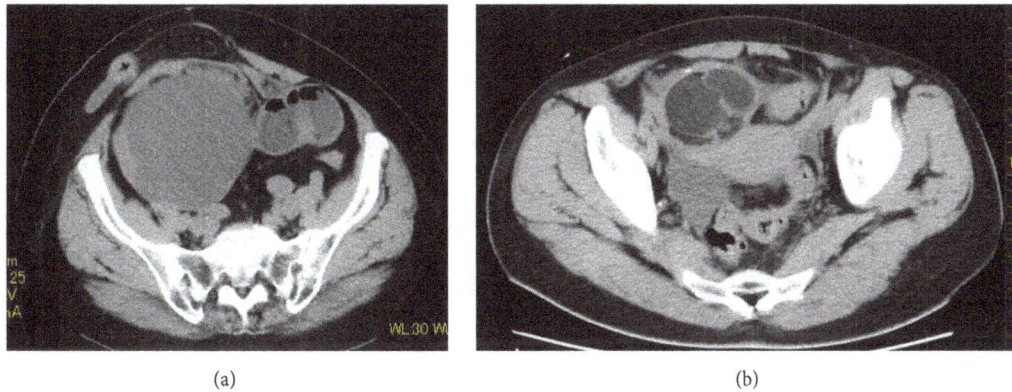

FIGURE 1: (a) Abdominal plain computed tomography (current). A huge mass measuring 21 cm in longest diameter can be seen in the right cranial portion of the uterine body. The mass is partially solid, suggesting malignancy. (b) Abdominal plain computed tomography (image obtained 10 years prior to the current admission). A mature cystic teratoma measuring 6 cm in diameter is observed on the right side. There are no findings suggestive of malignancy, such as a mural nodule or a solid component.

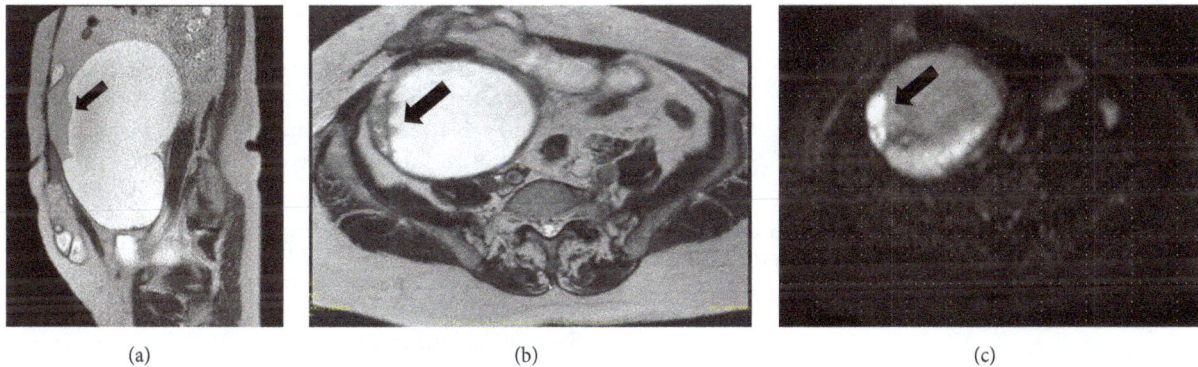

FIGURE 2: Pelvic plain magnetic resonance imaging. (a) T2-weighted image in the sagittal plane. A cyst measuring 21 × 19 × 12 cm is observed. It is partially solid. (b) T2-weighted image in the horizontal plane. (c) Diffusion-weighted image in the horizontal plane. The solid components observed on the T2-weighted image show high signal intensity on the diffusion-weighted image (←). The cyst is suspected to be a malignant lesion.

a right ovarian tumor measuring 6 cm in diameter (Figure 1(b)), which contained a part of calcification and fatty components; however, there had been no findings suggestive of malignancy, such as a solid component or a mural nodule. The right ovarian tumor was radiologically diagnosed with a mature cystic teratoma. After surgery for the acute perforated gastric ulcer, she had not been referred to the department of gynecology. No further examination of the right ovarian tumor was performed. She had not been followed up for the ovarian tumor. When the findings of abdominal plain CT performed during the current admission were compared to those of the abdominal CT obtained 10 years earlier, the ovarian tumor was noted to have grown markedly in size and to be partially solid. The CT performed during the current admission also revealed fatty components in the ovarian cyst. On the basis of these findings, malignant transformation of the mature cystic teratoma was suspected. Furthermore, pelvic plain magnetic resonance imaging (MRI) also showed a cyst measuring 21 cm in longest diameter that was partially solid on the right side of the uterine body (Figure 2(a)).

The solid components detected on T2-weighted images (Figure 2(b)) showed high signal intensity on diffusion-weighted images (Figure 2(c)) and low signal intensity on apparent diffusion coefficient maps, which suggested a malignant lesion. In addition, blood tests revealed tumor marker elevations: CEA, 7.1 ng/mL (<4.9 ng/mL); CA125, 58.3 U/mL (<35 U/mL); CA19-9, 405.8 U/mL (<37 U/mL); and SCC antigen, 6.2 ng/mL (<1.5 ng/mL). Based on the clinical course, imaging findings, and elevated tumor markers, malignant transformation of the previously recognized mature cystic teratoma was strongly suspected. Sixteen days after the initial examination, semiurgent surgery was performed. While neither lymphadenopathy nor distant metastasis was detected by imaging studies, the operation consisted of abdominal bilateral adnexectomy and repair of the abdominal incisional hernia in consideration of the patient's general condition. The intraoperative findings included slight accumulation of ascites with a pink tinge due to blood and swelling of the right ovary, which was larger than a newborn's head, whereas there were no signs of capsule rupture, torsion abnormality, and so on. We detected no macroscopic abnormalities in

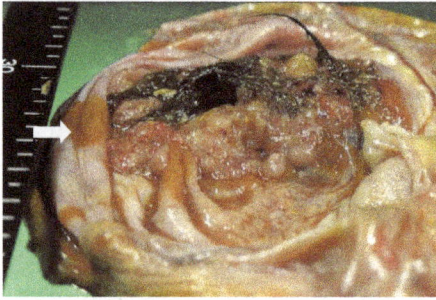

FIGURE 3: Resected specimen. Protruding lesions are observed on a portion of the wall of the right ovarian tumor.

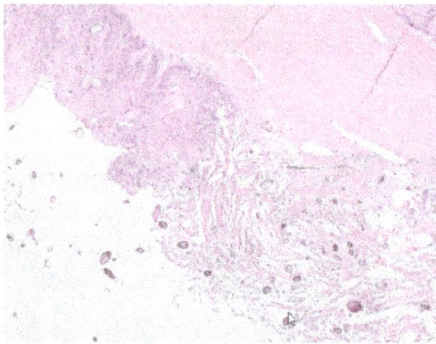

FIGURE 4: Histologically, squamous cell carcinoma was observed inside the cyst (left side of the picture). Granulation tissue containing hair was also found (right side of the picture) (H&E staining, ×100).

the uterus or the left adnexa. Neither disseminated lesions nor lymphadenopathy was observed in the peritoneal cavity. The tumor in the right ovary was unilocular and weighed 2960 g, containing both fatty components and hair. Moreover, protruding lesions were observed on a portion of the tumor wall (Figure 3). Cytology of ascites was negative. Histologically, cystic wall was lined by squamous epithelium and contained horny materials inside the cyst. Mature bone tissue and hair were also observed. Focally, granulation tissue was formed. Squamous cell carcinoma was found in the solid part protruding inside the cyst wall. There was a transition between squamous epithelium and squamous cell carcinoma (Figure 4). The postoperative clinical diagnosis was ovarian cancer FIGO stage IA, pT1aNxM0 due to malignant transformation of a mature cystic teratoma which had first been noted 10 years earlier. Given the history of allergy to multiple drugs, cardiopulmonary arrest, venous thrombosis of the lower limb, and pulmonary arterial embolism, postoperative chemotherapy was not planned. As of two years since surgery, no recurrence has been observed.

3. Discussion

Mature cystic teratoma, which is a commonly observed benign ovarian tumor in young women, is a germ cell tumor containing fat, hair, teeth, cartilage, and so forth. It is the most common type of benign ovarian tumor [1] accounting for approximately 20% of all ovarian tumors according to Hurwitz et al. [2]. A quarter of ovarian tumors are reportedly of the germ cell type, most of which are mature cystic teratomas [3]. Mature cystic teratoma is known to occasionally become malignant, and the majority of such transformations result in SCC. Malignant transformation was reported in 1.8% of 8000 patients with a mature cystic teratoma by Peterson [4] and 1% to 2% of such patients by Hurwitz et al. [2], while Kim et al. reported that malignant transformation was observed in 4 of 560 patients (0.6%) who underwent surgery for a mature cystic teratoma at their facility [5]. According to histological types, SCC accounts for the majority of cases, 80% to 90% according to Hurwitz et al. [2] and approximately 80% as reported by Hackethal et al. [3]. Adenocarcinoma [2, 6] and malignant melanoma [6] have also been reported. Kikkawa et al. reported that 42 cases with a mature cystic teratoma undergoing malignant transformation included 37 cases developing SCC, while the remaining cases had an adenocarcinoma or malignant melanoma [6]. According to a review of 277 cases with malignant transformation of a mature cystic teratoma into SCC described in 64 articles with sufficient data that were selected from among 126 articles published between 1978 and 2007, the mean age was 55 years, and the tumor diameter was 10 cm or longer in many cases [3, 7]. Moreover, Hackethal et al. reported that the diameter exceeded 100 mm in several cases with mature cystic teratoma undergoing malignant transformation [3]. Chen et al. reported that the cut-off value was 137 ± 57 mm [8], while Kikkawa et al. reported that it was 99 mm [9]. Regarding age, the reported mean ages were 48 [2] and 55 ± 14.4 years [8], whereas malignant transformation is reportedly common in patients 50 years of age or older [3]. As for diagnostic criteria, the reported cut-off values for age were 40 [5, 10] and 45 years [9].

Malignant transformation of a mature cystic teratoma is mainly detected by diagnostic imaging. It is considered to be important to focus on the presence or absence of solid components on pelvic MRI images [11]. In SCC cases, the SCC antigen is regarded as being a useful tumor marker [7]. Kikkawa et al. performed screening by measuring SCC antigen (<2.0 ng/mL), CA 125 (<35 U/mL), CA 19-9 (<37 U/mL), and CEA (<5.0 ng/mL) levels in cases with malignantly transformed mature cystic teratomas, reporting that diagnostic efficiencies were 63%, 50%, 28%, and 45%, respectively [9]. In our 67-year-old patient with SCC measuring 21 cm in diameter, these tumor markers (CEA, 7.1 ng/mL; CA 125, 58.3 U/mL; CA 19-9, 405.8 U/mL; and SCC antigen, 6.2 ng/mL) were elevated, and MRI revealed solid components suggestive of malignancy. Thus, in terms of age, histological type, tumor diameter, tumor marker elevations, and MRI findings, our case represents a typical example of the generally known features of patients with malignant transformation of a mature cystic teratoma. Although mature cystic teratoma is a frequently observed benign ovarian tumor, it may become malignant as seen in our case. Thus, these teratomas require continuous follow-up, and patients also need to be informed about the possibility of malignant transformation at the time of explanation.

Although the mechanism of malignant transformation of a mature cystic teratoma remains unknown, involvement of the human papilloma virus has been suggested [12, 13]. Moreover, no reports have mentioned how long it takes for a mature cystic teratoma to become malignant. In fact, it is difficult to estimate when malignant transformation occurred in our case. However, because the cancer was diagnosed as stage IA despite an interval of 10 years, we assume that malignant transformation had progressed very slowly. The peak age at diagnosis of mature cystic teratoma and the mean age of patients experiencing malignant transformation of a teratoma differ by at least 10 years, though there is one report describing an 85-year-old patient with a mature cystic teratoma that did not undergo malignant transformation [14]. Thus, malignant transformation appears to take a very long time. However, because it is difficult to predict or achieve early detection of malignant transformation, caution must be exercised when patients with mature cystic teratomas are followed up long-term.

We experienced a case with a mature cystic teratoma which underwent malignant transformation during an interval of 10 years since its initial detection. Although mature cystic teratoma is a benign tumor, surgery or regular follow-up needs to be planned after due consideration of the risk of malignant transformation.

References

[1] M. Fujimura, "Mature cystic teratoma," *Kanto San Fu Shi*, vol. 49, pp. 655–657, 2012.

[2] J. L. Hurwitz, A. Fenton, W. G. McCluggage, and S. McKenna, "Squamous cell carcinoma arising in a dermoid cyst of the ovary: a case series," *BJOG*, vol. 114, no. 10, pp. 1283–1287, 2007.

[3] A. Hackethal, D. Brueggmann, M. K. Bohlmann, F. E. Franke, H.-R. Tinneberg, and K. Münstedt, "Squamous-cell carcinoma in mature cystic teratoma of the ovary: systematic review and analysis of published data," *The Lancet Oncology*, vol. 9, no. 12, pp. 1173–1180, 2008.

[4] W. F. Peterson, "Malignant degeneration of benign cystic teratomas of the ovary. A collective review of the literature," *Obstetrical and Gynecological Survey*, vol. 12, no. 6, pp. 793–830, 1957.

[5] M. J. Kim, N. Y. Kim, D.-Y. Lee, B.-K. Yoon, and D. Choi, "Clinical characteristics of ovarian teratoma: age-focused retrospective analysis of 580 cases," *American Journal of Obstetrics and Gynecology*, vol. 205, no. 1, pp. 32–e4, 2011.

[6] F. Kikkawa, H. Ishikawa, K. Tamakoshi, A. Nawa, N. Suganuma, and Y. Tomoda, "Squamous cell carcinoma arising from mature cystic teratoma of the ovary: a clinicopathologic analysis," *Obstetrics and Gynecology*, vol. 89, no. 6, pp. 1017–1022, 1997.

[7] Japan Society of Gynecologic Oncology, "Treatment Guidelines for Ovarian Cancer 2015 Edition".

[8] R.-J. Chen, K.-Y. Chen, T.-C. Chang, B.-C. Sheu, S.-N. Chow, and S.-C. Huang, "Prognosis and treatment of squamous cell carcinoma from a mature cystic teratoma of the ovary," *Journal of the Formosan Medical Association*, vol. 107, no. 11, pp. 857–868, 2008.

[9] F. Kikkawa, A. Nawa, K. Tamakoshi et al., "Diagnosis of squamous cell carcinoma arising from mature cystic teratoma of the ovary," *Cancer*, vol. 82, no. 11, pp. 2249–2255, 1998.

[10] Y. Mori, H. Nishii, K. Takabe et al., "Preoperative diagnosis of malignant transformation arising from mature cystic teratoma of the ovary," *Gynecologic Oncology*, vol. 90, no. 2, pp. 338–341, 2003.

[11] M. Futagami, Y. Yokoyama, H. Mizunuma et al., "Is the malignant transformation of mature cystic teratoma predictable before operation?" *Aomori Rin San Fu Shi*, vol. 26, pp. 59–65, 2011.

[12] A.-J. Chiang, D.-R. Chen, J.-T. Cheng, and T.-H. Chang, "Detection of human papillomavirus in squamous cell carcinoma arising from dermoid cysts," *Taiwanese Journal of Obstetrics and Gynecology*, vol. 54, no. 5, pp. 559–566, 2015.

[13] I. B. D. O. Araujo, M. V. C. Pinheiro, P. H. Zanvettor, E. J. B. Studart, D. F. Filho, and S. E. Coupland, "High frequency of malignant transformation of ovarian mature teratoma into squamous cell carcinoma in young patients in northeast Brazil," *International Journal of Gynecological Pathology*, vol. 35, no. 2, pp. 176–184, 2016.

[14] K. Takahashi, T. Shinno, Y. Watanabe, H. Kurioka, and K. Miyazaki, "Benign teratoma in an 85-year-old woman," *Archives of Gynecology and Obstetrics*, vol. 263, no. 4, pp. 188–190, 2000.

14

Successful Spontaneous Pregnancy after Treatment for Ewing Sarcoma including Sacrectomy

T. Hockertz and M. Velickovic (iD)

Department of Orthopedic Surgery, Sports Traumatology and Trauma Surgery, Städtisches Klinikum Wolfenbüttel,
Alter Weg 80, 38302 Wolfenbüttel, Germany

Correspondence should be addressed to M. Velickovic; mirko.velickovic@gmx.de

Academic Editor: Seung-Yup Ku

Ewing sarcomas are highly malignant bone tumors and usually occur in childhood. Radiation therapy, chemotherapy, and surgical methods increase the survival rate of the affected patient, but infertility and reduced reproductive capacity are common late effects of pediatric cancer treatment.

1. Introduction

We report on the pregnancy of a patient with Ewing sarcoma treated at the age of 18 with chemo- and radiotherapy as well as total sacrectomy. In the course of time, a "neosacrum" developed and the patient gave birth to a boy at the age of 29. The course of pregnancy was uneventful. This was the second pregnancy of this patient. At the time of pregnancy, the patient was 29 years old.

2. Case Presentation

The patient was 18 years old at the time Ewing sarcoma of the sacrum was diagnosed. At the time when the patient consulted for the first time a doctor, she was already suffering from progressive pain in the lumbosacral region radiating into both legs with saddle block anesthesia, foot flexor paresis, and episodes of bladder and stool incontinence for four months. An initial MRI of the lower spine suggested a tethered cord syndrome and the patient was transferred and operated on in a neurosurgical clinic, but the patient did not benefit from the surgery. In an additional MRI of the pelvis, a large tumor was found. The tumor was partly intra-, partly extraosseous and involved the entire right sacrum wing and extended into the small pelvis and the dorsal pelvic soft parts. The histopathological examination of the sample biopsy confirmed Ewing sarcoma. Staging showed no evidence of metastasis of the tumor. The stage was documented with T3 N0 M0. We treated the patient with a combination of neoadjuvant chemotherapy, radiation therapy, and sacrectomy. In the first preoperative phase, the patient received 3-day blocks of polychemotherapy consisting of vincristine, etoposide, doxorubicin, and ifosfamide. This was performed preoperatively six times at intervals of 3 weeks. The tumor showed a marked reduction in size from 9 cm × 6.5 cm × 12 cm before the start of the therapy and 8 cm × 5,5 cm × 10,5 cm after 6 chemotherapy blocks (data in each case in width × depth × height). Total sacrectomy followed. In a first step, the position of the lumbar spine was secured with a lumbopelvic fixation from the ileum to the third lumbar vertebral body. The tumor could not be removed en bloc, so we performed an intralesional tumor resection. Before complete dissection of the sacrum was done, we placed an angular-stable ilioiliacal LCP plate sacrum in order to ensure an anatomical position of the pelvis (Figure 1). Postoperatively, we continued chemotherapy as well as radiation therapy due to the intralesional tumor resection. The radiation dose was 45 Gy. The follow-up period was 12 years. The radiological follow-up examinations over the course of time documented a nearly complete sacral osteoneogenesis including the neuroforamina with a stable fusion of the new sacrum with the posterior pelvic ring (Figures 2 and 3). The clinical outcome was very good, and the gait was almost normal; no crutches were needed anymore. Neurologically, an incomplete paraplegia remained, with preserved motor function and sensitivity below the spinal cord injury site L5/S1 with a clinically nonrelevant peroneal paresis on the right,

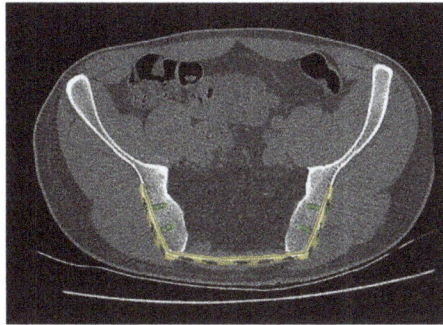

FIGURE 1: Schematic representation of the sacrectomy.

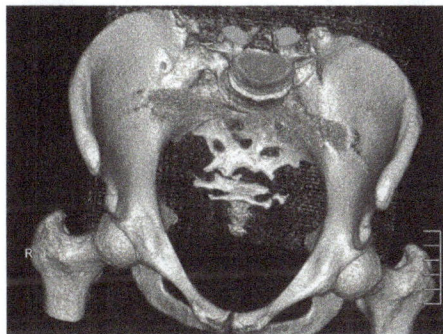

FIGURE 2: CT reconstruction of the pelvis showing the "neosacrum."

discrete paresthesia on the right lateral thigh and distal lower limbs, and a neurogenic bladder dysfunction.

3. Pregnancy

Contraception was done with birth control pills. The patient wanted to conceive so this medication was stopped. Three months later, the patient was pregnant at the age of 28 but lost the child in the 8th week of pregnancy. Curettage was necessary. The second pregnancy at the age of 29 was successful and she gave birth to a boy of 3460 g and 50 cm through a cesarean section at the 37 weeks' gestation by a community obstetrician. There were no birth complications (Figure 5).

4. Discussion

Ewing sarcoma is a highly malignant bone tumor which rapidly metastasizes at an early stage. Treatment options include radiation, chemotherapy, and operation. The combination of chemotherapy with both surgery and radiotherapy increases the survival rate by 15–20% as compared to chemotherapy with either local therapy alone [1, 2]. Prognosis has been improved in recent years. In the 1960s, the 2-year survival rate was only 21%. Due to modern treatments, long-term survival up to 70% to 80% can be reached among patients without metastases [3, 4]. The aim of treatment is to cure the patient with the least cost in terms of long-term morbidity.

A major fear among female survivors is the long-term effects of cancer therapy especially infertility. Family planning is for most people an essential part of life quality. In general, cancer survivors are less likely to become pregnant when compared to their siblings [5–7].

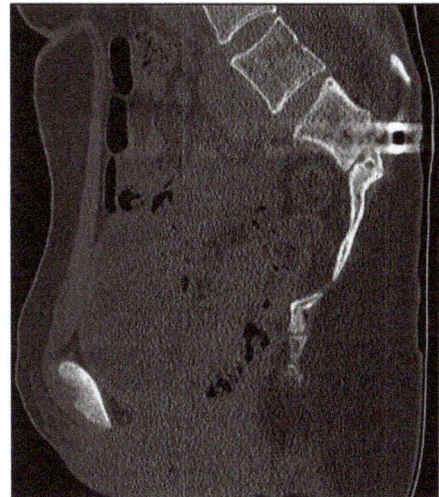

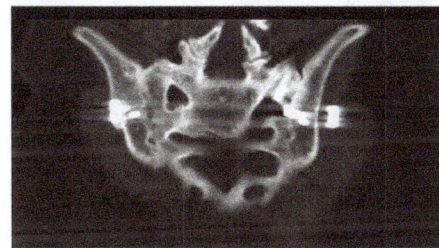

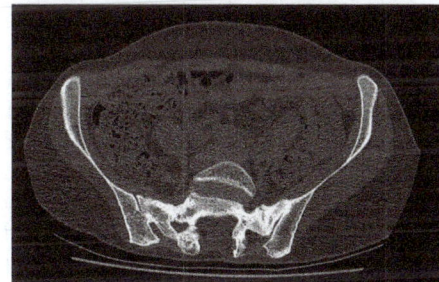

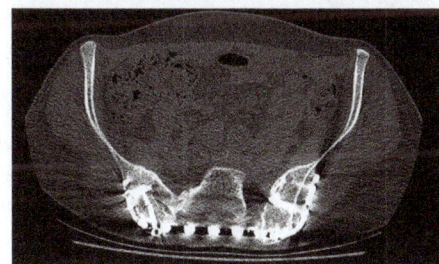

FIGURE 3: Selection of CT slices of the pelvis (CT and X-ray of the lower spine and pelvis were done in another hospital in 2015 due to lower back pain).

Ewing sarcoma occurs mainly in childhood. Strategies for preserving fertility are limited and should be planned before starting tumor therapy and discussed with the patient and family. However, this is often not possible due to the urge to start with the therapy. In general, we recommend an interdisciplinary team including a gynecologist in order to choose the best way to preserve fertility. Even in prepubertal girls, the physician should keep the possible wish to have children later on in mind. In our case, the patient was 18 years old when Ewing's sarcoma was diagnosed. There was no gynecologist involved and no pretreatment to preserve fertility was done.

According to Lee et al., there are several well established methods to preserve fertility, including gonadal shielding during radiotherapy, trachelectomy, and ovarian transposition. Methods like embryo cryopreservation are only useful in established stable partnership which is unlikely at the patient's age. Other methods like oocyte cryopreservation, ovarian cryopreservation and transplantation, and ovarian suppression with GnRH analogs or antagonists are experimental. But Lee et al. also highlighted that ovarian tissue cryopreservation and reimplantation is a main option to preserve fertility of cancer patients who need an immediate start of the cancer treatment. For patients in the prepubertal age, freezing is the only option to preserve fertility [8]. Up to now, a total of 17 babies from 12 patients have been born worldwide from ovarian tissue cryopreservation and reimplantation [8–10]. Three of them suffered from Ewing's sarcoma.

Treatment with multiagent chemotherapy, radiotherapy, and surgical procedures such as sacrectomy is associated with significant late effects and reduces the chance of pregnancy [11].

Radiation therapy leads to decreased fertility depending on the site irradiated. Ewing's sarcoma most commonly affects the femur and the pelvis in 20% of cases, so the female reproductive system is often affected. The younger the patient at the time of radiation, the greater the probability of infertility. The risk of pregnancy complications such as miscarriage, preterm delivery, and perinatal death is higher. There is also a higher risk of low birth weight less than 2500 g in infants born to patients treated with pelvic irradiation [12]. There is no known radiation dose threshold for uterine damage, but abdominal radiation with 20–30 Gy in childhood already leads to ovarian failure [13]. According to Teh et al., no successful pregnancy been reported after a direct radiation dose (>45 Gy) to the whole pelvis [14]. Our patient received a radiation dose of 45 Gy with no protective measures like ovarian transposition.

Haerr and Pratt recommend early chemotherapy in the course of many malignant sarcomas, despite pregnancy, to prevent the occurrence of metastases [15]. It is known that busulfan and high doses of lomustine are significantly associated with reduced pregnancy in female survivors of childhood cancer not exposed to pelvic or cranial radiotherapy. According to the same authors, chemotherapy-specific effects on pregnancy were generally few in patients without radiotherapy to the pelvis [16].

There is only one case in the literature which is similar to our case.

Kakogawa et al. reported a case of successful pregnancy in a patient who underwent sacrectomy combined with multiagent chemotherapy and radiotherapy for Ewing's sarcoma. The patient was diagnosed with Ewing's sarcoma of the sacrum at the age of 16. But in this case, pretreatment in order to protect the reproductive system was carried out, the ovaries were transposed, the uterus was shielded, and a gonadotropin-releasing hormone agonist was used during treatment to protect the ovarian function. The patient

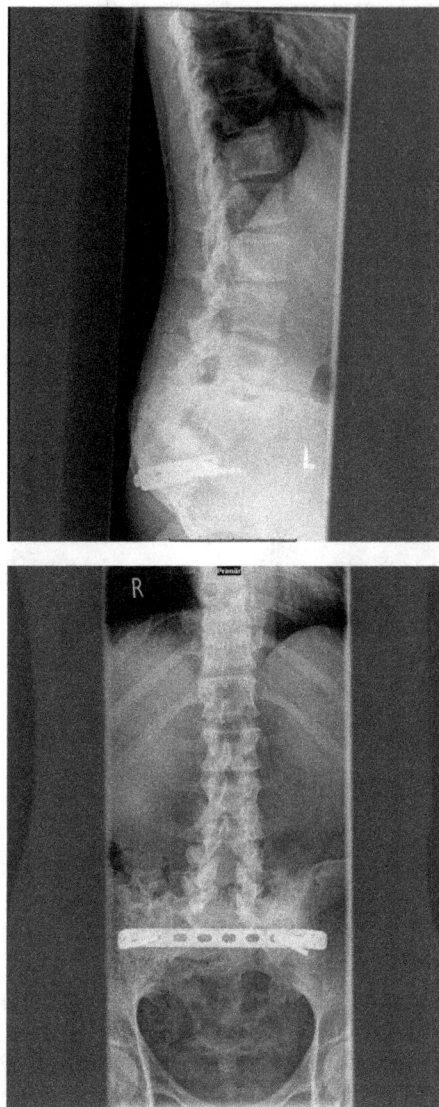

FIGURE 4: X-ray of the lower spine with ilioiliacal plate.

spontaneously conceived at the age of 27 [4, 17]. On the other hand, a spontaneous return of ovarian function and conception years after gonadal chemotherapy with evidence of ovarian failure is possible [18].

At the time the patient arrived at our hospital, she already suffered from severe neurologic symptoms. Due to the urgency to start with the therapy, no precautions were taken to maintain fertility.

This is the 6th reported case of pregnancy in a patient with Ewing's sarcoma [4, 19–21]. All women became naturally pregnant. The pregnancy course was in 4 cases uneventful; in one case only, an inadequate descent of the fetal head occurred due to pelvic distortion. In 3 cases, a caesarian section was done. In the other cases, the way of delivery is unknown. We also recommend a caesarian section. Biomechanically, the ilioiliacal pelvic plate acts as an internal fixator which prevents widening of the posterior pelvic ring at birth (Figure 4). In the case of a vaginal birth, the baby could be stuck in the birth canal or the pelvic ring may burst open.

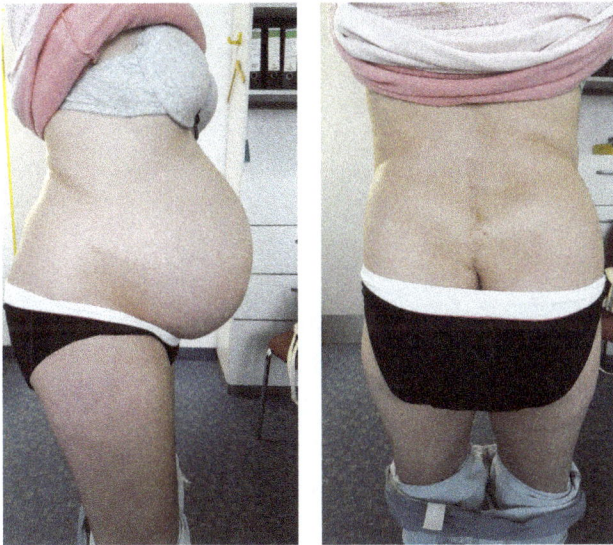

FIGURE 5

Both would put the mother and the child in unnecessary danger. Neurologically, an incomplete paraplegia remained, with preserved motor function and sensitivity below the spinal cord injury site L5/S1 with a clinically nonrelevant peroneal paresis on the right, discrete paresthesia on the right lateral thigh and distal lower limbs, and a neurogenic bladder dysfunction. Neurological deficits are not an absolute indication for cesarean delivery but caesarian section is recommended to reduce the risk for the baby.

Successful and uneventful pregnancy after sacrectomy combined with chemotherapy and radiotherapy can be achieved even without pretreatment for fertility preservation.

References

[1] "AWMF Interdisziplinäre Leitlinie der Deutschen Krebsgesellschaft und der Gesellschaft für Pädiatrischen Onkologie und Hämatologie, Ewing-Sarkome und PNET des Kindes- und Jugendalters," http://www.awmf.org/leitlinien/detail/ll/025-006.html.

[2] A. Schuck, S. Ahrens, M. Paulussen et al., "Local therapy in localized ewing tumors: results of 1058 patients treated in the CESS 81, CESS 86, and EICESS 92 trials," International Journal of Radiation Oncology, Biology, Physics, vol. 55, no. 1, pp. 168–177, 2003.

[3] U. Dirksen and H. Jürgens, "Approaching Ewing sarcoma," Future Oncology, vol. 6, no. 7, pp. 1155–1162, 2010.

[4] J. Kakogawa, T. Nako, K. Kawamura et al., "Successful Pregnancy After Sacrectomy Combined With Chemotherapy and Radiation for Ewing Sarcoma: Case Report and Literature Review," Journal of Pediatric & Adolescent Gynecology, vol. 28, no. 3, pp. e79–e81, 2015.

[5] H. Magelssen, K. K. Melve, R. Skjærven, and S. D. Fosså, "Parenthood probability and pregnancy outcome in patients with a cancer diagnosis during adolescence and young adulthood," Human Reproduction, vol. 23, no. 1, pp. 178–186, 2008.

[6] J. Y. Wo and A. N. Viswanathan, "Impact of radiotherapy on fertility, pregnancy, and neonatal outcomes in female cancer patients," International Journal of Radiation Oncology, Biology, Physics, vol. 73, no. 5, pp. 1304–1312, 2009.

[7] D. M. Green, T. Kawashima, M. Stovall et al., "Fertility of female survivors of childhood cancer: A report from the childhood cancer survivor study," Journal of Clinical Oncology, vol. 27, no. 16, pp. 2677–2685, 2009.

[8] S. Lee, J. Y. Song, S. Y. Ku, S. H. Kim, and T. Kim, "Fertility preservation in women with cancer," Clinical and Experimental Reproductive Medicine, vol. 39, no. 2, p. 46, 2012.

[9] R. Grundy, R. G. Gosden, M. Hewitt et al., "Fertility preservation for children treated for cancer (1): Scientific advances and research dilemmas," Archives of Disease in Childhood, vol. 84, no. 4, pp. 355–359, 2001.

[10] S. J. Silber, "Ovary cryopreservation and transplantation for fertility preservation," Molecular Human Reproduction, vol. 18, no. 2, Article ID gar082, pp. 59–67, 2012.

[11] L. E. Bath, W. Hamish, B. Wallace, and H. O. D. Critchley, "Late effects of the treatment of childhood cancer on the female reproductive system and the potential for fertility preservation," BJOG: An International Journal of Obstetrics & Gynaecology, vol. 109, no. 2, pp. 107–114, 2002.

[12] D. M. Green, C. A. Sklar, J. D. Boice Jr. et al., "Ovarian failure and reproductive outcomes after childhood cancer treatment: results from the childhood cancer survivor study," Journal of Clinical Oncology, vol. 27, no. 14, pp. 2374–2381, 2009.

[13] W. H. B. Wallace, S. M. Shalet, E. C. Crowne, P. H. Morris-Jones, and H. R. Gattamaneni, "Ovarian failure following abdominal irradiation in childhood: natural history and prognosis," Clinical Oncology, vol. 1, no. 2, pp. 75–79, 1989.

[14] W. T. Teh, C. Stern, S. Chander, and M. Hickey, "The impact of uterine radiation on subsequent fertility and pregnancy outcomes," BioMed Research International, vol. 2014, Article ID 482968, 2014.

[15] R. W. Haerr and A. T. Pratt, "Multiagent chemotherapy for sarcoma diagnosed during pregnancy," Cancer, vol. 56, no. 5, pp. 1028–1033, 1985.

[16] E. J. Chow, K. L. Stratton, W. M. Leisenring et al., "Pregnancy after chemotherapy in male and female survivors of childhood cancer treated between 1970 and 1999: A report from the Childhood Cancer Survivor Study cohort," The Lancet Oncology, vol. 17, no. 5, pp. 567–576, 2016.

[17] P. Hürmüz, D. Sebag-Montefiore, P. Byrne, and R. Cooper, "Successful spontaneous pregnancy after pelvic chemoradiotherapy for anal cancer," Clinical Oncology, vol. 24, no. 6, pp. 452–458, 2012.

[18] J. Nasir, C. Walton, S. W. Lindow, and E. A. Masson, "Spontaneous recovery of chemotherapy-induced primary ovarian failure: Implications for management," Clinical Endocrinology, vol. 46, no. 2, pp. 217–219, 1997.

[19] L. E. Bath, G. Tydeman, H. O. D. Critchley, R. A. Anderson, D. T. Baird, and W. H. B. Wallace, "Spontaneous conception in a young woman who had ovarian cortical tissue cryopreserved before chemotherapy and radiotherapy for a Ewing's sarcoma of the pelvis: case report," Human Reproduction, vol. 19, no. 11, pp. 2569–2572, 2004.

[20] I. G. Chihara, H. Osada, Y. Iitsuka, K. Masuda, and S. Sekiya, "Pregnancy after limb-sparing hemipelvectomy for Ewing's sarcoma: A case report and review of the literature," *Gynecologic and Obstetric Investigation*, vol. 56, no. 4, pp. 218–220, 2003.

[21] N. Sharon, Y. Neumann, G. Kenet, J. Schachter, G. Rechavi, and A. Toren, "Successful pregnancy after high-dose cyclophosphamide and ifosfamide treatment in two postpubertal women," *Pediatric Hematology and Oncology*, vol. 18, no. 4, pp. 247–252, 2001.

15

Recurrent Volvulus during Pregnancy: Case Report and Review of the Literature

Layan Alrahmani ⓘ,[1] **Jaclyn Rivington,**[2] **and Carl H. Rose**[1]

[1]*Mayo Clinic, Division of Maternal-Fetal Medicine, Department of Obstetrics and Gynecology, 200 First St. SW, Rochester, MN 55905, USA*
[2]*Metrohealth Medical Center, Department of Internal Medicine, 2500 Metrohealth Dr., Cleveland, OH 44109, USA*

Correspondence should be addressed to Layan Alrahmani; layan.md@gmail.com

Academic Editor: Maria Grazia Porpora

Introduction. Sigmoid colon volvulus (SV) represents the most common etiology of antepartum gastrointestinal obstruction, with repetitive antepartum episodes rarely reported. *Case Presentation.* A 25-year-old multiparous patient with history of SV at 26 weeks in her previous pregnancy presented with recurrent episodes of SV at 32 0/7, 32 4/7, 37 0/7, and 38 1/7 weeks successfully managed with colonoscopic decompression. Labor was successfully induced at 38 4/7 weeks, and she experienced two further episodes on postpartum days #1 and #32 also treated with colonoscopic decompression, followed by laparoscopic resection. *Conclusion.* Successful treatment of antepartum SV with colonoscopic decompression does not preclude recurrence later in gestation and in future pregnancies.

1. Background

Volvulus of the sigmoid colon represents the most common etiology of antepartum bowel obstruction [1, 2]. Circumferential torsion of an intestinal segment around its mesenteric origin produces symptoms of gastrointestinal colic, and if untreated may progress to bowel ischemia and perforation [1, 2]. The increase in uterine size accompanying advancing gestational age with subsequent cephalad displacement of pelvic segment of the colon has been proposed as a risk factor; most reported cases are isolated solitary occurrences, with recurrent episodes only rarely described. In this report, we present a case with recurrent sigmoid volvulus (SV) in two successive pregnancies treated with temporizing endoscopic decompression and elective postpartum sigmoid resection.

2. Case Presentation

A 25-year-old gravida 3, para 2002 at 32 0/7 weeks' gestation was referred with a 24-hour history of intermittent severe abdominal pain and obstipation. Her past medical history was significant for hypothyroidism, a microcytic anemia,

and sigmoid volvulus in her previous pregnancy two years prior requiring endoscopic reduction at 26 weeks' gestation. Physical examination revealed suprapubic and right lower quadrant tenderness, with normal bowel sounds on auscultation; peritoneal signs of rebound and/or guarding were absent. Obstetric ultrasound demonstrated a nonanomalous singleton fetus with biometry consistent with gestational age, no evidence of placental abruption, and normal cervix length. Due to gravid status, abdominal radiography was inconclusive but suggestive of colonic distention. Laboratory evaluation was remarkable for normal leukocyte count and lactate, amylase, and hepatic transaminase levels. Two tap water enemas were efficacious in prompting adequate stool output with alleviation of clinical symptoms, and she was discharged.

Subsequently, she returned at 32 4/7 weeks with similar complaints; the gastroenterology service was consulted, and magnetic resonance imaging confirmed a 90-degree twist of the colon 30 cm from the anal verge (Figure 1). Colonoscopic decompression followed by rectal tube placement for 24 hours was successful, and she was discharged home. Unfortunately, symptoms recurred at 37 0/7 weeks, and she

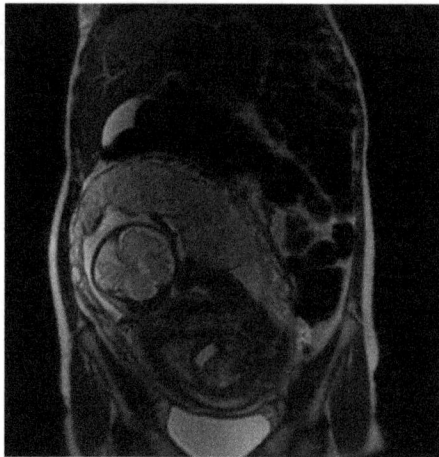

FIGURE 1: Magnetic resonance imaging without contrast performed at 32 weeks' gestation. There is marked distention of the sigmoid colon beginning at the level of the sigmoid along the left lateral aspect of the uterus where there appears to be a small, early (90 degree) twist of the sigmoid colon. The fetus may also be seen in this image.

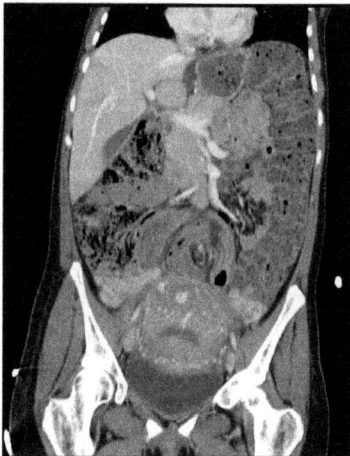

FIGURE 2: Computer tomography imaging with intravascular contrast performed on postpartum day 1. There is twisting of the mesentery and focal mesenteric edema in the mid lower abdomen. The findings are consistent with sigmoid volvulus.

underwent a second colonoscopy with decompression, with rectal tube left in place. At 38 1/7 weeks, she underwent a third colonoscopic decompression procedure, and the decision was made to proceed with delivery. Labor was induced, culminating in a spontaneous vaginal delivery of a healthy female infant. Unfortunately she again experienced worsening abdominal pain on the first day postpartum, with computer tomography imaging confirming sigmoid distention with recurrence of volvulus (Figure 2). A fourth colonoscopic decompression was performed, and she was discharged home on the second day postpartum. Symptoms again recurred on postpartum day 32 and were managed

by a fifth colonoscopic decompression followed by uncomplicated laparoscopic sigmoidectomy on postpartum day 34. Histopathologic evaluation of the excised specimen was benign.

3. Discussion and Conclusion

A literature search of the PubMed, Google Scholar, Scopus, and the Cochrane Library databases from January, 01, 1900, to January, 22, 2017, was performed using search terms "recurrent", "sigmoid volvulus", and "pregnancy" alone or in combination using the Boolean operator "AND". Only patients with recurrent sigmoid volvulus in pregnancy were considered for this review. The search initially yielded 8 articles, and after careful review by two of the authors (Jaclyn Rivington, Layan Alrahmani) only 3 met the inclusion criteria of multiple episodes of sigmoid volvulus recurring in the same pregnancy; specific characteristics are summarized in Table 1.

Intestinal obstruction in pregnancy is relatively rare, with an incidence of 1 in 1500 to 1 in 66,431 deliveries. To date, only 105 cases of volvulus have been reported during pregnancy [6], with only 3 authors describing repetitive episodes. Typical risk factors include older age, high fiber diet, constipation, and an elongated redundant sigmoid colon [7, 8]; the disproportionate incidence during pregnancy is theorized to occur due to the physical size of the enlarging gravid uterus displacing the colon out of the pelvis, perhaps explanatory of the frequency of third-trimester presentation. Furthermore, elevated gestational progesterone levels cause hypomotility of the gastrointestinal tract through smooth muscle relaxation, increasing constipation and volvulus risk [3]. Age and multigravidity do not appear to constitute significant factors [9]. Although in the nonpregnant population eventual recurrence of sigmoid volvulus is considered to be approximately 50%, it has only rarely been documented in pregnancy [10].

Management of sigmoid volvulus in pregnancy is similar to the nonpregnant state. The American Society of Colon and Rectal Surgeons suggest initial rigid or flexible endoscopy to assess for intestinal viability and to effect therapeutic detorsion and decompression (Grade 1c) [11]; this is reported to be successful in 75–95% of cases [11–13]. Definitive sigmoidectomy is considered in the acute setting if there is evidence of nonviable or perforated colon, or after the resolution of the acute phase of sigmoid volvulus to prevent recurrence (Grade 1c) [11]. A decompression tube is often placed for 1–3 days after the endoscopic procedure; however the utility of this intervention has not been established [14].

Alshawi suggests that elective sigmoidectomy be considered in the second trimester of recurrent cases of SV [4], due to the potential for continued recurrence with development of bowel necrosis later in gestation. However, due to the small cohort of patients actually reported to experience antepartum recurrence of SV, the optimal course of action is difficult to conclusively extrapolate. In our case, the patient was managed with repetitive endoscopic decompressions in the third trimester, which is considered to pose a low maternal

TABLE 1: Previously published cases of recurrent sigmoid volvulus during pregnancy.

Author (year)	Patient demographic	Initial episode (weeks gestation)	Intervention	Recurrence (weeks gestation)	Intervention	Delivery	Outcome
Bajaj et al. (2015) [3]	23 yo G3P2	5	Endoscopic decompression	36 5/7	Rigid sigmoidoscopy, only partial decompression	SVD at 36 weeks	Sigmoidectomy at 6 weeks postpartum
Alshawi (2005) [4]	22 yo G2P1	20	Sigmoidoscopic detorsion and rectal tube	28, 35	Colonoscopic detorsion and rectal tube	SVD at 38 weeks	Sigmoidectomy at 2 weeks postpartum
Bandler et al. (1964) [5]	28 yo G1P0	16	Laparotomy with derotation and pinning of sigmoid	37 1/7	Derotation during CD	CD at 37 weeks	Subtotal colectomy at 4 weeks postpartum
Our case	25 yo G3P2	32	Sigmoidoscopic detorsion and rectal tube	32 5/7, 37, 38 1/7	Endoscopic decompression and rectal tube	SVD at 38 weeks	Sigmoid colectomy at 4 weeks postpartum

CD, cesarean delivery; SVD, spontaneous vaginal delivery.

and fetal risk irrespective of gestational age [15]. The risk of elective or emergent surgical bowel resection must be weighed against the challenge of repeated endoscopic treatments; with anticipated reduction in uterine size following delivery, one could argue that the instigating factor would "resolve" postpartum, possibly eliminating the need for colon resection.

It is difficult to ascertain whether volvulus is more likely to recur in pregnancy. Since pregnancy is a predisposing factor, we can assume that since the enticing factor still exists, namely, pregnancy, the chance for recurrence is high. Time to recurrence of volvulus is variable. Prevention strategies for recurrence other than definitive surgery are unknown. Prevention of constipation with dietary modifications and stool softeners is safe but short-term efficacy is not determined.

Obstetrical management in these situations must be individualized; the authors would recommend a multi-disciplinary approach involving Obstetrics, Maternal-Fetal Medicine, Anesthesiology, Gastroenterology, and Colorectal Surgery. Vaginal delivery is not contraindicated, and cesarean delivery should be reserved for routine obstetrical indications; of note, in all reported cases of recurrent SV (including the current), vaginal delivery was accomplished. Monitoring for symptoms of intrapartum recurrence, particularly if neuraxial anesthesia is elected, is important; in the event that cesarean delivery is required, depending on preoperative preparation, concurrent elective bowel resection may be considered.

Reported prognosis of SV varies widely, with maternal mortality rates of 5–12% and fetal mortality of 20–26% [1]. Almost all maternal deaths occurred when patients presented more than 48 hours following onset of symptoms. Similarly, maternal mortality associated with viable bowel is only 5% but increases to greater than 50% once bowel perforation has occurred [6], underscoring the importance of timely diagnosis and intervention. Recurrence of SV in subsequent pregnancies and/or postpartum has not previously been described; interestingly the current case occurred at a similar gestational age in two successive pregnancies, suggesting the basic underlying anatomy with the additional uterine compression as the precipitating factor. Patients experiencing SV in pregnancy successfully treated with colonoscopic decompression should be counseled on the potential for recurrence both later in gestation and in future pregnancies.

Abbreviations

SV: Sigmoid volvulus.

Consent

The patient consented to participate in research. Consent for publication was obtained.

Authors' Contributions

Layan Alrahmani and Jaclyn Rivington reviewed the case and contributed to writing and editing the manuscript. Carl H. Rose reviewed and edited the manuscript.

References

[1] Z. Aftab, A. Toro, A. Abdelaal et al., "Endoscopic reduction of a volvulus of the sigmoid colon in pregnancy: case report and a comprehensive review of the literature," *World Journal of Emergency Surgery (WJES)*, vol. 9, p. 41, 2014.

[2] M. R. Khan and S. ur Rehman, "Sigmoid volvulus in pregnancy and puerperium: a surgical and obstetric catastrophe. Report of a case and review of the world literature," *World Journal of Emergency Surgery*, vol. 7, no. 1, article 10, 2012.

[3] M. Bajaj, C. Gillespie, and J. Dale, "Recurrent sigmoid volvulus in pregnancy," *ANZ Journal of Surgery*, 2 pages, 2015.

[4] J. S. Alshawi, "Recurrent sigmoid volvulus in pregnancy: Report of a case and review of the literature," *Diseases of the Colon & Rectum*, vol. 48, no. 9, pp. 1811–1813, 2005.

[5] M. Bandler, S. Freidman, and M. Roberts, "Recurrent volvulus of the sigmoid colon during pregnancy complicated by toxemia of pregnancy," *The American Journal of Gastroenterology*, vol. 42, pp. 447–453, 1964.

[6] A. M. Al Maksoud, A. K. Barsoum, and M. M. Moneer, "Surgery case reports signet ring cell carcinoma of the ampulla of vater?: report of a case and a review of the literature," *International Journal of Surgery Case Reports*, vol. 12, pp. 108–111, 2015.

[7] T. E. Madiba, C. Aldous, and M. R. Haffajee, "The morphology of the foetal sigmoid colon in the African population: A possible predisposition to sigmoid volvulus," *Colorectal Disease*, vol. 17, no. 12, pp. 1114–1120, 2015.

[8] S. A. Michael and S. Rabi, "Morphology of sigmoid colon in south indian population: a cadaveric study," *Journal of Clinical and Diagnostic Research*, vol. 9, no. 8, pp. AC04–AC07, 2015.

[9] W. B. Jr. Harer and W. B. Sr. Harer, "Volvulus complicating pregnancy and puerperium: report of three cases and review of literature," *Obstetrics & Gynecology*, vol. 12, no. 4, pp. 399–406, 1958.

[10] E. C. Mangiante, M. A. Croce, T. C. Fabian, O. F. Moore III, and L. G. Britt, "Sigmoid volvulus. A four-decade experience," *The American Surgeon*, vol. 55, no. 1, pp. 41–44, 1989.

[11] J. D. Vogel, D. L. Feingold, D. B. Stewart et al., "Clinical Practice Guidelines for Colon Volvulus and Acute Colonic Pseudo-Obstruction," *Diseases of the Colon and Rectum*, vol. 59, no. 7, pp. 589–600, 2016.

[12] S. S. Atamanalp, "Treatment of sigmoid volvulus: A single-center experience of 952 patients over 46.5 years," *Techniques in Coloproctology*, vol. 17, no. 5, pp. 561–569, 2013.

[13] J. R. Anderson and D. Lee, "The management of acute sigmoid volvulus," *British Journal of Surgery*, vol. 68, no. 2, pp. 1–4, 1981.

[14] M. E. Harrison, M. A. Anderson, and V. Appalaneni, "The role of endoscopy in the management of patients with known and suspected colonic obstruction and pseudo-obstruction," *Gastrointestinal Endoscopy*, vol. 71, no. 4, pp. 669–679, 2010.

[15] A. De Lima, B. Galjart, P. H. A. Wisse et al., "Does lower gastrointestinal endoscopy during pregnancy pose a risk for mother and child? - a systematic review," *BMC Gastroenterology*, vol. 15, no. 1, pp. 10–1186, 2015.

16

Expectant Management Leading to Successful Vaginal Delivery following Intrauterine Fetal Death in a Woman with an Incarcerated Uterus

Masafumi Yamamoto, Mio Takami, Ryosuke Shindo, Michi Kasai, and Shigeru Aoki

Perinatal Center for Maternity and Neonate, Yokohama City University Medical Center, Yokohama, Japan

Correspondence should be addressed to Mio Takami; takamimio@yahoo.co.jp

Academic Editor: Svein Rasmussen

Expectant management leads to successful vaginal delivery following intrauterine fetal death in a woman with an incarcerated uterus. Management of intrauterine fetal death in the second or third trimester of pregnancy in women with an incarcerated uterus is challenging. We report a case of successful vaginal delivery following intrauterine fetal death by expectant management in a woman with an incarcerated uterus. In cases of intrauterine fetal death in women with an incarcerated uterus, vaginal delivery may be possible if the incarceration is successfully reduced. If the reduction is impossible, expectant management can reduce uterine retroversion, thereby leading to spontaneous reduction of the incarcerated uterus. Thereafter, vaginal delivery may be possible.

1. Introduction

Uterine incarceration is a rare complication of pregnancy, where the enlarged retroflexed uterus becomes engaged into the small pelvis. Reported causes include pelvic adhesions resulting from a previous surgery, pelvic peritonitis, or endometriosis; uterine fibroids; and uterine malformation [1, 2]. Uterine incarceration is a rare condition, with an incidence of 1 in 3,000 to 10,000 pregnancies [3, 4].

In general, vaginal delivery is contraindicated in women with an incarcerated uterus, because this condition is associated with a high risk of intrapartum uterine rupture [5, 6]. In irreducible cases that persist close to delivery, cesarean delivery is recommended. However, in cases of intrauterine fetal death (IUFD), cesarean delivery offers no advantage; therefore, it is reasonable to attempt vaginal delivery, because cesarean delivery carries the risk of complications such as bleeding and physical and psychological burden for the pregnant woman. Thus, the management of IUFD in women with an incarcerated uterus poses a therapeutic dilemma for obstetricians.

Here, we report a case of successful vaginal delivery after IUFD by expectant management in a woman with an incarcerated uterus. We also describe a therapeutic strategy for the management of such cases.

2. Case Presentation

The patient was a 37-year-old primipara woman. She had a history of uterine fibroids and cystectomy due to rupture of ovarian endometrial cyst. Transvaginal ultrasound performed at 5 weeks of gestation revealed a 6 cm fibroid in the fundus of the uterus.

At 16 weeks and 6 days of gestation, the patient developed abdominal pain and genital bleeding and was admitted to our hospital. On speculum examination, the cervix was impossible to visualize, and slight bleeding was observed. On vaginal examination, a solid mass was palpated in the pouch of Douglas, and the external uterine orifice was displaced above the symphysis pubis. Based on these findings, uterine incarceration was suspected. To reduce the incarceration and relieve her symptoms, she was instructed to assume a knee-to-chest position after micturition. However, at 18 weeks and 4 days of gestation, the abdominal pain and genital bleeding persisted and the physical findings remained unchanged. At 18 weeks and 5 days of gestation, magnetic resonance

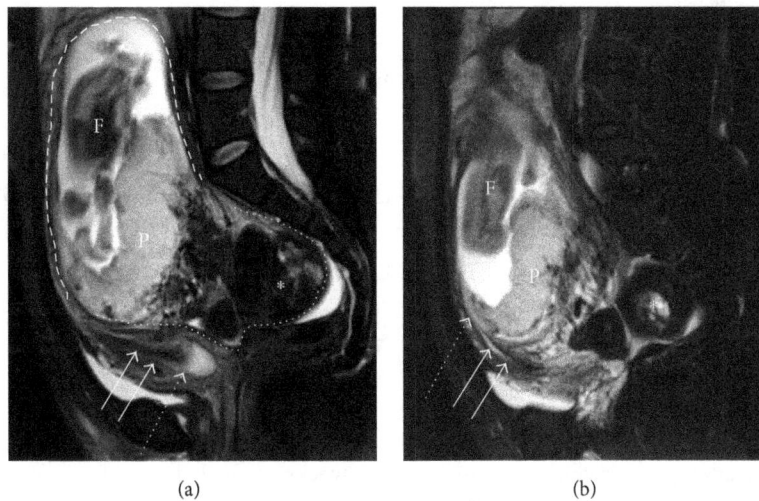

(a)   (b)

FIGURE 1: Sagittal T2-weighted magnetic resonance imaging (MRI) at 18 weeks of gestation shows a large fibroid (white asterisk) engaged in the pouch of Douglas. The cervix (white arrow) and the anterior wall of uterus (dashed line) are cranioventrally stretched. The fundus and the posterior wall of uterus (dotted line) were entrapped in the pelvis between the sacral promontory and pubic symphysis. Dashed arrows show external ostium of uterus (a) and internal one (b). F = fetus; P = placenta (a, b).

imaging (MRI) was additionally performed to obtain more detailed findings. MRI showed a large fibroid engaged in the pouch of Douglas and a cranioventrally stretched cervix. The uterus was strongly retroverted; therefore the fundus and the posterior wall of uterus were entrapped in the pelvis between the sacral promontory and pubic symphysis (Figure 1). Based on MRI findings, the patient was diagnosed with uterine incarceration and threatened abortion.

After that, she remained in the hospital and continued with the same management; however, the maneuver was unsuccessful. Therefore, manual reduction of the incarceration was planned. However, at 19 weeks and 5 days of gestation, IUFD occurred. Transvaginal and transrectal manual reduction was immediately attempted under general anesthesia to achieve vaginal delivery; however, the attempts were unsuccessful. An expectant management approach was planned, expecting a decrease in the uterine blood flow, leading to reduction in the size of the uterine cavity. We planned to follow up the patient once a week on an outpatient basis by speculum and pelvic examination for less than 4 weeks. Blood tests during the expectant management showed no signs of infection or coagulopathy. The minimum blood fibrinogen level before delivery was 335 mg/dl.

At 22 weeks and 3 days of gestation (19 days after IUFD), the cervix was visually recognized on speculum examination. On pelvic examination, the fibroid in the pouch of Douglas was still palpated, but the external uterine orifice was palpated in the normal position. At 23 weeks and 5 days of gestation (28 days after IUFD), the incarcerated uterus of the patient resolved spontaneously with reduction of the uterus; subsequently, labor was induced with gemeprost vaginal suppository after mechanical dilatation of the uterine cervix. The macerated fetus was successfully delivered. The patient had a favorable course after delivery and was discharged uneventfully. MRI performed 3 months after delivery showed a large fibroid in the fundus of the uterus (Figure 2). Uterine

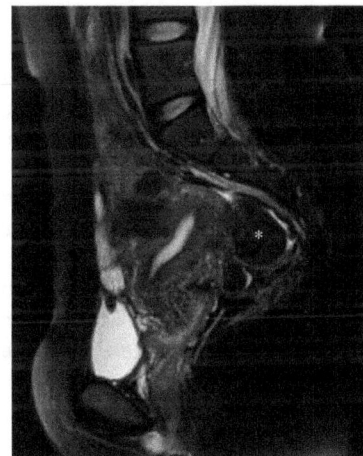

FIGURE 2: Sagittal T2-weighted MRI after delivery shows a large fibroid (white asterisk) located in fundus.

fibroid may cause recurrence of an incarcerated uterus on the next pregnancy; hence, we performed laparoscopic myomectomy and adhesiolysis of the adhesion between the uterine posterior wall and the rectum.

3. Discussion

We reported a case of successful vaginal delivery following IUFD by expectant management in a woman with an incarcerated uterus. Based on the findings of this case and those of previously reported cases, we propose a therapeutic strategy for the management of IUFD in the second or third trimester in women with an incarcerated uterus.

To the best of our knowledge, there are three case reports on IUFD in the second or third trimester in women with an incarcerated uterus. Our case is the fourth one (Table 1).

TABLE 1: Summary of cases of IUFD in the second or third trimester in women with an incarcerated uterus.

Number	Author	Year	Age (years)	Gravida/para	GA at IUFD	Result of manual reduction	Delivery method
1	Van Beekhuizen	2003	40	0/0	23	Unsuccessful	Vaginal delivery after spontaneous rupture of the membranes
2	Van Beekhuizen	2003	33	0/0	28	Unsuccessful	Cesarean delivery
3	Matsushita	2014	36	0/0	21	Successful	Vaginal delivery after successful manual reduction
4	Current case	2016	37	0/0	19	Unsuccessful	Vaginal delivery after spontaneous reduction by expectant management

GA, gestational age (weeks); IUFD, intrauterine fetal death.

In the first case, the patient was diagnosed with IUFD at 23 weeks of gestation. An attempt to reduce the uterus failed. Subsequently, vaginal delivery was induced despite the presence of her incarcerated uterus, but this attempt also failed. Finally, vaginal delivery was achieved after spontaneous rupture of the membranes [7]. In the second case, the patient was diagnosed with IUFD at 28 weeks of gestation. Several attempts of manual reduction were unsuccessful. Finally, cesarean delivery was performed [7]. In the third case, the patient was diagnosed with IUFD at 21 weeks of gestation. Vaginal delivery was induced despite the presence of her retroverted uterus but was unsuccessful. Subsequently, manual reduction of the uterus was performed, resulting in successful uterine reduction, after which induction of delivery was attempted again; this resulted in a successful vaginal delivery [8]. A case of induced abortion in the second trimester in a woman with an incarcerated uterus has also been reported. Manual reduction was attempted but was unsuccessful; finally, cesarean delivery was performed [9]. However, these reports lack information regarding gestational age at delivery or the time between the diagnosis of IUFD and delivery. These reports have not mentioned the cause of IUFD.

Complications of an incarcerated uterus include miscarriage and IUFD [3, 10, 11]. Although the cause of IUFD is unknown, decreased uterine arterial blood flow by malposition of the uterus may play a role [3, 10]. The reason for fetal demise in the present case is also unclear. However, the reduction of blood flow may be one of the factors associated with IUFD.

The findings of these cases suggest that vaginal delivery may be possible after successful reduction of the incarceration. If the reduction is impossible, expectant management can be an option to enable spontaneous reduction of the incarcerated uterus, so as to achieve vaginal delivery.

There are two advantages of expectant management. First, blood flow to the uterus decreases after IUFD, leading to softening and loosening of fetal tissues and reduction in the placenta size. The reduction in the uterine volume decreases uterine flexion, which may lead to spontaneous resolution of the incarcerated uterus. In addition, amniocentesis, which was not performed in this case, may be effective for reducing the uterine volume. Second, expectant management allows spontaneous onset of labor and subsequent vaginal delivery.

It is known that spontaneous labor usually begins within 3 weeks of fetal death in approximately 90% of the cases [12]. If patients go into spontaneous labor during expectant management, they are allowed a trial of vaginal delivery without medical intervention. However, careful monitoring is required when labor begins in women with an incarcerated uterus. If the delivery does not progress as expected, an increased risk of uterine rupture should be considered. Accordingly, cesarean delivery is necessary.

Complications of expectant management include intrauterine infection and coagulation disorder [13–15]. Pritchard reported that coagulation disorder (blood fibrinogen level < 150 mg/dl) did not occur within 5 weeks of IUFD [16]. However, he also reported that coagulation disorder (blood fibrinogen level < 100 mg/dl) was possible to occur after 6 weeks of IUFD [14]. Therefore, one may assume that expectant management for less than 4 weeks can be safely performed with a regular blood test. In the present case, the patient was followed up with blood tests once a week, and there were no signs of infection or coagulopathy during the remaining pregnancy.

No change in the retroflexion of the uterus after 4-week expectant management indicates that the risk of intrapartum uterine rupture still persists; in such cases, cesarean delivery should be considered. The possibility of spontaneous reduction of the uterus decreases as the fetus grows, probably making vaginal delivery difficult. Therefore, the effectiveness of expectant management is to be evaluated separately for cases of IUFD in women in the latter stage of the second trimester and those in the third trimester.

4. Conclusion

In summary, in cases of IUFD in women with an incarcerated uterus, vaginal delivery may be possible after successful reduction of the uterus. If the reduction is impossible, expectant management can be an option for reduction of the incarcerated uterus, in order to achieve vaginal delivery. However, careful and individualized management of IUFD is required in women with an incarcerated uterus.

References

[1] L. Lettieri, J. F. Rodis, D. A. McLean, W. A. Campbell, and A. M. Vintzileos, "Incarceration of the Gravid Uterus," *Obstetrical & Gynecological Survey*, vol. 49, no. 9, pp. 640–646, 1994.

[2] B. Jacobsson and D. Wide-Swensson, "Incarceration of the retroverted gravid uterus - A review," *Acta Obstetricia et Gynecologica Scandinavica*, vol. 78, no. 8, pp. 665–668, 1999.

[3] J. M. Gibbons and W. B. Paley, "The incarcerated gravid uterus," *Obstetrics and Gynecology*, vol. 33, no. 6, pp. 842–845, 1969.

[4] L. W. Hess, T. E. Nolan, R. W. Martin, J. N. Martin, W. L. Wiser, and J. C. Morrison, "Incarceration of the retroverted gravid uterus: Report of four patients managed with uterine reduction," *Southern Medical Journal*, vol. 82, no. 3, pp. 310–312, 1989.

[5] M. N. Singh, J. Payappagoudar, J. Lo, and S. Prashar, "Incarcerated retroverted uterus in the third trimester complicated by postpartum pulmonary embolism," *Obstetrics and Gynecology*, vol. 109, no. 2, pp. 498–501, 2007.

[6] M. C. Renaud, S. Bazin, and P. Blanchet, "Case condensations: Asymptomatic uterine incarceration at term," *Obstetrics and Gynecology*, vol. 88, no. 4, p. 721, 1996.

[7] H. J. Van Beekhuizen, H. W. Bodewes, E. M. Tepe, H. P. Oosterbaan, R. Kruitwagen, and R. Nijland, "Role of magnetic resonance imaging in the diagnosis of incarceration of the gravid uterus," *Obstetrics and Gynecology*, vol. 102, no. 5, pp. 1134–1137, 2003.

[8] H. Matsushita, K. Watanabe, and A. Wakatsuki, "Management of a second trimester miscarriage in a woman with an incarcerated retroverted uterus," *Journal of Obstetrics and Gynaecology*, vol. 34, no. 3, pp. 272-273, 2014.

[9] L. Wang, J. Wang, and L. Huang, "Incarceration of the retroverted uterus in the early second trimester performed by hysterotomy delivery," *Archives of Gynecology and Obstetrics*, vol. 286, no. 1, pp. 267–269, 2012.

[10] J. T. Van Winter, P. L. Ogburn Jr., J. A. Ney, and D. J. Hetzel, "Uterine incarceration during the third trimester: A rare complication of pregnancy," *Mayo Clinic Proceedings*, vol. 66, no. 6, pp. 608–613, 1991.

[11] I. Dierickx, L. J. Meylaerts, C. D. Van Holsbeke et al., "Incarceration of the gravid uterus: Diagnosis and preoperative evaluation by magnetic resonance imaging," *European Journal of Obstetrics Gynecology and Reproductive Biology*, vol. 179, pp. 191–197, 2014.

[12] V. Tricomi and S. G. Kohl, "Fetal death in utero," *American Journal of Obstetrics and Gynecology*, vol. 74, no. 5, pp. 1092–1097, 1957.

[13] F. G. Cunningham, *Williams' Obstetrics*, McGraw-Hill Professional, 24rd edition, 2014, p. 808–814.

[14] J. A. Pritchard, "Hematological problems associated with delivery, placental abruption, retained dead fetus and amniotic fluid embolism," *Clinical Haematology*, vol. 2, pp. 563–586, 1973.

[15] J. Trinder, P. Brocklehurst, R. Porter, M. Read, S. Vyas, and L. Smith, "Management of miscarriage: expectant, medical, or surgical? Results of randomised controlled trial (miscarriage treatment (MIST) trial)," *The British Medical Journal*, vol. 332, no. 7552, pp. 1235–1238, 2006.

[16] J. A. Pritchard, "Fetal death in utero," *Obstetrics and Gynecology*, vol. 14, pp. 573–580, 1959.

17

Long-Acting Luteinizing Hormone-Releasing Hormone Agonist for Ovarian Hyperstimulation Induced by Tamoxifen for Breast Cancer

Nobue Kojima [iD],[1] **Yui Yamasaki,**[1] **Houu Koh,**[1] **Masaru Miyashita,**[2] **and Hiroki Morita**[1]

[1]*Department of Obstetrics and Gynecology, Rokko Island Konan Hospital, Kobe, Japan*
[2]*Department of Surgery, Konan Hospital, Kobe, Japan*

Correspondence should be addressed to Nobue Kojima; nbeko10-kojima@yahoo.co.jp

Academic Editor: Kyousuke Takeuchi

Tamoxifen treatment for breast cancer may induce ovarian cysts and supraphysiological levels of serum estrogen. We report successful management with luteinizing hormone-releasing hormone (LHRH) agonist of ovarian hyperstimulation induced by tamoxifen. A 49-year-old woman was operated on for invasive ductal carcinoma of the right breast. She received breast irradiation and adjuvant tamoxifen therapy. After 2 years, she had a cystic ovarian mass, and her serum concentration of estradiol was 1280 pg/mL. She was treated with an injection of 11.25 mg leuprolide acetate, a long-acting LHRH agonist, without abandoning tamoxifen therapy. The levels of estradiol decreased to <10 pg/mL and the cystic mass disappeared 2 months later. Three-month depot treatment with LHRH agonists can be useful for patients receiving tamoxifen for breast cancer who have ovarian cysts and supraphysiological levels of estrogen.

1. Introduction

Tamoxifen is a selective estrogen receptor modulator (SERM), which is widely used as hormone therapy for estrogen-receptor-positive breast cancer. It is effective for both adjuvant therapy after surgery and treatment of metastatic cancer [1, 2].

Women treated with tamoxifen have increased risks of endometrial hyperplasia and uterine cancer [3]. Moreover, tamoxifen treatment sometimes induces ovarian hyperstimulation, which causes ovarian cysts and supraphysiological levels of serum estrogen [4, 5]. Tamoxifen-induced ovarian cysts are observed in premenopausal women or in women who have amenorrhea after chemotherapy.

Some studies have shown that cotreatment with luteinizing hormone-releasing hormone (LHRH) agonists and continuation of tamoxifen resolves ovarian hyperstimulation and that LHRH agonists are given by monthly injections for 3 or 6 months [4, 5]. Three-month depot formulation of LHRH agonists may reduce the injection times if it is effective.

This report presents a rare case of a perimenopausal woman diagnosed with tamoxifen-induced ovarian hyperstimulation who had amenorrhea for 8 months, without chemotherapy for breast cancer. To the best of our knowledge, this is the first report to treat ovarian hyperstimulation with 3-month depot LHRH agonists. In addition, there are few reports about tamoxifen-induced ovarian hyperstimulation in Japanese women, and this is the first report to treat ovarian hyperstimulation without abandoning tamoxifen in Japanese women with breast cancer.

2. Case Presentation

A 49-year-old Japanese woman, gravid 3 para 3, was referred to our hospital with a diagnosis of right ovarian cyst. She had amenorrhea for 5 months. Transvaginal ultrasonography demonstrated two cystic lesions in the right ovary (ovarian size was 49 × 33 mm). Color Doppler ultrasonography did not show neovascularity in the right ovary (Figure 1).

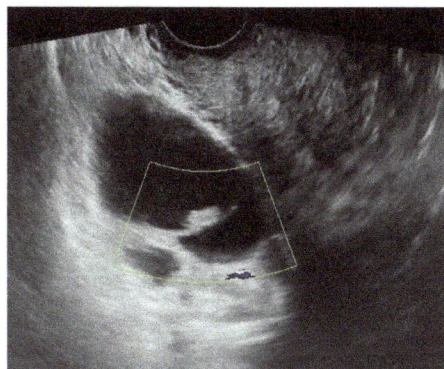

FIGURE 1: Ultrasonography demonstrated two cystic lesions in the right ovary. Color Doppler ultrasonography did not show neovascularity in the right ovary.

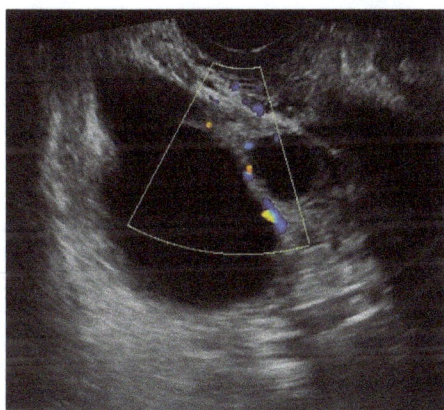

FIGURE 2: The cystic tumor of the right ovary had neovascularity demonstrated by color Doppler ultrasonography.

Three months later, there were four cystic lesions, whereas the ovarian size had not increased. At that time, color Doppler ultrasonography demonstrated neovascularity in the tumor (Figure 2). No evidence of ascites was observed. Tumor markers, cancer antigen- (CA-) 125, CA19-9, and carcinoembryonic antigen (CEA) were within the normal range. Pelvic enhanced magnetic resonance imaging (MRI) showed no evidence of malignancy.

Her medical history revealed that she was operated on for invasive ductal carcinoma of the right breast 2 years and 6 months before her first visit. Immunohistochemical test revealed that her breast cancer was estrogen receptor- (ER-) positive, progesterone receptor- (PgR-) positive, and human epidermal growth receptor 2- (HER2-) negative. After surgery, she received breast irradiation and adjuvant tamoxifen therapy (20 mg/day) without LHRH agonists. The duration of tamoxifen treatment was 2 years and 4 months. She had received gynecological check-up, and her uterus and both ovaries were normal 9 months before her first visit in the other clinic.

As the patient had received tamoxifen therapy, ovarian hyperstimulation was suspected to be the reason for ovarian enlargement. The serum concentration of estradiol and follicle-stimulating hormone (FSH) were 1280 pg/mL and 7.93 mIU/mL, respectively.

The patient had amenorrhea for 8 months, and the thickness of the endometrium was 3 mm. The right ovary (51 × 40 mm) had four follicles (the largest was 44 × 29 mm), and the left ovary (24 × 11 mm) had two follicles (both <10 mm diameter).

Informed consent for continuation of tamoxifen therapy and additional LHRH agonist therapy was received. She was treated with an injection of 11.25 mg leuprolide acetate, a long-acting LHRH agonist, without abandoning tamoxifen therapy. The levels of estradiol decreased to 51 pg/mL 4 weeks later and then to <10 pg/mL 2 months later. The ultrasonography revealed that the right ovary decreased in size, containing one follicle (27 × 20 mm) 4 weeks later, and it became normal 2 months later. These findings continued for 6 months at least.

Written informed consent was obtained from the patient for publication of this case.

3. Discussion

Ovarian hyperstimulation, ovarian cysts, and supraphysiological levels of serum estrogen have been reported as adverse effects of tamoxifen in 11–17% women treated with tamoxifen for breast cancer [6–8]. Tamoxifen may increase the levels of estrogen by interfering with the normal negative pituitary feedback mechanism [9] and by its direct effect with ovarian granulosa cells [10].

Tamoxifen-induced ovarian cysts are observed more frequently in premenopausal women than postmenopausal women [7]. Supraphysiological estrogen concentration is observed only in premenopausal women whose menstrual cycles in the last 3 months were regular or irregular or in women who have chemotherapy-induced menopause [8, 11]. In the present case, the patient was treated with tamoxifen without chemotherapy, and she had amenorrhea for 8 months. She seemed to be in transition to menopause; however, ovarian cysts and supraphysiological estrogen concentration were observed. It is reported that, in patients receiving tamoxifen, women with oligomenorrhea sometimes have high levels of estradiol [11] and that no relation between estradiol levels and endometrial thickness was found [12], and amenorrhea is an insufficient parameter to define menopausal status, similar to our findings.

Tamoxifen-induced ovarian hyperstimulation may cause ovarian cysts and supraphysiological levels of serum estrogen. Ovarian cysts may result from functional cysts, primary ovarian tumor including ovarian cancer, or metastasis of breast cancer. It is reported that some patients with tamoxifen-induced cysts need surgical intervention because of vascular torsion [13], cystic necrosis without vascular torsion [14], or ovarian hyperstimulation syndrome [15], or to rule out the possibility of malignant tumor. Elevated levels of serum estrogen may cause thrombotic events, endometrial hyperplasia, and uterine cancer [16]. Although the effect of supraphysiological levels of estrogen on breast cancer is unknown, increased estrogen may cause poor prognosis in women with estrogen-receptor-positive breast cancer.

When ovarian hyperstimulation is observed, the following management options can be selected: observation, surgical intervention, cessation of tamoxifen treatment, or LHRH agonist without abandoning tamoxifen treatment.

In women with breast cancer treated with tamoxifen but with no treatment for ovarian cysts, 32% of ovarian cysts increased in size and 68% decreased or completely disappeared [6]. Metastatic breast cancer and ovarian endometrioid adenocarcinoma are also reported in patients treated with tamoxifen for breast cancer [17]. If the ovarian tumor is malignant, it may progress during observation.

Surgical intervention may be needed to rule out the malignancy of ovarian tumors. Some report showed that there were malignant ovarian tumors in patients treated with tamoxifen for breast cancer [17]. On the other hand, another report showed that tamoxifen might reduce the risk of ovarian cancer in patients with breast cancer [18]. As oophorectomy reduces estrogen levels completely, it may cause long-term side-effects, including cardiovascular disease. In the present case, the possibility of ovarian cancer was considered and the results of pelvic enhanced MRI and serum tumor markers revealed that the ovarian cysts were unlikely to be malignant. In addition, after beginning the treatment of LHRH agonist, we observed ovarian cysts every 4 weeks until the cysts completely disappeared.

About 72% of tamoxifen-associated ovarian cysts disappear after cessation of tamoxifen treatment [7]. However, cessation of tamoxifen treatment might lead to poor prognosis in women with breast cancer. Ovarian cyst torsion after cessation of tamoxifen has also been reported [13].

Ovarian suppression such as LHRH agonist therapy seems to be one of the best ways to resolve ovarian hyperstimulation promptly. Three or six monthly injections of LHRH agonists can cause regression of the cysts and enable continuation of tamoxifen treatment [5]. It was reported that, within 3 weeks of the first LHRH agonist injection, serum estradiol levels fell to menopausal levels, and ovarian cysts completely disappeared within 2 months [4]. Following discontinuation of LHRH agonist cotreatment, serum estradiol levels remained at physiological levels and the ovaries remained their normal size in 64% of patients [4].

The 3-month depot formulation of 11.25 mg leuprorelin acetate produced similar pharmacodynamic effects of hormonal suppression to those achieved with monthly injections of 3.75 mg leuprorelin acetate [19]. Three-month depot leuprorelin with oral tamoxifen can suppress serum estradiol to the menopausal level within 4 weeks after injection in premenopausal women [20]. In the present case, after treatment with 3-month depot LHRH agonist, ovarian cysts and increased estrogen levels disappeared within 2 months. As LHRH agonist was needed only once, the patient could avoid receiving extra surgery.

In conclusion, ovarian cysts in women treated with tamoxifen for breast cancer may result from ovarian hyperstimulation even if she is in transition to menopause. And 3-month depot treatment with LHRH agonists can be useful in patients with ovarian cysts and supraphysiological levels of estrogen resulting from tamoxifen treatment.

References

[1] Early Breast Cancer Trialists' Collaborative Group (EBCTCG), "Relevance of breast cancer hormone receptors and other factors to the efficacy of adjuvant tamoxifen: patient-level meta-analysis of randomised trials," *The Lancet*, vol. 378, no. 9793, pp. 771–784, 2011.

[2] M. Crump, C. A. Sawka, G. DeBoer et al., "An individual patient-based meta-analysis of tamoxifen versus ovarian ablation as first line endocrine therapy for premenopausal women with metastatic breast cancer," *Breast Cancer Research and Treatment*, vol. 44, no. 3, pp. 201–210, 1997.

[3] W. E. Hoogendoorn, H. Hollema, H. H. Van Boven et al., "Prognosis of uterine corpus cancer after tamoxifen treatment for breast cancer," *Breast Cancer Research and Treatment*, vol. 112, no. 1, pp. 99–108, 2008.

[4] I. Cohen, R. Tepper, A. Figer, D. Flex, J. Shapira, and Y. Beyth, "Successful co-treatment with LHRH-agonist for ovarian over-stimulation and cystic formation in premenopausal tamoxifen exposure," *Breast Cancer Research and Treatment*, vol. 55, no. 2, pp. 119–125, 1999.

[5] A. Shushan, T. Peretz, and S. Mor-Yosef, "Therapeutic approach to ovarian cysts in tamoxifen-treated women with breast cancer," *International Journal of Gynecology and Obstetrics*, vol. 52, no. 3, pp. 249–253, 1996.

[6] M. J. E. Mourits, E. G. E. De Vries, P. H. B. Willemse et al., "Ovarian cysts in women receiving tamoxifen for breast cancer," *British Journal of Cancer*, vol. 79, no. 11-12, pp. 1761–1764, 1999.

[7] A. Shushan, T. Peretz, B. Uziely, A. Lewin, and S. Mor-Yosef, "Ovarian cysts in premenopausal and postmenopausal tamoxifen-treated women with breast cancer," *American Journal of Obstetrics & Gynecology*, vol. 174, no. 1, pp. 141–144, 1996.

[8] R. Yamazaki, M. Inokuchi, S. Ishikawa et al., "Tamoxifen-induced ovarian hyperstimulation during premenopausal hormonal therapy for breast cancer in Japanese women," *SpringerPlus*, vol. 4, no. 1, article no. 425, pp. 1–5, 2015.

[9] P. M. Ravdin, N. Fritz, and D. C. Tormey, "Endocrine status of premenopausal node-positive breast cancer patients following adjuvant chemotherapy and long-term tamoxifen," *Cancer Research*, vol. 48, no. 4, pp. 1026–1029, 1988.

[10] M. Knecht, C.-H. Tsai-Morris, and K. J. Catt, "Estrogen dependence of luteinizing hormone receptor expression in cultured rat granulosa cells. inhibition of granulosa cell development by the antiestrogens tamoxifen and keoxifene," *Endocrinology*, vol. 116, no. 5, pp. 1771–1777, 1985.

[11] M. Berliere, F. P. Duhoux, F. Dalenc et al., "Tamoxifen and Ovarian Function," *PLoS ONE*, vol. 8, no. 6, Article ID e66616, 2013.

[12] C. Buijs, P. H. B. Willemse, E. G. E. De Vries et al., "Effect of tamoxifen on the endometrium and the menstrual cycle of premenopausal breast cancer patients," *International Journal of Gynecological Cancer*, vol. 19, no. 4, pp. 667–681, 2009.

[13] A. Taran, H. Eggemann, S.-D. Costa, B. Smith, and J. Bischoff, "Ovarian cyst torsion and extreme ovarian stimulation in a premenopausal patient treated with tamoxifen for ductal carcinoma in situ of the breast," *American Journal of Obstetrics & Gynecology*, vol. 195, no. 4, pp. e5–e6, 2006.

[14] C. J. Jolles, D. Smotkin, K. L. Ford, and K. P. Jones, "Cystic ovarian necrosis complicating tamoxifen therapy for breast cancer in a premenopausal woman. A case report," *Obstetrics, Gynaecology and Reproductive Medicine*, vol. 35, no. 3, pp. 299-300, 1990.

[15] A. Baigent and H. Lashen, "Ovarian hyperstimulation syndrome in a patient treated with tamoxifen for breast cancer," *Fertility and Sterility*, vol. 95, no. 7, pp. 2429–e7, 2011.

[16] C. Madeddu, G. Gramignano, P. Kotsonis, F. Paribello, and A. Macciò, "Ovarian hyperstimulation in premenopausal women during adjuvant tamoxifen treatment for endocrine-dependent breast cancer: A report of two cases," *Oncology Letters*, vol. 8, no. 3, pp. 1279–1282, 2014.

[17] I. Cohen, Y. Beyth, R. Tepper, and et al, "Ovarian tumors in postmenopausal breast cancer patients treated with tamoxifen," *International Journal of Gynecology & Obstetrics*, vol. 54, no. 2, pp. 208-209, 1996.

[18] K. F. McGonigle, S. A. Vasilev, T. Odom-Maryon, and J. F. Simpson, "Ovarian histopathology in breast cancer patients receiving tamoxifen," *Gynecologic Oncology*, vol. 73, no. 3, pp. 402–406, 1999.

[19] U.S. Food and Drug Administration, "LUPRON DEPOT®-3 Month 11.25 mg (leuprolide acetate for depot suspension) 3-month formulation," 2012, https://www.accessdata.fda.gov/drugsatfda_docs/label/2012/020708s033lbl.pdf.

[20] J. Kurebayashi, T. Toyama, S. Sumino, E. Miyajima, and T. Fujimoto, "Efficacy and safety of leuprorelin acetate 6-month depot, TAP-144-SR (6M), in combination with tamoxifen in postoperative, premenopausal patients with hormone receptor-positive breast cancer: a phase III, randomized, open-label, parallel-group comparative study," *Breast Cancer*, vol. 24, no. 1, pp. 161–170, 2017.

18

Unsuspected Diagnosis of Uterine Leiomyosarcoma after Laparoscopic Myomectomy in an Isolated Bag

Süleyman Salman, Fatma Ketenci Gencer, Bülent Babaoğlu, Melih Bestel, Serkan Kumbasar ⓘD, Guray Tuna, Esra Güzel, Durkadın Elif Yıldız, Tuba Kotancı, Ali Selçuk Yeniocak, and Özlem Sögüt

Gaziosmanpaşa Taksim Eğitim ve Araştırma Hastahanesi, Kadın Hastalıkları ve Doğum Bölümü, İstanbul, Turkey

Correspondence should be addressed to Serkan Kumbasar; doktor1977@hotmail.com

Academic Editor: Yoshio Yoshida

Minimally invasive techniques are generally applied for patients suspected of having benign fibroids if medical treatment is insufficient. On the other hand, sometimes some occult carcinomas of uterus like leiomyosarcomas may be reported for the patients' applied morcellation. This condition is rare but outcomes are clinically significant. Fragmentation of occult sarcoma in the abdominal cavity without isolation bag results in widespread and poor survival. In this article, we report a case of 37-year-old woman suffering from pain due to unexpected leiomyosarcoma. Laparoscopic myomectomy was performed with power morcellation in an isolated bag. Although isolation bag is generally reported to be preventive, recurrence of sarcoma was seen at 5th month of follow-up. Even though morcellation within a bag seems to block wide spreading, dispersion of tumor cannot be stopped and more investigations have to be done.

1. Introduction

Uterine sarcomas comprise 3% of uterine malignancies and leiomyosarcoma (LMS) accounts one-third of all uterine sarcomas [1]. LMS is a significant reason for uterine cancer deaths and its five-year overall survival rates range from 30% to 42% [1, 2]. The patient age is the major risk factor and patients older than 55 are at increased risk [1]. On the other hand LMS cannot be diagnosed accurately by ultrasound, computed tomography (CT), and magnetic resonance imaging (MRI) without diffuse weighted imaging [3]. Patients may undergo surgical procedure due to supposed benign fibroids which are in fact malignant. Minimally invasive techniques such as laparoscopic myomectomy or hysterectomy with morcellation for supposed benign leiomyosarcomas are nowadays controversial according to US Food and Drug Administration Safety communication initially issued in April 2014 and updated in November 2014[4].

We report a case of 37-year-old young women with presumed benign leiomyoma treated with laparoscopic myomectomy with morcellation within an isolated morcellation bag reported as leiomyosarcoma at paraffin section (Figure 1).

2. Case Report

37-year-old woman presented to the emergency room with headache. Bilateral pelvic sensitivity and a mass painful to touch in a plastic texture that filled the Douglas' pouch were detected during the examination; the mass was evaluated in favor of leiomyoma. ß-hcg was negative, wbc was 9800/mm^3, hgb was 12 g/dl, htc was 35%, plt was 282000/mm^3, and no unusual characteristics was found in complete urinalysis. Ultrasonography revealed a mass consistent with a degenerated myoma measuring 77x82mm, of which subserous component was greater in the posterior wall and endometrial thickness was 7-8 mm, which was concordant with the cycle. The left ovary of the patient was normal, but since the right ovary could not be fully evaluated, computerized tomography (CT) was requested for possible adnexal pathologies. CT

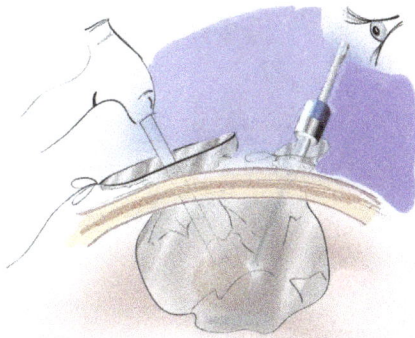

FIGURE 1: Isolated bag.

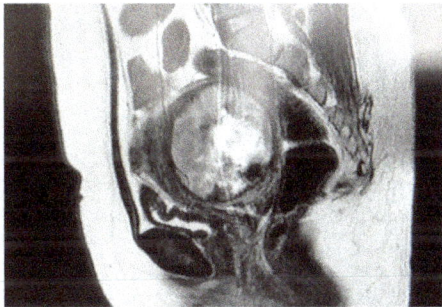

FIGURE 2: MRI image of myoma before surgery.

demonstrated a hypodense nodular lesion with a diameter of 75 mm that extended to the right adnexal region and MRI with contrast was performed on the patient. MRI revealed a mass with a hypovascular appearance following a heterogeneous and hypointense IV contrast material with a diameter of 8 mm, which appeared to displace the posterior cervix.

It is seen that myoma included by central necrosis depleted by cervix in the posterior part of the uterus. Also the development of necrosis was seen and myomatosis was evaluated in favor of degeneration (Figure 2).

In addition, since the patient's pain regressed spontaneously during the follow-up, surgical operation was postponed to perform in elective conditions. After making necessary preparations for the operation, laparoscopic myomectomy was performed. Myoma was not considered suspicious apart from being degenerated. It was removed by morcellating in an isolated bag (Figures 3(a), 3(b), 3(c), and 3(d)).

No complication or hemorrhage occurred during surgery. As there was not any problem observed during the post-op follow-up, the patient was discharged from the hospital on condition that the pathology report was brought on the second day of post-op. The subsequent report revealed marked cellularity and pleomorphism, extensive necrosis, mitosis >5/10BBA, KI67 proliferation index > %50, weak positivity for p53, and LMS with no detectable lymphovascular invasion.

The patient was informed about the pathology report and interned again to perform transabdominal hysterectomy and bilateral salphingoopherectomy. The pathology report revealed "atypical pleomorphic fusiform cell proliferation area" measuring 3x2 mm in a focal area within the cavity consistent with residual LMS when evaluated together with laparoscopic myomectomy material.

To follow-up the patient was referred to radiotherapy and medical oncologists. After 3 months from her 1st surgery, positron emission tomographic scan (PET-CT) was performed and fluoro-2-deoxyglucose (FDG) uptake is noted in the area above rectosigmoid mesentery towards the left abdominal wall in pelvic floor (Figure 4).

She was referred to gynecologic oncologist and 3rd operation was performed. A mass about 4-5 cm of size in defined localization was excised; there were not any other mass and lymphadenopathy detected during the surgery. The pathology result was high grade malign mesenchymal tumor with high cellularity, extensive necrosis, mitosis 40/10 BBA, and moderate atypia. There was no tumor in surgical margin. She is now being followed up by the gynecologic oncologist with appropriate medical treatment.

3. Discussion

Myomectomy is a surgical approach for uterine fibroids for young patients unresponsive to medical treatment [4]. Uterine fibroids, in other words leiomyomas, affect not only women's health but also quality of life and fertility [5]. Minimally invasive procedures with morcellation which means fragmentation into small pieces make taking out large leiomyomas or uterine specimens easier [6]. LMS is reported after surgery for supposed benign leiomyoma in 1 case per 1960-8300 fibroid surgeries [7]. Risk of occult malignancy is 20 times higher between 50 and 59 aged women when compared to those younger than 40 [8]. In our case the patient is 37 years old that is in low risk category. If the tumor is larger than 7 cm, the risk of malignancy is about 40%, while for those smaller than 7 cm the risk is about 16% [7]. According to this, our case of 77x82 mm size is borderline.

This soft tissue sarcoma is rare but aggressive and highly resistant malignancy with poor survival. This can be potentiated by power morcellation due to dispersion of tumor [9]. As proven in MITO retrospective group study, power morcellation is the only independent factor associated with survey and increases 3 times the risk of death [10]. To prevent this, morcellation within a bag is much more important as applied in our patient despite her young age. On the other hand, power morcellation decreases survey without illness but the overall survey is not significantly different [10]. In our case the bag was not perforated during the surgery and there was no leakage of sarcoma material into the abdominal cavity. Even morcellation within a bag could not block the dispersion as FDG uptake detected in PET-CT after her second operation. We assumed that one of the main factors associated with dispersion is the myomectomy procedure. Myomectomy may be questioned as a treatment modality because it can be the reason for direct inoculation.

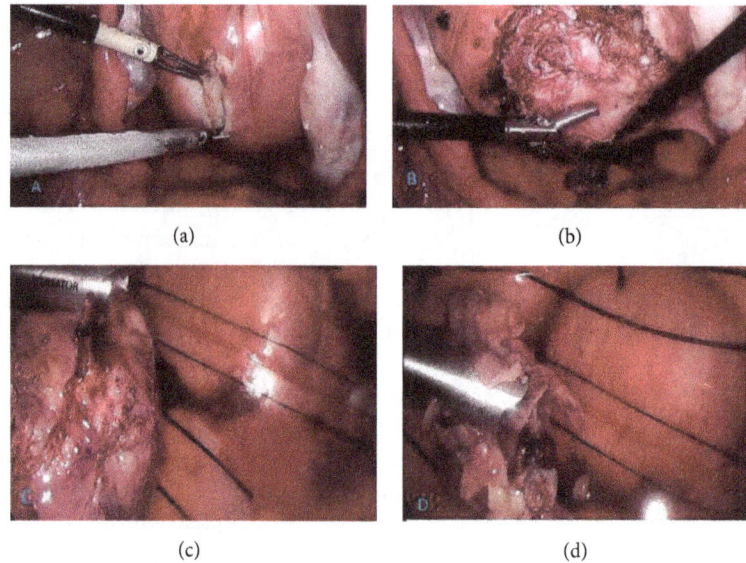

(a)

(b)

(c)

(d)

FIGURE 3: (a, b, c, d) Laparoscopic morcellation of fibroid in isolated bag.

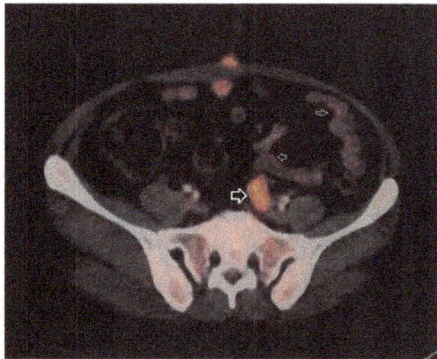

FIGURE 4: Abdominal positron emission tomographic (PET-CT) scan. Axial view shows variable-sized heterogeneous contrast-enhancing above rectosigmoid mesentery towards the left abdominal wall in pelvic floor (arrowheads). Arrow shows the lateral port site deposit.

Degenerated leiomyomas may be more carefully evaluated and also morcellation may be avoided for especially young patients as in our case.

Although this type of cancer is rarely seen, morcellating it within an isolated bag is important to prevent the worsening of its already adverse consequences. There was no known risk factor involved in this case; however, it is worth noting that any leiomyoma could have a potential risk for cancer. The patient must be informed in detail about this cancer risk even all the risk factors are excluded.

Morcellation within a bag seems to prevent dispersion but even in a benign suggestive case, like ours, dispersion could not be prevented and that again reminds us about myomectomy procedure's role contributing to dispersion before putting the tumor into bag. We assume that only wide dispersion may be prevented with morcellation within a bag as in our case. Using bag may not be preventive due

to inoculation during myomectomy via bleeding or seeding with local transmission by touching malign mass.

References

[1] S. Kaya, H. B. Bacanakgil, Z. Soyman, İ. Öz, S. Battal Havare, and B. Kaya, "Myxoid leiomyosarcoma of the cervix: A case report," *Journal of Obstetrics & Gynaecology*, vol. 36, no. 8, pp. 989–991, 2016.

[2] C. Garcia, J. S. Kubat, R. S. Fulton et al., "Clinical outcomes and prognostic markers in uterine leiomyosarcoma: a population-based cohort," *International Journal of Gynecological Cancer*, vol. 25, no. 4, pp. 622–628, 2015.

[3] K. Gaetke-Udager, K. McLean, A. P. Sciallis et al., "Diagnostic accuracy of ultrasound, contrast-enhanced CT, and conventional mri for differentiating leiomyoma from leiomyosarcoma," *Academic Radiology*, vol. 23, no. 10, pp. 1290–1297, 2016.

[4] B. Carranza-Mamane, J. Havelock, R. Hemmings et al., "The management of uterine fibroids in women with otherwise unexplained infertility," *Journal of Obstetrics and Gynaecology Canada*, vol. 37, no. 3, pp. 277–285, 2015.

[5] M. A. Lumsden and E. M. Wallace, "Clinical presentation of uterine fibroids," *Baillière's Clinical Obstetrics and Gynaecology*, vol. 12, no. 2, pp. 177–195, 1998.

[6] V. Leren, A. Langebrekke, and E. Qvigstad, "Parasitic leiomyomas after laparoscopic surgery with morcellation," *Acta Obstetricia et Gynecologica Scandinavica*, vol. 91, no. 10, pp. 1233–1236, 2012.

[7] S. L. Cohen, E. Hariton, Y. Afshar, and M. T. Siedhoff, "Updates in uterine fibroid tissue extraction," *Current Opinion in Obstetrics and Gynecology*, vol. 28, no. 4, pp. 277–282, 2016.

[8] J. D. Wright, A. I. Tergas, W. M. Burke et al., "Uterine pathology in women undergoing minimally invasive hysterectomy using

morcellation," *Journal of the American Medical Association*, vol. 312, no. 12, pp. 1253–1255, 2014.

[9] US Food and Drug Administration, "Updated laparoscopic uterine power morcellation in hysterectomy and myomectomy: FDA safety communication," 2014, http://www.fda.gov/MedicalDevices/Safety/AlertsandNotices/ucm424443.htm.

[10] F. Raspagliesi, G. Maltese, G. Bogani et al., "Morcellation worsens survival outcomes in patients with undiagnosed uterine leiomyosarcomas: A retrospective MITO group study," *Gynecologic Oncology*, vol. 144, no. 1, pp. 90–95, 2017.

19

A Postmenopausal Woman with Giant Ovarian Serous Cyst Adenoma: A Case Report with Brief Literature Review

Nishat Fatema ⓘ and Muna Mubarak Al Badi

Department of Gynaecology & Obstetric, Ibri Regional Hospital, Ministry of Health, Ibri, Oman

Correspondence should be addressed to Nishat Fatema; nishat.doc.om@gmail.com

Academic Editor: Seung-Yup Ku

Giant (>10 cm) ovarian cyst is a rare finding. In the literature, a few cases of giant ovarian cysts have been mentioned sporadically, especially in elderly patients. We report a 57-year-old postmenopausal woman with a giant left ovarian cyst measuring $43 \times 15 \times 9$ cm. She was referred to us from the local health center in view of palpable pelvic mass for six-month period. Considering the age and menopausal state, we performed a total abdominal hysterectomy and bilateral salpingo-oophorectomy with excision of the giant left ovarian cyst intact and successfully without any significant complication. On histopathological examination, the cyst was confirmed as benign serous cystadenoma of the ovary. During the management of these high-risk cases of multidisciplinary approach, intraoperative and postoperative strict vigilance is necessary to avoid unwanted complications.

1. Background

Giant ovarian tumor has become rare, because of the early detection of adnexal pathology with the advent of routine imaging modalities in the recent era of medical practice [1, 2].

In previous studies, the definition of large or giant ovarian cysts was described as cysts measuring more than 10 cm in diameter in the radiological scan or those cysts reaching above the umbilicus [1].

Cystadenoma, adenofibroma, and surface papillomas are the benign serous tumors. These tumors occur in about 25% of all benign ovarian neoplasms and 58% of all ovarian serous tumors [2].

Serous tumors are commonly seen during the reproductive period and 50% of them occur before the age of 40 years. Most of these cysts are benign in nature with the chance of malignancy being only 7%–13% in premenopausal and 8%–45% in postmenopausal women [3, 4].

Huge size ovarian serous cystadenoma is rare. In the literature, a few cases of giant ovarian cysts have been mentioned sporadically, primarily in elderly patients [2, 3].

We report a 57-year-old postmenopausal woman with a giant left ovarian cyst ($43 \times 15 \times 9$ cm). Considering the age and menopausal state, we performed the total abdominal hysterectomy (TAH) and bilateral salpingo-oophorectomy (BSO) with cystectomy for the patient. On histopathological examination, the cyst was confirmed as benign serous cyst adenoma of the ovary.

2. Case

A 57-year-old, para 04 postmenopausal woman was referred to our hospital from the local health center with a palpable pelvic mass for the last six months. She had been menopausal for the 7 years with the last childbirth occurring 17 years ago. She is a known case of hypothyroidism and on Tab. Thyroxin 50 microgram once daily. No significant surgical history was obtained.

On presentation, she was asymptomatic and had no complaints of anorexia, nausea vomiting, weight loss, or any postmenopausal bleeding. Her bowel and bladder habit was normal.

On general examination, she was found to be average built and weighing 62 kg. Abdominal examination revealed a pelvic mass extending beyond the umbilicus, corresponding to 26-week gravid uterus. The mass was mobile, firm, and

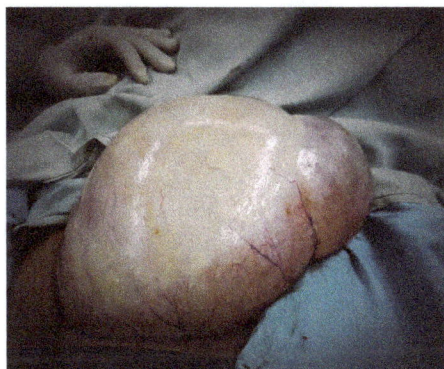

FIGURE 1: Left ovarian cyst (40 × 15 cm).

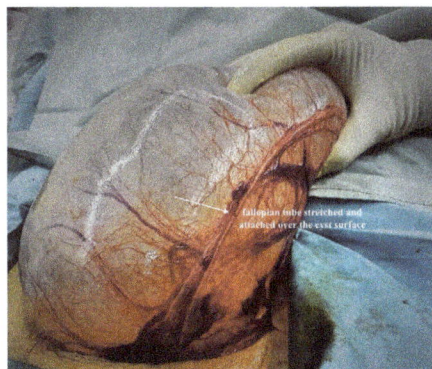

FIGURE 2: The left fallopian tube: adherent and stretched over the cyst.

nontender on palpation. On vaginal examination, cervix was found normal and fornixes were obliterated due to presence of the mass.

Laboratory tests were unremarkable except that the TFT value-TSH was 35.5 mIU/Li and free T4 was 6.9 pico mol/Li. Tumor markers were within normal limit, and CA 125 revealed 12 U/ml. Cervical PAP smear showed no evidence of dyskaryotic or malignant cells.

Radiological ultrasound revealed normal sized and shaped uterus with endometrial thickness 7 mm. A large left adnexal cyst was seen which was bilocular, thin smooth walled with clear anechoic contents measuring around 17.5 × 17.3 × 9.5 cm.

We did not conduct computerized tomography (CT) scans or magnetic resonance imaging (MRI) as the ultrasound scan findings were highly suggestive of a benign cyst, that is, a unilateral cyst with no solid areas or irregular surface and no ascites.

The calculated RMI (risk of malignancy index) was $1 \times 3 \times 12 = 36$. Total score was USG score × menopausal score × Ca_{125} (U/Ml). USG score was as follows: 0, no risk factor; 1, one risk factor; 3, 2–5 risk factors. High-risk factors in USG were multilocular cysts, solid areas, bilateral lesions, ascites, and evidence of metastasis. Menopausal status was as follows: 1, premenopausal; 3, postmenopausal. Score < 200 indicates low risk (risk of ovarian malignancy is 0.15 times). Score > 200 indicates high risk (risk of ovarian malignancy is 42 times) [3].

We planned for TAH with BSO considering her age and menopausal status. After normalization of thyroid hormones value, we performed TAH with BSO.

The abdomen was opened by a low transverse incision. Intraoperative around 40 × 15 cm sized left ovarian cyst (Figure 1) was seen; no healthy ovarian tissue was seen separately. The left tube was adherent and stretched over the cyst (Figure 2). Right tube, ovary, and the uterus were found healthy (Figure 3). There were no intraoperative complications and delay in total operative procedure. The blood loss was minimal.

On histopathology examination, the cyst was bilocular with smooth thin walled measuring 43 × 15 × 9 cm and lined by a single layer of bland flattened epithelial cells with occasional cuboidal epithelial cells. The cyst was filled with

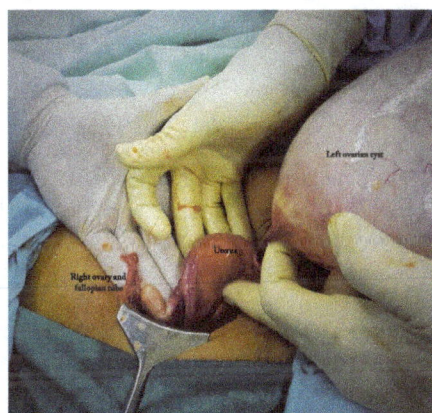

FIGURE 3: Healthy uterus, right fallopian tube, and ovary.

clear serous fluid. No malignant cells or nuclear atypia were observed. The histopathology was suggestive of benign serous cystadenoma of the ovary.

Her postoperative period was unremarkable. Oral feeding and ambulation were started 12 hours after the surgery. She was discharged on the fourth postoperative day in good condition.

3. Discussion

Large/giant ovarian cysts are benign in most of the cases and histopathologically these cysts are either serous or mucinous [4].

Serous tumors secrete serous fluids and are originated by invagination of the surface epithelium of ovary. Serous tumors are commonly benign (70%); 5–10% have borderline malignant potential, and 20–25% are malignant. Only 10% cases of all serous tumors are bilateral [3].

Serous cystadenomas are multilocular. In some instances, they include papillary projections. Giant ovarian serous cyst adenoma is a rare finding. In the literature, a few cases of giant ovarian cysts have been mentioned sporadically and especially in elderly postmenopausal women [2, 3].

Our presented case was a 57-year-old postmenopausal para 4 woman who experienced a palpable pelvic mass for

TABLE 1: Giant ovarian cysts in postmenopausal women: literature review.

Study (year)	Age	Symptom	Site	Size of the cyst	Tumor marker CA 125 (U/ml)	Type of the cyst	Surgery
Sujatha and Babu (2009) [2]	66	Vague abdominal pain, anorexia	Unilateral	60 × 47 × 30 cm	46.61	Serous cyst adenoma	TAH + BSO
Alobaid et al. (2013) [4]	69	Abdominal distention and discomfort	Unilateral	Max diameter 20 cm	Normal	Serous cyst adenoma	LAVH + BSO
Madhu et al. (2013) [5]	55	Mechanical discomfort due to distended abdomen	Unilateral	50 × 39 × 47 cm	---	Mucinous cyst adenoma	TAH + BSO
Bhasin et al. (2017) [6]	85	Diffuse abdominal pain	Unilateral	58 × 46 cm	---	Mucinous cyst adenoma	Total excision of the cyst
Agrawal et al. 2015 [1]	65	Dull aching pain in the lower back, shortness of breath	Unilateral	25 × 28 × 15 cm	31.31	Serous cyst adenoma	TAH + BSO
Kim et al. 2016 [7]	52	Abdominal distention	Unilateral	36 × 21 × 30 cm	109.5I	Benign cystic lesion with hemorrhage	Total excision of the cyst

six-month period without any other associated symptoms. We performed the total abdominal hysterectomy and bilateral salpingo-oophorectomy with the removal of an intact giant left ovarian serous cyst adenoma measuring 43 × 15 × 9 cm successfully.

Previous studies mentioned that the patients with huge adnexal mass are commonly presented with diffuse abdominal pain and distension, sometimes associated with anorexia and mechanical discomfort (Table 1). In this context, our patient had no significant symptoms except palpable pelvic mass for six-month period. In a reported case of mucinous cystadenoma, Madhu et al. mentioned that a patient was presented to them with the history of abdominal distention for the past 13 years and she sought medical management when her daily activity became restricted due to overdistension of abdomen [5]. Some other reported cases in previous studies were presented within a short period of time ranging from six months to two years, similar to our case (Table 1). In recent studies, the size of giant serous cyst adenoma of ovary was found in postmenopausal women measuring maximum 60 × 47 × 30 cm [2]. In most of the studies, tumor marker CA 125 was within normal range or mildly increased (Table 1). In this context, our patient's CA 125 level was also observed within the normal limit, 12 U/ml.

For the diagnosis of ovarian tumors, various imaging techniques are used. Pelvic ultrasonography, computed tomography, and magnetic resonance are the choice of imaging modalities that are used for the diagnosis of larger adnexal masses and metastatic involvement. Besides these, the serial measurements of the tumor marker CA-125 can be helpful [1].

We diagnosed the cyst by ultrasonography and the preoperative estimation of RMI (risk of malignancy index) to exclude malignancy. We did not conduct computerized tomography (CT) scans or magnetic resonance imaging (MRI), as the ultrasound scan findings were highly suggestive of a benign cyst, that is, a unilateral cyst with no solid areas or irregular surface and no ascites.

Large benign ovarian cysts are usually of two varieties— serous or mucinous—and because of their enlarged size and associated symptoms, they almost always require surgical intervention [4].

Extremely large ovarian cysts are traditionally managed by laparotomy. But the recent advances in endoscopic surgery have offered alternative choice by laparoscopic treatment of such extremely large ovarian cysts [8].

However, laparotomy and total excision of cysts are the choice of treatment in case of large ovarian cyst cases, until or unless prior to laparoscopic surgery ultrasound guided decompression or aspiration of the cyst is done [6].

As a first-line treatment modality for giant adnexal cysts, laparoscopy is still limited [9]. Due to technical difficulties, like restricted space, only a few surgeons practice laparoscopic management of extremely large ovarian cysts. In addition, there is a risk of cyst rupture and intra-abdominal spillage and trocar site implantation of malignant cells [4, 8].

In a review, Bellati and colleagues mentioned laparoscopically guided minilaparotomy (LGML) in case of benign large adnexal masses, with no other risk factor for malignancy, other than size. They concluded that in terms of safety and feasibility LGML is a better option in comparison to laparoscopy [10].

Excision of large ovarian cyst in women at reproductive age may damage ovarian reserve. In a literature review, the authors mentioned that bilateral cystectomies compared to unilateral cystectomy cause more damage to the ovarian reserve, but they observed recovery of ovarian reserve in both groups. Another study comparing unilateral cystectomy/ovariectomy with other abdominal and pelvic surgical interventions did not find any statistical difference in terms of long-term postoperative fertility [11, 12].

Regarding skin incision during excision of the large cysts, Madhu et al. noted that a low transverse incision associated with low risk of ventral hernia formation allows restoration of normal rectus abdominis muscle function.

In contrast, vertical elliptical incision does not allow for adequate resection of the skin in the vertical plane [5, 13]. For our case, we opened the abdominal skin with a low transverse incision and successfully excised the cyst in intact condition without any complication.

Surgery is essential for large ovarian tumors even if benign [1]. Until now, there has been no randomized controlled trial for the laparoscopic management of ovarian cysts >20 cm, so laparotomy remained the ideal method for the excision of the giant ovarian cysts [4].

During surgical removal of large ovarian tumors, various intraoperative complications are reported in previous studies like splanchnic dilatation and venous pooling after the sudden removal of large intra-abdominal masses, and hypotension can occur due to decreased venous return resulting from obstructed inferior vena cava and pulmonary edema due to sudden reexpansion of a chronically collapsed lung, which occurred due to compression by the enlarged abdomen [1].

Hence, during the management of these high-risk cases of multidisciplinary approach, intraoperative and postoperative strict vigilance is necessary to avoid unwanted complications.

References

[1] S. P. Agrawal, S. K. Rath, G. S. Aher, and U. G. Gavali, "Large ovarian tumor: A case report," *International Journal of Scientific Study*, 2015, http://www.ijss-sn.com/uploads/2/0/1/5/20153321/ijss_jun_cr08.pdf.

[2] V. V. Sujatha and S. C. Babu, "Giant ovarian serous cystadenoma in a postmenopausal woman: A case report," *Cases Journal*, vol. 2, no. 7, 2009.

[3] M. Dey and N. Pathak, "Giant serous papillary cystadenoma," *Medical Journal Armed Forces India*, vol. 67, no. 3, pp. 272-273, 2011.

[4] A. Alobaid, A. Memon, S. Alobaid, and L. Aldakhil, "Laparoscopic Management of Huge Ovarian Cysts," *Obstetrics and Gynecology International*, vol. 2013, pp. 1-4, 2013.

[5] Y. Madhu, K. Harish, and P. Gotam, "Complete resection of a giant ovarian tumour," *Gynecologic Oncology Reports*, vol. 6, pp. 4-6, 2013.

[6] S. K. Bhasin, V. Kumar, and R. Kumar, "Giant Ovarian Cyst," *Case Report*, vol. 16, no. 3, 2017.

[7] H. Y. Kim, M. K. Cho, E. H. Bae, S. W. Kim, and S. K. Ma, "Hydronephrosis caused by a giant ovarian cyst," *International Brazilian Journal of Urology*, vol. 42, no. 4, pp. 848-849, 2016.

[8] R. Sagiv, A. Golan, and M. Glezerman, "Laparoscopic management of extremely large ovarian cysts," *Obstetrics & Gynecology*, vol. 105, no. 6, pp. 1319-1322, 2005.

[9] G. H. Eltabbakh, A. M. Charboneau, and N. G. Eltabbakh, "Laparoscopic surgery for large benign ovarian cysts," *Gynecologic Oncology*, vol. 108, no. 1, pp. 72-76, 2008.

[10] F. Bellati, M. L. Gasparri, I. Ruscito, J. Caccetta, and P. Benedetti Panici, "Minimal invasive approaches for large ovarian cysts: A careful choice," *Archives of Gynecology and Obstetrics*, vol. 287, no. 3, pp. 615-616, 2013.

[11] R. Alammari, M. Lightfoot, and H. Hur, "Impact of cystectomy on ovarian reserve: Review of the literature," *Journal of Minimally Invasive Gynecology*, vol. 24, no. 2, pp. 247-257, 2017.

[12] F. Bellati, I. Ruscito, M. L. Gasparri et al., "Effects of unilateral ovariectomy on female fertility outcome," *Archives of Gynecology and Obstetrics*, vol. 290, no. 2, pp. 349-353, 2014.

[13] W. E. Matory, R. G. Pretorius, R. E. Hunter, and F. Gonzalez, "A new approach to massive abdominal tumors using immediate abdominal wall reconstruction," *Plastic and Reconstructive Surgery*, vol. 84, no. 3, pp. 442-448, 1989.

20

Sequence and Timing of Intracranial Changes in Cytomegalovirus in Pregnancy: A Case Report and Literature Review

Cynthia O'Sullivan,[1] Shankari Arulkumaran,[2] Lorin Lakasing,[2] Eric Jauniaux,[3] and Karl Murphy[2]

[1]*Department of Urology, Wellington Hospital, Wellington, New Zealand*
[2]*Department of Obstetrics and Gynaecology, St. Mary's Hospital, Imperial College London NHS Trust, Praed Street, London W2 1NY, UK*
[3]*Academic Department of Obstetrics and Gynaecology, Institute for Women's Health, University College London, 86-96 Chenies Mews, London WC1E 6HX, UK*

Correspondence should be addressed to Shankari Arulkumaran; shankari.arulkumaran@imperial.nhs.uk

Academic Editor: Giampiero Capobianco

Cytomegalovirus (CMV) is the most common cause of intrauterine infection, occurring in up to 2% of all live births. Most women are asymptomatic or experience nonspecific symptoms, which can lead to long-term sequelae in newborns including neurological impairment, hearing loss, and mental retardation. A 41-year-old woman (G6 P2), with a medical history of epilepsy, presented for her routine anomaly scan at 20 + 4/40. A single finding of echogenic bowel was noted on ultrasound which prompted a full investigation. A repeat ultrasound only five days later demonstrated progressive changes, which included bilateral ventriculomegaly with oedema of the posterior ventricular wall, periventricular hyperechogenicity, and enlargement of the cisterna magna. CMV DNA was detected at amniocentesis. Ultrasound findings are not diagnostic for CMV with only 11–15% of at-risk fetuses being identified. Unfortunately, these findings may be the only indication of an abnormality. There is a well-documented lack of awareness surrounding CMV and screening is not routinely offered. Given the risk to the pregnancy of CMV and to subsequent pregnancies, simple education at the start of a pregnancy could significantly reduce the incidence of maternal CMV.

1. Introduction

CMV is the most common cause of intrauterine infection [1–3] with an incidence of 0.3–2% in all live born infants [1, 2, 4–6]. Infected women often present with nonspecific signs and symptoms, but the majority are asymptomatic [6]. Approximately 10% of newborns show symptoms at birth [1, 3–5] but this increases to 20–30% if their mothers were infected in the first trimester [7]. There is a 30% mortality in the affected infants and 90% will have long-term neurological impairment [4, 5]. Of the asymptomatic neonates, 10% will develop permanent sequelae, including hearing loss and mental retardation [1, 3–5].

CMV infection can be a result of a primary infection, a reinfection with a new strain, or a reactivation of the residing virus [1, 5, 7]. The rate of primary infection from mother to child is approximately 40% (range 24–75%), as opposed to 1–2.2% in the case of reinfection (secondary) with a new strain [6]. The impact of primary infection on the fetus however is more significant [1, 3, 4]. The latency between primary and secondary infection and the detection of these differences on ultrasound are still under debate [1]. It appears that the fetal infection is more common when maternal infection occurs later in pregnancy, but the severity of the infection is higher before 18 weeks of gestation [5]. Transmission of the virus to the fetus can, however, occur weeks after maternal primary or secondary infection [7].

The ultrasound findings in CMV are not diagnostic as many features are shared with other conditions [1]. In addition, some studies have demonstrated that these findings

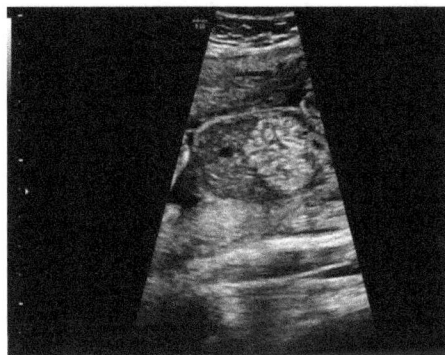

FIGURE 1: Echogenic bowel.

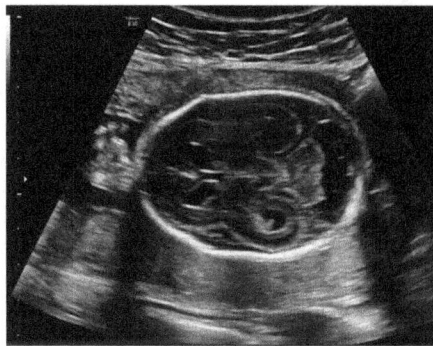

FIGURE 2: Bilateral ventriculomegaly with oedema of the posterior ventricular wall and periventricular hyperechogenicity.

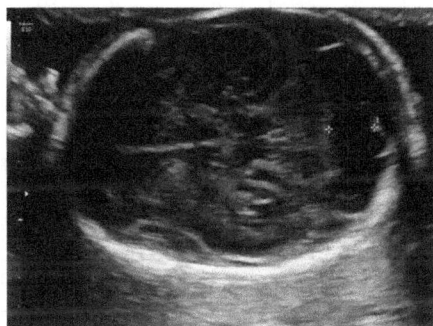

FIGURE 3: Enlargement of the cisterna magna.

are only present in up to one-third of the cases [1]. Lazzarotto et al. [6], in fact, only found that ultrasound detected not more than 5% of the infected fetuses. Furthermore, new ultrasound features to help in the diagnosis of intrauterine CMV have not been identified yet [1]. As most countries do not offer universal CMV screening in pregnancy, ultrasound monitoring is important as it is currently the only way of monitoring and assessing the prognosis of a fetus infected by CMV [2–4, 6]. Around 50% of the infected fetuses after a primary infection will be affected and present with both extracerebral and cerebral features on ultrasound and up to one-third demonstrate cerebral features only [1].

Anti-CMV IgG avidity is currently the most reliable test to identify primary infection in a pregnant woman [6]. Low avidity indicates an acute or primary infection as opposed to high avidity which indicates no current or recent infection [6]. Anti-CMV IgG avidity performed before the 16–18th week of pregnancy will identify all women at risk to have an infected fetus with a reported 100% sensitivity. After 20 weeks of gestation, the sensitivity is drastically reduced [6]. Amniocentesis is recommended between 21 and 22 weeks of gestation; CMV is a slow replication virus and will take up to 6–9 weeks before it is excreted in the fetal urine, in amounts large enough to be detected in the amniotic fluid [1, 6]. Conducting an invasive procedure too early could in fact result in a false negative result [1]

Ultrasound is therefore a useful adjunct in predicting the likelihood of postnatal disease. It can also be used as a prognostic parameter as the positive predictive value of ultrasound increases 2-fold when results from invasive testing indicate fetal infection [1, 4]. We present an unusual case where ultrasound was essential to guide the diagnosis of congenital CMV.

2. Case Study

A 41-year-old Gravida 6, Para 2, presented in her first trimester with an unremarkable blood serology and a low combined screening risk for trisomy. Her obstetric history included 3 first-trimester miscarriages and a caesarean section and vacuum delivery, both at term. She was on medication for epilepsy but otherwise fit and well. Echogenic bowel was detected at her routine anomaly scan at 20 weeks

and 4 days. She was referred to the Fetal Medicine Unit, where a repeat ultrasound, performed the following day, confirmed the findings of an isolated echogenic bowel with no other obvious structural anomalies (Figure 1). She was offered screening for a number of conditions known to be associated with echogenic bowel, including fetal aneuploidy, cytomegalovirus, toxoplasmosis, parvovirus, and cystic fibrosis. The couple declined an amniocentesis at this point.

The blood tests revealed that the couple were both carriers for the cystic fibrosis gene. In addition, the CMV IgG was positive, whilst the IgM was negative. This was checked retrospectively against her stored booking bloods, which revealed a positive IgG and IgM. The IgG antibody avidity was investigated and found to be low. Following these results, the couple proceeded with an amniocentesis at 22 weeks of gestation. The scan at this gestation still only revealed isolated echogenic bowel. The karyotype was normal but CMV DNA was detected in the amniotic fluid.

However, only 5 days later, a further scan revealed new findings which included bilateral ventriculomegaly with oedema of the posterior ventricular wall, periventricular hyperechogenicity (Figure 2), and enlargement of the cisterna magna (Figure 3). The progressive changes on ultrasound indicated a poor prognosis for the fetus, and the couple terminated the pregnancy at 24 weeks of gestation. They declined a postmortem, but histopathology of the placenta demonstrated extensive lymphocyte infiltration with occasional CMV inclusions suggestive of chronic villitis due to the virus.

3. Discussion

3.1. Effect of Gestational Age. Information regarding the effect of gestational age on the outcome of the congenital infection is important as it is helpful in determining strategies for prevention, diagnosis, and treatment of infection in pregnancy [7]. As in our case, echogenic bowel and ventriculomegaly are the most common findings, but, despite this, they may only be identified in 11.8–15% of fetuses at risk [7]. Borderline ventriculomegaly is most common, but severe cases have been reported [4]. Lissencephaly is often described from 24 weeks of gestation and mega cisterna magna from 26 weeks of gestation [2, 4]. Other common features include periventricular hyperechogenicity, also identified in this case [2, 4]. Intraventricular synechia are seen in 50% of the cases, as well as intercranial calcifications in the periventricular area, brain parenchyma, cerebellum, and the corpus callosum [7]. Most report punctiform calcifications in the cerebellum, but linear calcifications have also been described [4]. In the transverse cerebellar plane, vermian defects can be identified [4]. Another classic feature of CMV in pregnancy is thalamic hyperechogenicity secondary to vasculitis, which is commonly referred to as the "candlestick sign" [2, 4]. Picone et al. [3] describe an occipital horn cyst, which has not been demonstrated in any other infective process, and they speculate that this may be unique to CMV infection in utero.

3.2. Pathogenesis. Understanding the development of the brain in utero is crucial to correlating findings seen on ultrasound scan with the exact time that maternal infection has occurred. The CMV virus, which is a double-stranded DNA virus, has a predisposition for the neuroblasts of the germinal matrix. This forms in the seventh week of gestation [8–10]. Infection before the eighth week of gestation leads to lissencephaly, when CMV interferes with neuronal migration [4], whereas infection between 18 and 24 weeks of gestation results in focal dysplastic cortices [2]. The cerebellum ends its formation by 18 weeks of gestation, and, therefore, the presence of cerebellar anomalies is suggestive of maternal infection prior to this [2]. Periventricular cysts and germinal matrix necrosis are seen in the second trimester, whereas fetuses with normal gyral patterns and periventricular echogenicities are probably injured in the third trimester [2]. Neuronal growth is complete by 26 weeks of gestation, so infections later in pregnancy have a little effect [10]. Similar to our case, Malinger et al. [2] described one case of rapid changes occurring within a week, from solely intraventricular adhesions to periventricular irregular patterns in the germinal matrix adjacent to the occipital horns.

Subependymal cystic lesions or calcifications, which develop during the second trimester, are thought to be the result of the necrotizing inflammatory effect of CMV on the subependymal germinal matrix of the lateral ventricles [2, 8]. Furthermore, it is thought that the scattered cerebral calcifications seen in the basal ganglia and thalami may correlate to the severity of the disease [8]. The encephaloclastic effect of the virus disturbs the cell proliferation in the developing brain, causing brain atrophy, and dilated ventricles may be seen as a result. Ventriculomegaly may also be a result of vasculitis or inflammatory exudates obstructing the flow of cerebrospinal fluid [8, 9].

3.3. Prognosis. It appears that children with congenital CMV infection were more likely to have serious sequelae if their mothers were infected earlier in the pregnancy. 23% of the infants were symptomatic when CMV infection occurred in the first trimester, compared to 11.4% in mothers infected after the first trimester [7]. There was also a trend towards greater abnormal neurological ultrasound findings being identified in those mothers infected in the first trimester. 26% of the cases of CMV diagnosed in pregnancy showed abnormal findings if the mothers were infected before 20 weeks of gestation, as opposed to 6.2% after 20 weeks of gestation [11]. Romanelli et al. [5] did not find any correlation between ultrasound findings and fetal infection, and Guerra et al. [1] stated that only fetuses with a severe disease will demonstrate obvious ultrasound abnormalities. The authors, however, do agree with Malinger et al. [2] that any combination of features on ultrasound do indicate a poorer prognosis. Unfortunately, because of the pathophysiology of CMV, several weeks can elapse before ultrasound features become obvious, and sometimes this may be the case until the third trimester [1]. It is therefore recognised that fetal cerebral features on ultrasound may not appear until significantly after maternal infection has occurred [4].

The findings on fetal MRI are fairly well correlated with ultrasound features [5], but the MRI is considered better in detecting abnormal gyration [1]. It may be useful if ultrasound imaging is inconclusive or difficult secondary to an unfavourable fetal lie or maternal habitus [12]. When there are no cerebral findings, MRI is not indicated [3], and, in our case, the findings were so severe, and MRI would not have changed management.

3.4. Subsequent Pregnancies. When counseling the parents following a primary CMV infection, it is important to provide information regarding the risks of CMV in subsequent pregnancies; the transmission rate can vary from 0.2% to 7% [13–15]. Of those infected, up to 8% of the infants may have neurological sequelae [15]. Reinfection with a different strain of CMV can occur in up to 62% of the seropositive mothers [16]. This is complicated by the fact that infected infants born to mothers with recurrent CMV infection are rarely symptomatic at birth making it more difficult to diagnose clinically [14, 15]. Transmission of CMV often occurs through saliva and the urine of infected children; therefore, although the risk cannot be eliminated, education on hygiene and behavioural measures should be provided to all women regardless of the serological status [6].

3.5. Prevention and Treatment. It is important to prevent CMV to reduce the burden of morbidity associated with congenital infection [12]. However, neither the Royal College of Obstetricians and Gynaecologists nor the National Collaborating Centre for Women's and Children's Health recommends routine CMV screening of all pregnant women. At present, treatment has been focused on reducing the adverse outcomes in the infected children after birth [12].

Studies using Ganciclovir following birth to prevent late-onset hearing loss have been controversial, as there have been high losses to follow-up and serious side effects, including haematological toxicity, have been demonstrated [12]. Oral Valaciclovir has been used to try and treat symptomatic CMV in utero, but no significant benefits with treatment have been demonstrated [12]. Similarly, research has been carried out into the antenatal administration of hyperimmune globulin therapy to try and reduce either the rate of transmission or the severity of the disease in an infected fetus [5]. This preparation uses pooled human plasma from screened donors to provide a therapeutic alternative for congenital CMV to termination of pregnancy or conservative management, whilst avoiding the potential fetal toxicity of antivirals such as Ganciclovir [12]. However, its efficacy has not been proven in any randomised controlled trials, and there have not been any long-term follow-up studies to look at adverse sequelae to the neonates in mothers who have been treated with the immunoglobulin [1, 12].

3.6. Awareness Campaigns. There is a well-documented lack of awareness surrounding CMV; Cannon et al. [17] found that only 7% of men and 13% of women had heard of CMV infection and mean to prevent the spread of the disease [18, 19]. Due to the asymptomatic nature of CMV infection and lack of public awareness, the mechanisms of prevention are currently centred around education and hygiene. Studies have shown that simple education at the start of a pregnancy could significantly reduce the incidence of maternal CMV [18, 20, 21]. CMV Action [22] is one of the nonprofit organisations based in the United Kingdom to raise the public's awareness of congenital CMV and publicise any new CMV research findings through their website and social media. They offer support to families that may have been affected by the condition and are working with medical professionals with an interest in the field.

Disclosure

This study was carried out at St. Mary's Hospital, Imperial College London NHS Trust, Praed Street, London W2 1NY, United Kingdom.

References

[1] B. Guerra, G. Simonazzi, C. Puccetti et al., "Ultrasound prediction of symptomatic congenital cytomegalovirus infection," *American Journal of Obstetrics and Gynecology*, vol. 198, no. 4, pp. 380.e1–380.e7, 2008.

[2] G. Malinger, D. Lev, N. Zahalka et al., "Fetal cytomegalovirus infection of the brain: the spectrum of sonographic findings," *American Journal of Neuroradiology*, vol. 24, no. 1, pp. 28–32, 2003.

[3] O. Picone, N. Teissier, A. G. Cordier et al., "Detailed in utero ultrasound description of 30 cases of congenital cytomegalovirus infection," *Prenatal Diagnosis*, vol. 34, no. 6, pp. 518–524, 2014.

[4] Y. Dogan, A. Yuksel, I. H. Kalelioglu, R. Has, B. Tatli, and A. Yildirim, "Intracranial ultrasound abnormalities and fetal cytomegalovirus infection: report of 8 cases and review of the literature," *Fetal Diagnosis and Therapy*, vol. 30, no. 2, pp. 141–149, 2011.

[5] R. M. Romanelli, J. F. Magny, and F. Jacquemard, "Prognostic markers of symptomatic congenital cytomegalovirus infection," *Brazilian Journal of Infectious Diseases*, vol. 12, no. 1, pp. 38–43, 2008.

[6] T. Lazzarotto, B. Guerra, M. Lanari, L. Gabrielli, and M. P. Landini, "New advances in the diagnosis of congenital cytomegalovirus infection," *Journal of Clinical Virology*, vol. 41, no. 3, pp. 192–197, 2008.

[7] R. F. Pass, K. B. Fowler, S. B. Boppana, W. J. Britt, and S. Stagno, "Congenital cytomegalovirus infection following first trimester maternal infection: symptoms at birth and outcome," *Journal of Clinical Virology*, vol. 35, no. 2, pp. 216–220, 2006.

[8] A. Kapilivsky, W. B. Garfinkle, H. K. Rosenberg et al., "US case of the day. Congenital cytomegalovirus (CMV) brain infection," *Radiographics*, vol. 15, no. 1, pp. 238–242, 1995.

[9] W. Butt, R. J. Mackay, L. C. De Crespigny, L. J. Murton, and R. N. Roy, "Intracranial lesions of congenital cytomegalovirus infection detected by ultrasound scanning," *Pediatrics*, vol. 73, no. 5, pp. 611–614, 1984.

[10] A. J. Barkovich and C. E. Lindan, "Congenital cytomegalovirus infection of the brain: imaging analysis and embryologic considerations," *American Journal of Neuroradiology*, vol. 15, no. 4, pp. 703–715, 1994.

[11] C. Liesnard, C. Donner, F. Brancart, F. Gosselin, M.-L. Delforge, and F. Rodesch, "Prenatal diagnosis of congenital cytomegalovirus infection: prospective study of 237 pregnancies at risk," *Obstetrics and Gynecology*, vol. 95, no. 6, part 1, pp. 881–888, 2000.

[12] F. P. McCarthy, C. Jones, S. Rowlands, and M. Giles, "Primary and secondary cytomegalovirus in pregnancy," *The Obstetrician & Gynaecologist*, vol. 11, no. 2, pp. 96–100, 2009.

[13] G. Nigro, M. Mazzocco, M. M. Anceschi, R. La Torre, G. Antonelli, and E. V. Cosmi, "Prenatal diagnosis of fetal cytomegalovirus infection after primary or recurrent maternal infection," *Obstetrics and Gynecology*, vol. 94, no. 6, pp. 909–914, 1999.

[14] G. J. Demmler, "Congenital cytomegalovirus infection and disease," *Advances in Pediatric Infectious Diseases*, vol. 11, pp. 135–162, 1996.

[15] K. B. Fowler, S. Stagno, R. F. Pass, W. J. Britt, T. J. Boll, and C. A. Alford, "The outcome of congenital cytomegalovirus infection in relation to maternal antibody status," *The New England Journal of Medicine*, vol. 326, no. 10, pp. 663–667, 1992.

[16] S. B. Boppana, L. B. Rivera, K. B. Fowler, M. Mach, and W. J. Britt, "Intrauterine transmission of cytomegalovirus to infants of women with preconceptional immunity," *New England Journal of Medicine*, vol. 344, no. 18, pp. 1366–1371, 2001.

[17] M. J. Cannon, K. Westbrook, D. Levis, M. R. Schleiss, R. Thackeray, and R. F. Pass, "Awareness of and behaviors related to child-to-mother transmission of cytomegalovirus," *Preventive Medicine*, vol. 54, no. 5, pp. 351–357, 2012.

[18] C. Vauloup-Fellous, O. Picone, A.-G. Cordier et al., "Does hygiene counseling have an impact on the rate of CMV primary

infection during pregnancy? Results of a 3-year prospective study in a French hospital," *Journal of Clinical Virology*, vol. 46, supplement 4, pp. S49–S53, 2009.

[19] J. Johnson, B. Anderson, and R. F. Pass, "Prevention of maternal and congenital cytomegalovirus infection," *Clinical Obstetrics and Gynecology*, vol. 55, no. 2, pp. 521–530, 2012.

[20] S. P. Adler, J. W. Finney, A. M. Manganello, and A. M. Best, "Prevention of child-to-mother transmission of cytomegalovirus among pregnant women," *Journal of Pediatrics*, vol. 145, no. 4, pp. 485–491, 2004.

[21] M. G. Revello, C. Tibaldi, G. Masuelli et al., "Prevention of primary cytomegalovirus infection in pregnancy," *EBioMedicine*, vol. 2, no. 9, pp. 1205–1210, 2015.

[22] http://cmvaction.org.uk.

21

Intramural Hematoma of the Esophagus Complicating Severe Preeclampsia

Simone Garzon,[1] **Giovanni Zanconato,**[1] **Nicoletta Zatti,**[1]
Giuseppe Chiarioni,[2] **and Massimo Franchi**[1]

[1]Department of Surgical, Odontostomatological and Maternal and Child Sciences, University of Verona, Piazzale L.A. Scuro 10, 37134 Verona, Italy
[2]Department of Medicine and Gastroenterology, University of Verona, Piazzale L.A. Scuro 10, 37134 Verona, Italy

Correspondence should be addressed to Giovanni Zanconato; giovanni.zanconato@univr.it

Academic Editor: Akihide Ohkuchi

Intramural hematoma of the esophagus is a rare injury causing esophageal mucosal dissection. Forceful vomiting and coagulopathy are common underlying causes in the elderly population taking antiplatelets or anticoagulation agents. Acute retrosternal pain followed by hematemesis and dysphagia differentiates the hematoma from other cardiac or thoracic emergencies, including acute myocardial infarction or aortic dissection. Direct inspection by endoscopy is useful, but chest computed tomography best assesses the degree of obliteration of the lumen and excludes other differential diagnoses. Intramural hematoma of the esophagus is generally benign and most patients recover fully with conservative treatment. Bleeding can be managed medically unless in hemodynamically unstable patients, for whom surgical or angiographic treatment may be attempted; only rarely esophageal obstruction requires endoscopic decompression. We report an unusual case of esophageal hematoma, presenting in a young preeclamptic woman after surgical delivery of a preterm twin pregnancy, with a favorable outcome following medical management.

1. Introduction

Intramural hematoma of the esophagus (IHE) is a rare condition in which bleeding starts within the submucosal layer causing the hematoma formation and the dissection of the esophageal wall [1, 2].

IHE is considered part of a spectrum of esophageal injuries that include local mucosal tears (Mallory-Weiss syndrome), full-thickness rupture (Boerhaave's syndrome), and dissecting intramural hematoma [3]. Although these syndromes are usually associated with severe vomiting, dissecting IHE is not always associated with an increase in intraesophageal pressure. Other underlying causes of submucosal bleeding can be any one of the following: coagulopathy and abnormal hemostasis, trauma, and portal hypertension. IHE has severe implications but an excellent prognosis when managed conservatively [4, 5].

We report the case of a dissecting intramural hematoma of the esophagus acutely complicating a preeclamptic woman shortly after Cesarean section.

2. Case Presentation

A 37-year-old G2P1 woman of Indian origin was admitted in the Obstetrical Department of the University Hospital of Verona with a 32-week dichorionic twin gestation. She complained of moderate dyspnea (SpO2 98%) and sudden ankle swelling; her blood pressure was high and had significant proteinuria (>30 mg/mmol on spot protein-creatinine). Obstetric history included a term vaginal delivery and a laparoscopic salpingectomy for ectopic pregnancy. She had conceived the index pregnancy after an in vitro fertilization and embryo transfer (IVF-ET) in India. In her country of origin, she had gone through regular antenatal visits, receiving vaginal progesterone, anticoagulant therapy with LMWH for multiple venous thromboembolism risk factors, and levothyroxine due to a pregestational autoimmune hypothyroidism. Prophylactic cerclage had also been placed in India at 14 weeks where she was started on a daily low-dose aspirin regimen.

At admission, treatment was started with oral labetalol 100 mg every 8 hours and a 2-day betamethasone course

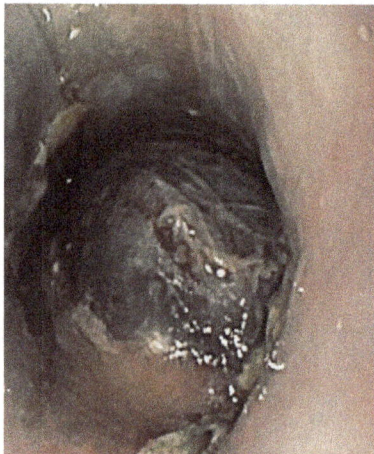

FIGURE 1: Endoscopic view of a bluish mass obliterating the lumen of the proximal esophagus.

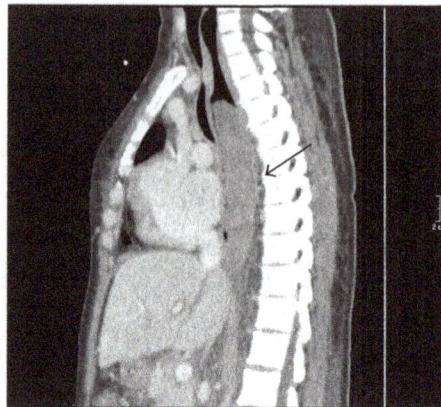

FIGURE 2: Second post-C-section day chest CT sagittal view of the esophageal hematoma (black arrow) infiltrating the posterior wall.

for fetal lung maturation. Aspirin was discontinued, while LMWH was kept, due to multiple risk factors: age (37 years), twin pregnancy, IVF/ART, and preeclampsia. Twenty-four-hour proteinuria was 2,1 g/d and preeclampsia was confirmed. Platelet count showed a reduction from 125×10^9/L at admission to 98×10^9/L. Ultrasound evaluation showed a normal growth, normal amniotic fluid, and Doppler indices of uterine blood flow for both fetuses.

At 33 weeks of gestation, the patient was delivered with a C-section under general anesthesia due to an uncontrolled rise of the blood pressure failing to respond to treatment (160/100 mmHg) and a further platelet count reduction (91,000/dL). Bleeding amounted to 600 mL. After C-section, no evidence of coagulopathy was observed with stable platelet count. Hemoglobin levels (11.5 g/dL) as well as other coagulation indexes remained in the normal range. The newborns weighted 2090 g and 1830 g and were transferred to the Neonatology Intensive Care unit to be treated for prematurity.

After Cesarean, a sudden increase of blood pressure (175/110 mmHg) was observed and intravenous labetalol was started along with magnesium sulphate for eclampsia prevention. LMWH was continued to prevent postpartum and postoperative DVT. Treatment effectively lowered the blood pressure and obtained a stable condition, with the patient only complaining of moderate heartburn and occasional vomiting. Accordingly, H2 receptor antagonists therapy was started. On the first postoperative day, the patient suddenly complained of a right side retrosternal pain extending to the shoulder blade, nausea, vomiting, and dysphagia. Occurrence of HELLP syndrome was ruled out since platelet count and liver enzymes were normal and no signs of hemolysis were recorded. ECG and chest X-ray were both negative. The following day hematemesis was observed which warranted the indication of a gastroscopy. In the initial phase of the endoscopic evaluation, an eccentric mass was seen, completely obliterating the lumen of the esophagus, which prompted the end of the procedure (Figure 1).

A chest CT scan showed bilateral pleural effusion and confirmed an intramural hematoma of the posterior

esophageal wall, extending 15 cm caudally (Figure 2); no active bleeding was seen.

The patient was transferred to ICU where she remained hemodynamically stable, with no sign of perforation and no mediastinal involvement. A conservative management was chosen: supportive care and parenteral nutrition, administration of proton pump inhibitors to decrease gastric acid production, and broad-spectrum antibiotic therapy.

The chest CT control two days later showed no modification of the hematoma with no active bleeding and improvement of the pleural effusion.

Nine days after the initial diagnosis and eleven days after C-section, a new episode of hematemesis required a repeat CT scan. This time a reduction of the hematoma was seen with concomitant blood collection in the stomach. Gastroscopy was indicated, blood content aspirated, and the active bleeding controlled with local therapy. The patient was transfused with 2 units of packed red cells.

After this episode, the patient was discharged from ICU and transferred to a surgical ward where conservative treatment was continued until restarting of food intake; the subsequent course was uncomplicated.

A control chest CT, 17 days after C-section, showed an open lumen, a reduction of the thickness of the esophageal wall, and an almost complete resolution of the parietal hematoma (Figure 3).

The patient was discharged asymptomatic 20 days after the initial diagnosis under antihypertensive and antacid therapy. A detailed chart including medications, laboratories results, images, and procedures throughout hospitalization is presented in Table 1.

3. Discussion

Pathogenesis of intramural esophageal bleeding leading to hematoma formation and submucosal dissection is often unclear. Several causes have been proposed: emetogenic, traumatic, related to aortic disease, and coagulopathic; in few instances, the cause remains undetermined. Severe bleeding results in proximal or distal intramural dissection, as

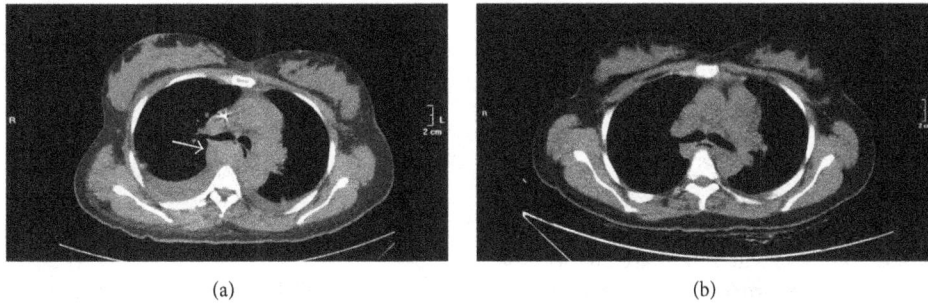

FIGURE 3: Chest CT transverse view of (a) hematoma (white arrow) displacing the esophageal lumen on 2nd day after C-section. (b) Normal esophageal anatomy and lumen patency after full recovery, 17 days after C-section.

TABLE 1: Time chart of the entire hospitalization period.

	Admission			C-section	Pain symptoms	IHE diagnosis		Bleeding episode		Discharge
Treatment										
Aspirin	Stop									
HLMW		•	•	•	•	•	•			
Mg				•	•					
Betamethasone		•	•							
Laboratory										
Hb (gr/dL)	11.7	12.1	12.2	11.2	9.5	8.7	7.8	6.5	8.4	11.2
INR		0.84	0.83	0.84	0.79	0.87	0.94	1	1.06	1.01
PLT (10^3/dL)	125	114	122	91	103	131	127	264	307	353
AST/ALT (UI/L)	—/39	46/35	—/36	—/39	—/24	—/18		—/16		38/43
BP	140/95	130/90	140/90	160/100	175/110	120/80	<140/90	<140/90	<140/90	<140/90
24 h U proteins		2.1 gr								0.89 gr
Imaging/procedures										
Chest CT						•	•	•	•	
Endoscopy						•		•		
Blood transfusion								•		
Day	1	2	3	8	9	10	12	19	25	30

the hematoma develops concentrically or eccentrically, as in the present case [5]. About one-fifth of patients appear to have a spontaneous origin, although this may be associated with an underlying predisposition: abnormal pressure changes within the esophagus or a coagulation disorder [6].

Although the direct cause was not clear, we do not consider emesis a relevant contributing factor in the present case. The patient complained of little vomiting, not strong enough, in our opinion, to raise the intrathoracic pressure and to produce intramural trauma and hemorrhage. Instead, we believe the following were precipitating factors: coagulopathy secondary to LMWH treatment and platelet reduction in association with high blood pressure during the episode of severe preeclampsia. Even though no case of IHE in association with gestational hypertension has ever been described, it is a well-known fact that preeclampsia carries an increased risk of bleeding and of several hemorrhagic complications such as liver, renal, and intracranial hematoma [7–10].

We also tend to exclude the iatrogenic trauma from intubation during general anesthesia since no abnormal manoeuver was reported by the anesthesiologist.

Clinical presentation of this case with chest pain and dysphagia matches the observations of other authors: gradually increasing chest pain (66–84%) localized in the retrosternal or epigastric region and odynophagia/dysphagia (26–59%), exacerbated by swallowing [5]. Differently from the Mallory-Weiss syndrome where the debut symptom is usually hematemesis, this complaint is an infrequent initial manifestation of IHE. According to other studies, the clinical triad of retrosternal pain, difficulty in swallowing, and hematemesis is present in just one-third of cases [11]. Hematemesis occurs when the intramural hematoma expands and the mucosa ruptures. Blood loss is usually moderate, and only 10% of the patients will require a transfusion [12].

In any preeclamptic woman presenting with chest pain, other complications which need to be ruled out are HELLP syndrome, congestive cardiac failure, liver hematoma, or liver rupture. The association of chest pain with dysphagia and hematemesis helps the clinician in reaching the correct diagnosis of this rare situation which has a 2:1 female preponderance and a mortality rate of 7–9% after either surgical or medical treatment [13].

Endoscopy is considered the first-line diagnostic tool and it revealed the esophageal lesion in our case. However, this technique has some disadvantages when compared with chest CT scan since it is an invasive procedure which may not reveal the abnormality in the absence of a mucosal tear and may further damage the esophageal wall. Chest CT has the advantage of being noninvasive and finds indication to confirm the diagnosis and to exclude active bleeding; besides the esophageal wall, it explores the aorta and other mediastinal structures, thus excluding other thoracic processes [5].

After the diagnostic confirmation, the hematoma was treated conservatively and resolved in less than 3 weeks, a length of time necessary to obtain the spontaneous drainage, the complete healing of the mucosal tear, and the recovery of a normal esophageal peristalsis [5, 14]. Although most bleeding in IHE can be managed medically, surgical drainage and repair of the laceration or therapeutic angiography may become an urgent indication in those cases of massive hemorrhage and hemodynamically unstable patients [15].

In conclusion, although a rare event, IHE may unexpectedly complicate the pregnant state. Diagnosis is not always simple, since chest pain is a presenting symptom found in other conditions, particularly in a preeclamptic woman. Medical treatment is associated with full recovery in most cases and surgical or endoscopic interventions are rarely required.

References

[1] A. Jalihal, A. Z. F. Jamaludin, S. Sankarakumar, and V. H. Chong, "Intramural hematoma of the esophagus: a rare cause of chest pain," *American Journal of Emergency Medicine*, vol. 26, no. 7, pp. 843.e1-843.e2, 2008.

[2] V. S. Katabathina, C. S. Restrepo, S. Martinez-Jimenez, and R. F. Riascos, "Nonvascular, nontraumatic mediastinal emergencies in adults: a comprehensive review of imaging findings," *Radiographics*, vol. 31, no. 4, pp. 1141–1160, 2011.

[3] P. Modi, A. Edwards, B. Fox, and J. Rahamim, "Dissecting intramural haematoma of the oesophagus," *European Journal of Cardio-Thoracic Surgery*, vol. 27, no. 1, pp. 171–173, 2005.

[4] Y.-H. Chiu, J.-D. Chen, C.-Y. Hsu, C.-K. How, D. H.-T. Yen, and C.-I. Huang, "Spontaneous esophageal injury: esophageal intramural hematoma," *Journal of the Chinese Medical Association*, vol. 72, no. 9, pp. 498–500, 2009.

[5] C. S. Restrepo, D. F. Lemos, D. Ocazionez, R. Moncada, and C. R. Gimenez, "Intramural hematoma of the esophagus: a pictorial essay," *Emergency Radiology*, vol. 15, no. 1, pp. 13–22, 2008.

[6] M. Sanaka, Y. Kuyama, S. Hirama, R. Nagayama, H. Tanaka, and M. Yamanaka, "Spontaneous intramural hematoma localized in the proximal esophagus: truly 'spontaneous'?" *Journal of Clinical Gastroenterology*, vol. 27, no. 3, pp. 265-266, 1998.

[7] P. Vigil-De Gracia and L. Ortega-Paz, "Pre-eclampsia/eclampsia and hepatic rupture," *International Journal of Gynecology and Obstetrics*, vol. 118, no. 3, pp. 186–189, 2012.

[8] T. Diallo, I. Amiel, E. Lira et al., "Sub-capsular renal hematoma during severe preeclampsia: clinical case and review of the literature," *Annales Françaises d'Anesthésie et de Réanimation*, vol. 33, no. 9-10, pp. 536–539, 2014.

[9] S. A. Shainker, J. A. Edlow, and K. O'Brien, "Cerebrovascular emergencies in pregnancy," *Best Practice and Research: Clinical Obstetrics and Gynaecology*, vol. 29, no. 5, pp. 721–731, 2015.

[10] B. O. Djoubairou, J. Onen, A. K. Doleagbenou, N. El Fatemi, and M. R. Maaqili, "Chronic subdural haematoma associated with pre-eclampsia: case report and review of the literature," *Neurochirurgie*, vol. 60, no. 1-2, pp. 48–50, 2014.

[11] S. N. Cullen and A. S. McIntyre, "Dissecting intramural haematoma of the oesophagus," *European Journal of Gastroenterology & Hepatology*, vol. 12, pp. 1151–1162, 2000.

[12] R. Enns, J. A. Brown, and L. Halparin, "Intramural esophageal hematoma: a diagnostic dilemma," *Gastrointestinal Endoscopy*, vol. 51, no. 6, pp. 757–759, 2000.

[13] G. Biagi, G. Cappelli, L. Propersi, and A. Grossi, "Spontaneous intramural haematoma of the oesophagus," *Thorax*, vol. 38, no. 5, pp. 394-395, 1983.

[14] C. Steadman, P. Kerlin, F. Crimmins et al., "Spontaneous intramural rupture of the oesophagus," *Gut*, vol. 31, no. 8, pp. 845–849, 1990.

[15] J. Shim, J. Y. Jang, Y. Hwangbo et al., "Recurrent massive bleeding due to dissecting intramural hematoma of the esophagus: treatment with therapeutic angiography," *World Journal of Gastroenterology*, vol. 15, no. 41, pp. 5232–5235, 2009.

22

Uterine Fibroid Torsion during Pregnancy: A Case of Laparotomic Myomectomy at 18 Weeks' Gestation with Systematic Review of the Literature

Annachiara Basso,[1] Mariana Rita Catalano,[1] Giuseppe Loverro,[1]
Serena Nocera,[1] Edoardo Di Naro,[1] Matteo Loverro,[1]
Mariateresa Natrella,[2] and Salvatore Andrea Mastrolia[1]

[1]Department of Obstetrics and Gynecology, Azienda Ospedaliera Universitaria Policlinico di Bari, School of Medicine,
 Università degli Studi di Bari "Aldo Moro", Bari, Italy
[2]School of Nursing, Azienda Ospedaliera Universitaria Policlinico di Bari, School of Medicine,
 Università degli Studi di Bari "Aldo Moro", Bari, Italy

Correspondence should be addressed to Salvatore Andrea Mastrolia; mastroliasa@gmail.com

Academic Editor: Maria Grazia Porpora

Uterine myomas are the most common benign growths affecting female reproductive system, occurring in 20–40% of women, whereas the incidence rate in pregnancy is estimated from 0.1 to 3.9%. The lower incidence in pregnancy is due to the association with infertility and low pregnancy rates and implantation rates after in vitro fertilization treatment. Uterine myomas, usually, are asymptomatic during pregnancy. However, occasionally, pedunculated fibroids torsion or other superimposed complications may cause acute abdominal pain. There are many controversies in performing myomectomy during cesarean section because of the risk of hemorrhage. Nevertheless, the majority of indication arises before labor and delivery due to acute symptoms leading to a discussion regarding the need for intervention during pregnancy. Therefore, we present a case of successful multiple laparotomic myomectomy at 17 + 2 weeks of gestational age and a systematic review of the literature in order to clarify the approach to this pathologic condition and its effect on pregnancy outcome.

1. Introduction

Uterine myomas are the most common benign growths affecting female reproductive system, occurring in 20–40% of women [1], whereas the incidence rate in pregnancy is estimated from 0.1 to 3.9%. The lower incidence in pregnancy is due to the association with infertility and low pregnancy rates and implantation rates after in vitro fertilization treatment [2]. Uterine myomas, usually, are asymptomatic during pregnancy. However, occasionally, pedunculated fibroids torsion or other superimposed complications may cause acute abdominal pain. Urinary and gastroenteric symptoms may occur due to the rapid increase in size in reason of hyperestrogenic environment and, consequently, compression and displacement of surrounding organs. Additionally, fibroids predispose to pregnancy complications, including early miscarriage, antepartum bleeding, preterm labor, premature rupture of membranes, fetal malpresentations, labor dystocia, and postpartum hemorrhage.

Conservative management with anti-inflammatory therapy is considered a gold standard, and surgery is generally avoided during pregnancy because of the risks of hysterectomy secondary to severe hemorrhage, pregnancy injury, and pregnancy loss [3]. The main conditions that induce inevitably the surgical procedure are the torsion of pedunculated fibroids or rare cases of necrosis, resultant inflammatory peritoneal reaction, and, finally, if symptoms persist after 72 hours of pharmacological therapy [4–7]. Therefore, the diagnosis needs a particular attention for the appropriate management choice. Surgical removal fibroids in pregnancy can be performed by laparotomy or laparoscopy technique taking into account the volume and location of nodules [1, 8].

Laparoscopy can be considered in selected cases such as small, subserous, pedunculated myomas.

There are many controversies in performing myomectomy during cesarean section because of the risk of hemorrhage [3]. Nevertheless, the majority of indication arises before labor and delivery due to acute symptoms leading to a discussion regarding the need for intervention during pregnancy.

Therefore, we present a case of successful multiple laparotomic myomectomy at 17 + 2 weeks of gestational age and a systematic review of the literature in order to clarify the approach to this pathologic condition and its effect on pregnancy outcome.

2. Case Report

Uterine myomas are usually asymptomatic during pregnancy. However, pedunculated fibroids torsion may occasionally cause acute abdominal pain [1].

Most cases of laparotomic myomectomy described in literature have been performed during a cesarean section due to the risk of managing them surgically at low gestational age [2–4]. We present a case of a successful multiple laparotomic myomectomy during the second trimester of pregnancy.

A 36-year-old, morbidly obese primigravida presented at our emergency room at 17 + 0 weeks of gestational age complaining of abdominal pain. At clinical examination, the uterus appeared to be of higher volume compared to the gestational age, the abdomen was painful but treatable, and the obstetrical examination was normal. The patient was then referred to US Unit of our Department for further evaluation. The sonographic assessment revealed the presence of three subserous uterine myomas located on anterior wall (maximum diameter: 13.2 cm), the right wall (maximum diameter: 12.6 cm), and the left wall (maximum diameter: 11.7 cm) of the uterus, respectively. All myomas were vacuolated inside as for suspected necrosis. The scan also showed other multiple myomas less than 3 cm in size. Vital signs were monitored (blood pressure 140/90 mmHg, maternal heart rate 124 bmp, SO2 94%, apyretic). Amniotic fluid was normal and fetal well-being was preserved. Thus, the patient was admitted to the High-Risk-Pregnancy Unit. When collecting the medical history, the first trimester ultrasound scan, performed at 11 weeks' gestation, revealed the presence of the same lesions with a size of 10.8 cm, 10.2 cm, and 6.14 cm, respectively.

Laboratory studies demonstrated rising inflammatory markers (C-reactive protein: 354 mg/L; WBC: $16.92 \times 10^3 \mu L$).

Due to the persistence of the symptoms, despite of two days of analgesic, antispastic, and antibiotic therapy, after multidisciplinary discussion, and a thorough counseling to inform the parents of the surgical and postoperative risks connected with uterine surgery during the gestation, the patient underwent surgery. Laparotomy approach by longitudinal skin incision, considering the volume and the position of the myomas, was performed under general anesthesia. Three huge bulky subserous pedunculated myomas were evidenced, the largest located at the uterine fundus, with a maximum diameter of 15 cm and a torsion of its pedicle (Figure 1). Furthermore, intra-abdominal adhesions were found within

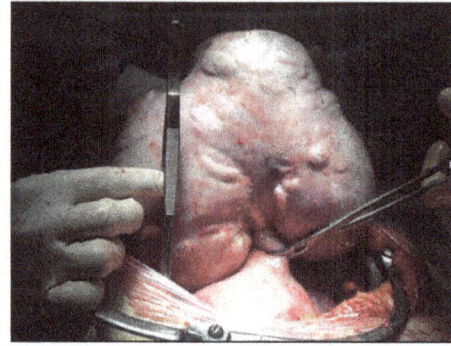

FIGURE 1: Myoma of the uterine fundus with evidence of torsion of its pedicle.

peritoneal cavity. Blunt dissection was undertaken to free the omentum and look for the appendix, which was normal. The three large myomas evidenced by ultrasound were removed and sent for pathologic examination. A pelvic drainage was left and removed 24 hours postoperatively. Pathology showed widespread phenomena of necrosis, especially in the myoma with torsion of its pedicle.

During the following nine days, the patient received antibiotics, low molecular heparin, and progesterone, and fetal heartbeat was checked daily. Considering the improvement in clinical condition, the patient was discharged with an indication to treatment with progesterone and low molecular heparin.

Three weeks later, at 21 weeks' gestation, the patient was admitted again due to abdominal pain. Obstetrical evaluation revealed cervical effacement and the transvaginal ultrasound scan showed a reduction of cervical length (18 mm), funneling, and sludge. An ultrasound scan was performed showing good fetal variables. Consequently, the therapy with progesterone was increased. The patient had a positive vaginal culture for *Staphylococcus haemolyticus*, urine culture was negative, and C-reactive protein resulted to be positive. Therefore, antibiotic therapy with macrolides was given, according to antibiogram result. A cervical cerclage was proposed to the patient, but she refused to undergo the procedure.

Hospitalization lasted for seven days; then the woman was discharged due to an improvement of her clinical condition. The patient underwent obstetric evaluation every two weeks until she presented in labor and delivered vaginally at 38 + 1 weeks' gestation a healthy female newborn of 2940 g, appropriate for gestational age according to national growth curves [9]. Apgar score was 9/10 at 1′ and 5′ respectively.

3. Data Source and Literature Search

To identify potentially eligible studies, we searched PubMed, Scopus, and Cochrane Library (all from inception to 16 March 2017). No language restrictions were initially applied. We used a combination of key words and text words represented by "myomectomy," "myoma," and "pregnancy."

Two reviewers (Annachiara Basso and Mariana Rita Catalano) independently screened the titles and abstracts of

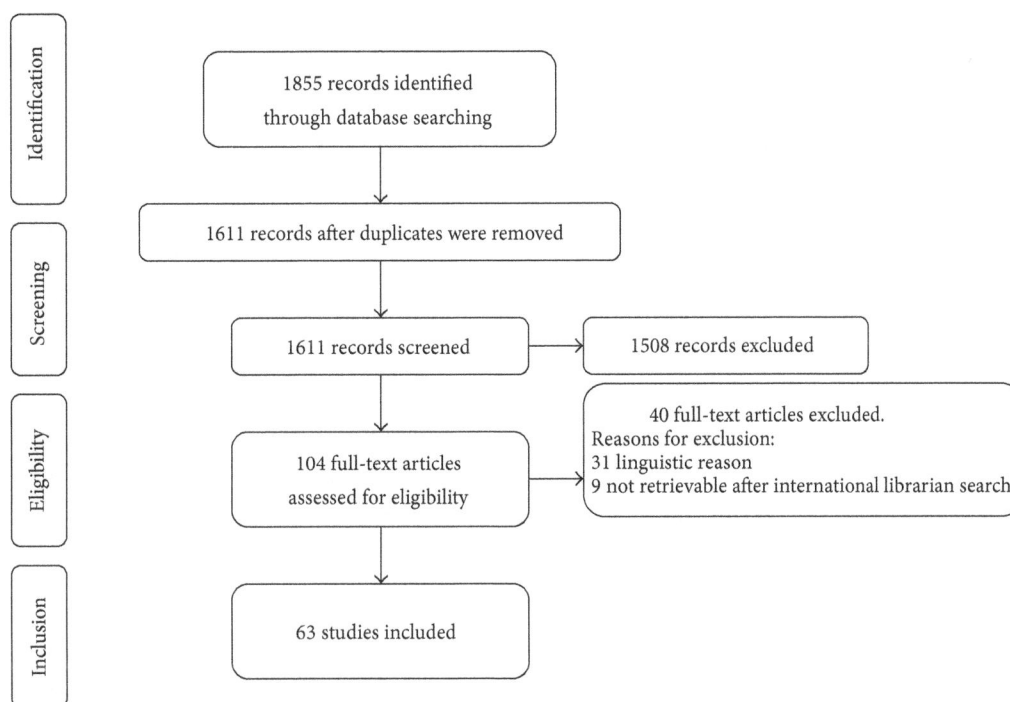

FIGURE 2: Study selection process.

records retrieved through database searches. Both reviewers recommended studies for the full-text review. The screen of full-text articles recommended by at least one reviewer was done independently by the same two reviewers and assessed for inclusion in the systematic review. Disagreements between reviewers were resolved by consensus. For all full-text manuscripts, reference lists were analyzed in order to find additional eligible studies.

4. Results

The electronic database search provided a total of 1855 results. After duplicate exclusion, there were 1611 citations left. Of these, 1508 were not relevant to the review based on title and abstract screening. 103 studies were considered for full-text assessment, of which 40 were excluded for the following reasons: we could not translate 31 articles, while nine papers could not be retrieved even after international librarian search.

Overall, 63 [3–6, 10–67] articles were incorporated for further assessment. The study selection process is shown in Figure 2. The main characteristics of the selected studies are included in Table 1.

5. Discussion

Our review included 197 women undergoing myomectomy during pregnancy. The procedure was successful in 184 women, while in the remaining 13 cases a miscarriage or fetal demise happened after the myomectomy.

In 14 cases, a laparoscopic approach was chosen; in one case there was a vaginal surgery, while all the other cases for which the surgical information was available underwent laparotomy. These data confirm that the most used surgical intervention for myomas during pregnancy is the laparotomy route.

Maternal outcomes were favorable after myomectomy, with only two episodes of hemoperitoneum [33, 67], one uterine abscess [39], and only one woman requiring perioperative blood transfusion [61].

Moreover, the analysis of all reports was limited by two factors: (1) the heterogeneity of diagnostic information as well as descriptive data connected to operation and pathology examination which did not allow clear categorization of the pathology preoperatively and postoperatively and (2) the large amount of missing or unreported data.

6. Conclusion

Myomectomy is a feasible procedure if performed during pregnancy. Candidates need to be chosen carefully among those with symptomatic myomas, since abdominal surgery during pregnancy can be associated with an increased risk for the development of the great obstetrical syndromes, especially preterm labor and delivery.

Disclosure

This paper has been presented in part at the 19th National Congress of the Italian Society of Perinatal Medicine (Società

TABLE 1: Characteristics of the relevant studies.

Reference	Number of patients	Gestational age at diagnosis (weeks)	Gestational age at myomectomy (weeks)	Type of surgery	Fibroid maximum volume (cm)	Mode of delivery	Gestational age at delivery	Neonatal outcome (Apgar, birthweight, pH)
De Carolis et al., 2001	18	nd	13	LPT	8	CS	39	8/8, 3150 g
		nd	23	LPT	40	CS	38	8/8, 2670 g
		nd	19	LPT	14	VD	36	8/9, 3080 g
		nd	17	LPT	21	CS	38	8/9, 3060 g
		nd	19	LPT	15	\multicolumn{2}{Fetal demise at 19 weeks}		
		nd	20	LPT	6	VD	41	9/9, 2970 g
		nd	19	LPT	12	CS	39	7/9, 3180 g
		nd	8	LPT	9	CS	40	9/9, 3300 g
		nd	12	LPT	8	CS	38	9/10, 2780 g
		nd	17	LPT	24	CS	38	9/9, 3900 g
		nd	15	LPT	10	CS	40	8/10, 3170 g
		nd	17	LPT	13	CS	39	9/10, 3100 g
		nd	6	LPT	15	nd	nd	nd
		nd	20	LPT	8	CS	39	9/10, 2860 g
		nd	10	LPT	16	CS	40	9/10, 3500 g
		nd	16	LPT	10	CS	39	9/10, 3930 g
		nd	13	LPT	14	CS	39	9/9, 3180 g
		nd	7	LPT	15	CS	38	9/10 - 2550 g
Domenici et al., 2014	1	16	16	LPT	20	CS	38	8/9 - 3250 g
Michalas et al., 1995	1	14	15	LPT	20	CS	39	2800 g
Danzer et al., 2001	1	12	12	LPT	10	CS	37	9/10, 3235 g; 9/10, 2810 g
Lozza et al., 2011	1	12	16	LPT	18	CS	36	9/9, 2280 g
Joó et al., 2001	1	8	25	LPT	12	CS	40	3600 g
Çelik et al., 2002	5	nd	22	LPT	13	CS	38.6 +/- 1.1	10, 3200 g
		nd	18	LPT	10	CS	38.6 +/- 1.1	9, 3400 g
		nd	20	LPT	12	CS	38.6 +/- 1.1	10, 3600 g
		nd	16	LPT	15	CS	38.6 +/- 1.1	8, 3100 g
		nd	13	LPT	20	CS	38.6 +/- 1.1	9, 2800 g
Hasbargen et al., 2002	1	18	18	LPT	15	CS	36	8/9, 2495 g
Umezurike and Feyi-Waboso, 2005	1	19	19	LPT	32	VD	38	8/10, 3500 g
Usifo et al., 2007	1	13	13	LPT	17	CS	38	3990 g
Suwandinata et al., 2009	1	nd	18	LPT	nd	CS	37	8/9, 2950 g

TABLE 1: Continued.

Reference	Number of patients	Gestational age at diagnosis (weeks)	Gestational age at myomectomy (weeks)	Type of surgery	Fibroid maximum volume (cm)	Mode of delivery	Gestational age at delivery	Neonatal outcome (Apgar, birthweight, pH)
Bhatla et al., 2009	1	8	19	LPT	28	VD	38	2740 g
Leite et al., 2009	1	1st trimester	17	LPT	10	CS	39	9/10, 3315 g
Isabu et al., 2010	1	14	14	LPT	nd	CS	37	2700 g
Leach et al., 2011	1	11	11	LPT	14	CS	40	9/9, 4356 g
Doerga-Bachasingh et al., 2012	1	9	10	LPT	15	CS	37	nd
Jhalta et al., 2016	1	13	13	LPT	16	VD	39	8/10, 3000 g
Kosmidis et al., 2015	1	10	10	LPS	8	nd	nd	nd
Saccardi et al., 2015	1	9	15	LPS	24	CS	41	4460 g, 7.2
Obara et al., 2014	1	6	13	VAG	6	VD	40	2775 g
Currie et al., 2013	1	11	11	LPS	8	nd	nd	nd
Kobayashi et al., 2013	1	21	21	LPT	8	CS	37	2730 g
MacCiò et al., 2012	3	8	19	LPS	11	CS	39	3150 g
		20	20	LPS	10	VD	40	3310 g
		20	20	LPS	nd	CS	39	3050 g
Shafiee et al., 2012	1	15	21	LPS	15	CS	38	nd
Ardovino et al., 2011	1	14	14	LPS	6	VD	40	3216 g
Müller Vranjes et al.	1	14	18	LPT	35	CS	33	10/10, 1750 g, 7.28
Son et al., 2011	1	18	18	LPS	9	VD	39	3740 g
Kasum 2010	1	15	15	LPT	9	VD	38	nd
Fanfani et al., 2010	1	25	25	LPS	9	VD	40	2950 g
Adeyemi et al., 2007	1	19	19	LPT	30	VD	39	7/10, 3500 g
Okonkwo and Udigwe, 2007	1	19	24	LPT	nd	CS	nd	nd
Dracea and Codreanu, 2006	1	12	13	LPT	24	VD	nd	nd
Melgrati et al., 2005	1	24	24	LPS	7	VD	39	9/9

TABLE 1: Continued.

Reference	Number of patients	Gestational age at diagnosis (weeks)	Gestational age at myomectomy (weeks)	Type of surgery	Fibroid maximum volume (cm)	Mode of delivery	Gestational age at delivery	Neonatal outcome (Apgar, birthweight, pH)
Sentilhes et al., 2003	1	17	17	LPS	5	CS	37	3530 g
Lolis et al., 2003	13	nd	16	LPT	nd	CS	37	3340 g
		nd	15	LPT	nd	CS	39	3600 g
		nd	19	LPT	nd	CS	37	2970 g
		nd	16	LPT	nd	CS	36	3000 g
		nd	15	LPT	nd	CS	Fetal demise at 15 weeks	
		nd	15	LPT	nd	CS	37	2740 g
		nd	16	LPT	nd	CS	38	3180 g
		nd	16	LPT	nd	CS	39	3515 g
		nd	16	LPT	nd	CS	39	3190 g
		nd	19	LPT	nd	CS	38	2920 g
		nd	17	LPT	nd	CS	38	3520 g
		nd	16	LPT	nd	CS	38	3000 g
		nd	15	LPT	nd	CS	29	1606 g
Donnez et al., 2002	1	Before pregnancy	25	LPT	22	CS	35	2280 g
Williamson, 1908	1	22	22	LPT	32	VD	23	Neonatal death
Stewart, 1906	1	20	20	LPT	24	VD	40	nd
Wittich et al., 2000	1	12	15	LPT	20	CS	37	9/9, 3275 g
Majid et al., 1997	1	17	18	LPT	24		Fetal demise 19 weeks	
Algara et al., 2015	1	18	18	LPS	7	VD	24	nd
Lockyer, 1914	1	21	21	LPT	nd	VD	40	2300 g
von Hoffmann, 1911	3	16	16	LPT	nd	VD	40	3630 g
		22	25	LPT	nd		Fetal demise at 25 weeks	
		14	15	LPT	nd	VD	40	nd
Andrews, 1910	1	Before pregnancy	9	LPT	nd	VD	40	nd
Swayne, 1908	2	20	20	LPT	nd	nd	nd	nd
		16	16	LPT	nd	VD	24	nd
Doran, 1906	1	20	21	LPT	10	VD	40	nd
Evans, 1899	1	20	20	LPT	7	nd	nd	nd
Exacoustòs and Rosati, 1993	13	nd	<26	nd	nd	N.G	40 (8), preterm > 32 (5)	nd
Burton et al., 1989	8	nd	13	LPT	18	VD	40	nd
		nd	15	LPT	14	VD	Fetal demise 15 weeks	nd
		nd	nd	LPT	5	VD	40	nd
		nd	nd	LPT	5	VD	40	nd
		nd	nd	LPT	5	VD	40	nd
		nd	nd	LPT	5	VD	40	nd
		nd	nd	LPT	5	VD	40	nd
		nd	nd	LPT	5	nd	nd	nd
Rella et al., 1980	1	10	12	LPT	nd	VD	27	Neonatal death

Table 1: Continued.

Reference	Number of patients	Gestational age at diagnosis (weeks)	Gestational age at myomectomy (weeks)	Type of surgery	Fibroid maximum volume (cm)	Mode of delivery	Gestational age at delivery	Neonatal outcome (Apgar, birthweight, pH)
Pelosi et al., 1995	1	13	15	LPS	6	CS	39	nd
Pelissier-Komorek et al., 2012	1	10	13	LPT	22	VD	35	2280 g
Mollica et al., 1996	18	8–17	10–19	LPT	>10	CS (17), VD (1)	nd	>7 (18), >2500 g (17), <2500 g (1)
Febo et al., 1997	3	nd	12–19	LPT	N.G.	CS (2), abortion (1)	37–38	nd
Bonito et al., 2007	5	nd	9–15	LPT	3.5–14.5	CS (2), VD (3)	38.2	9 +/− 0.83, 3200–4072 g
Vázquez Camacho et al., 2009	1	7	16	LPT	6.2	VD	40	9/9
Makar et al., 1989	1	12	17	LPT	13,500 g	CS	38	9/9, 3950 g
Horno Liria, 1962	1	16	16	LPT	nd	VD	40	3600 g
Alanis et al., 2008	1	7	12	LPT	30	VD	38	2330 g
Ardizzone, 1955	27	8	8	LPT	nd	nd	nd	nd
		8	8	LPT	nd	nd	nd	nd
		8	8	LPT	nd	nd	Miscarriage at 9 weeks	
		24	24	LPT	nd	nd	Fetal demise at 25 weeks	
		8	8	LPT	nd	nd	Miscarriage at 8 weeks	
		16	16	LPT	nd	nd	nd	nd
		8	8	LPT	nd	nd	nd	nd
		8	8	LPT	nd	nd	nd	nd
		12	12	LPT	nd	nd	Fetal demise at 14 weeks	
		20	20	LPT	nd	nd	nd	nd
		16	16	LPT	nd	nd	nd	nd
		20	20	LPT	nd	nd	nd	nd
		20	20	LPT	nd	nd	nd	nd
		12	12	LPT	nd	nd	nd	nd
		12	12	LPT	nd	nd	Fetal demise at 13 weeks	
		8	8	LPT	nd	nd	nd	nd
		8	8	LPT	nd	nd	nd	nd
		12	12	LPT	nd	nd	Fetal demise at 13 weeks	
		12	12	LPT	nd	nd	nd	nd
		16	16	LPT	nd	nd	Fetal demise at 17 weeks	
		8	8	LPT	nd	nd	nd	nd
		12	12	LPT	nd	nd	nd	nd
		12	12	LPT	nd	nd	nd	nd
		12	12	LPT	nd	nd	nd	nd
		8	8	LPT	nd	nd	Fetal demise at 12 weeks	
		12	12	LPT	nd	nd	nd	nd
		12	12	LPT	nd	nd	nd	nd

TABLE 1: Continued.

Reference	Number of patients	Gestational age at diagnosis (weeks)	Gestational age at myomectomy (weeks)	Type of surgery	Fibroid maximum volume (cm)	Mode of delivery	Gestational age at delivery	Neonatal outcome (Apgar, birthweight, pH)
		nd	12	LPT	nd	VD	40	nd
		nd	12	LPT	nd	VD	40	nd
		nd	8	LPT	nd	VD	40	nd
		nd	8	LPT	nd	VD	40	nd
		nd	16	LPT	nd	VD	38	nd
		nd	8	LPT	nd	VD	40	nd
		nd	12	LPT	nd	VD	38	nd
Cozzi, 1967	16	nd	8	LPT	nd	VD	40	nd
		nd	16	LPT	nd	VD	40	nd
		nd	20	LPT	nd	VD	36	nd
		nd	8	LPT	nd	VD	40	nd
		nd	12	LPT	nd	VD	40	nd
		nd	12	LPT	nd	VD	40	nd
		nd	12	LPT	nd	VD	40	nd
		nd	16	LPT	nd	VD	40	nd
		nd	8	LPT	nd	VD	40	nd
Rochet et al., 1964	14	nd	nd	LPT	10	nd	nd	nd
Sciannameo et al., 1996	1	20	20	LPT	4	nd	nd	nd

nd, not determined; CS, cesarean section; VD, vaginal delivery; LPT, laparotomy; LPS, laparoscopy; VAG, vaginal surgery.

Italiana di Medicina Perinatale, SIMP), Naples (Italy), 19–21 January 2017.

References

[1] S. G. Vitale, A. Tropea, D. Rossetti, M. Carnelli, and A. Cianci, "Management of uterine leiomyomas in pregnancy: review of literature," *Updates in Surgery*, vol. 65, no. 3, pp. 179–182, 2013.

[2] S. K. Sunkara, M. Khairy, T. El-Toukhy, Y. Khalaf, and A. Coomarasamy, "The effect of intramural fibroids without uterine cavity involvement on the outcome of IVF treatment: a systematic review and meta-analysis," *Human Reproduction*, vol. 25, no. 2, pp. 418–429, 2010.

[3] V. Lozza, A. Pieralli, S. Corioni, M. Longinotti, and C. Penna, "Multiple laparotomic myomectomy during pregnancy: a case report," *Archives of Gynecology and Obstetrics*, vol. 284, no. 3, pp. 613–616, 2011.

[4] L. Domenici, V. Di Donato, M. L. Gasparri, F. Lecce, J. Caccetta, and P. B. Panici, "Laparotomic myomectomy in the 16th week of pregnancy: a case report," *Case Reports in Obstetrics and Gynecology*, 5 pages, 2014.

[5] D. E. Lolis, S. N. Kalantaridou, G. Makrydimas et al., "Successful myomectomy during pregnancy," *Human Reproduction*, vol. 18, no. 8, pp. 1699–1702, 2003.

[6] S. De Carolis, G. Fatigante, S. Ferrazzani et al., "Uterine myomectomy in pregnant women," *Fetal Diagnosis and Therapy*, vol. 16, no. 2, pp. 116–119, 2001.

[7] N. Bhatla, B. B. Dash, A. Kriplani, and N. Agarwal, "Myomectomy during pregnancy: a feasible option," *Journal of Obstetrics and Gynaecology Research*, vol. 35, no. 1, pp. 173–175, 2009.

[8] A. Cagnacci, D. Pirillo, S. Malmusi, S. Arangino, C. Alessandrini, and A. Volpe, "Early outcome of myomectomy by laparotomy, minilaparotomy and laparoscopically assisted minilaparotomy. A randomized prospective study," *Human Reproduction*, vol. 18, no. 12, pp. 2590–2594, 2003.

[9] F. Parazzini, S. Cipriani, G. Bulfoni et al., "Centiles of weight at term birth according to maternal nationality in a northern Italian region," *Italian Journal of Gynaecology and Obstetrics*, vol. 28, no. 2, pp. 52–56, 2016.

[10] S. P. Michalas, F. V. Oreopoulou, and J. S. Papageorgiou, "Myomectomy during pregnancy and caesarean section," *Human Reproduction*, vol. 10, no. 7, pp. 1869–1870, 1995.

[11] E. Danzer, W. Holzgreve, D. Batukan, P. Miny, S. Tercanli, and I. Hoesli, "Myomectomy during the first trimester associated with fetal limb anomalies and hydrocephalus in a twin pregnancy," *Prenatal Diagnosis*, vol. 21, no. 10, pp. 848–851, 2001.

[12] J. G. Joó, J. Inovay, M. Silhavy, and Z. Papp, "Successful enucleation of a necrotizing fibroid causing oligohydramnios and fetal postural deformity in the 25th week of gestation. A case report," *Journal of Reproductive Medicine*, vol. 46, no. 10, pp. 923–925, 2001.

[13] Ç. Çelik, A. Acar, N. Çiçek, K. Gezginc, and C. Akyürek, "Can myomectomy be performed during pregnancy?" *Gynecologic and Obstetric Investigation*, vol. 53, no. 2, pp. 79–83, 2002.

[14] U. Hasbargen, A. Strauss, M. Summerer-Moustaki et al., "Myomectomy as a pregnancy-preserving option in the carefully selected patient," *Fetal Diagnosis and Therapy*, vol. 17, no. 2, pp. 101–103, 2002.

[15] C. Umezurike and P. Feyi-Waboso, "Successful myomectomy during pregnancy: a case report," *Reproductive Health*, vol. 2, no. 1, 2005.

[16] F. Usifo, R. Macrae, R. Sharma, I. O. Opemuyi, and B. Onwuzurike, "Successful myomectomy in early second trimester of pregnancy," *Journal of Obstetrics and Gynaecology*, vol. 27, no. 2, pp. 196–197, 2007.

[17] F. S. Suwandinata, S. E. Gruessner, C. O. Omwandho, and H. R. Tinneberg, "Pregnancy-preserving myomectomy: preliminary report on a new surgical technique," *European Journal of Contraception and Reproductive Health Care*, vol. 13, no. 3, pp. 323–326, 2008, Erratum in: *European Journal of Contraception and Reproductive Health Care*, vol. 13, no. 4, article 438, 2008.

[18] G. K. Leite, H. A. Korkes, T. Viana Ade, A. Pitorri, G. Kenj, and N. Sass, "Myomectomy in the second trimester of pregnancy: case report," *Revista Brasileira De Ginecologia E Obstetricia*, vol. 32, no. 4, pp. 198–201, 2010.

[19] P. Isabu, J. Eigbefoh, F. Okogbo, S. Okunsanya, and R. Eifediyi, "Myomectomy during second trimester pregnancy: a case report," *The Nigerian Postgraduate Medical Journal*, vol. 17, no. 4, pp. 324–326, 2010.

[20] K. Leach, L. Khatain, and K. Tocce, "First trimester myomectomy as an alternative to termination of pregnancy in a woman with a symptomatic uterine leiomyoma: a case report," *Journal of Medical Case Reports*, vol. 5, article 571, 2011.

[21] S. Doerga-Bachasingh, V. Karsdorp, G. Yo, R. Van Der Weiden, and M. Van Hooff, "Successful myomectomy of a bleeding myoma in a twin pregnancy," *JRSM Short Reports*, vol. 3, no. 2, article 13, 2012.

[22] P. Jhalta, S. G. Negi, and V. Sharma, "Successful myomectomy in early pregnancy for a large asymptomatic uterine myoma: case report," *Pan African Medical Journal*, vol. 13, no. 24, article 228, Article ID 228, 2016.

[23] C. Kosmidis, G. Pantos, C. Efthimiadis, I. Gkoutziomitrou, E. Georgakoudi, and G. Anthimidis, "Laparoscopic excision of a pedunculated uterine leiomyoma in torsion as a cause of acute abdomen at 10 weeks of pregnancy," *American Journal of Case Reports*, vol. 16, pp. 505–508, 2015.

[24] C. Saccardi, S. Visentin, M. Noventa, E. Cosmi, P. Litta, and S. Gizzo, "Uncertainties about laparoscopic myomectomy during pregnancy: a lack of evidence or an inherited misconception? A critical literature review starting from a peculiar case," *Minimally Invasive Therapy and Allied Technologies*, vol. 24, no. 4, pp. 189–194, 2015.

[25] M. Obara, Y. Hatakeyama, and Y. Shimizu, "Vaginal myomectomy for semipedunculated cervical myoma during pregnancy," *American Journal of Perinatology Reports*, vol. 4, no. 1, pp. 37–40, 2014.

[26] A. Currie, E. Bradley, M. McEwen, N. Al-Shabibi, and P. D. Willson, "Laparoscopic approach to fibroid torsion presenting as an acute abdomen in pregnancy," *Journal of the Society of Laparoendoscopic Surgeons*, vol. 17, no. 4, pp. 665–667, 2013.

[27] F. Kobayashi, E. Kondoh, J. Hamanishi, Y. Kawamura, K. Tatsumi, and I. Konishi, "Pyomayoma during pregnancy: a case report and review of the literature," *Journal of Obstetrics and Gynaecology Research*, vol. 39, no. 1, pp. 383–389, 2013.

[28] A. MacCiò, C. Madeddu, P. Kotsonis et al., "Three cases of laparoscopic myomectomy performed during pregnancy for

pedunculated uterine myomas," *Archives of Gynecology and Obstetrics*, vol. 286, no. 5, pp. 1209–1214, 2012.

[29] M. Shafiee, M. Nor Azlin, and D. Arifuddin, "A successful antenatal myomectomy," *Malaysian Family Physician*, vol. 31, no. 7(2-3), pp. 42–45, 2012.

[30] M. Ardovino, I. Ardovino, M. A. Castaldi, A. Monteverde, N. Colacurci, and L. Cobellis, "Laparoscopic myomectomy of a subserous pedunculated fibroid at 14 weeks of pregnancy: a case report," *Journal of Medical Case Reports*, vol. 5, article 545, 2011.

[31] A. Müller Vranjes, S. Sijanović, D. Vidosavljević, Z. Kasac, and K. Abicic Zuljević, "Surgical treatment of large smooth muscle tumor of uncertain malignant potential during pregnancy," *Medicinski Glasnik Journal*, vol. 8, no. 2, pp. 290–292, 2011.

[32] C. E. Son, J. S. Choi, J. H. Lee, S. W. Jeon, J. W. Bae, and S. S. Seo, "A case of laparoscopic myomectomy performed during pregnancy for subserosal uterine myoma," *Journal of Obstetrics and Gynaecology*, vol. 31, no. 2, pp. 180–181, 2011.

[33] M. Kasum, "Hemoperitoneum caused by a bleeding myoma in pregnancy," *Acta Clinica Croatica*, vol. 49, no. 2, pp. 197–200, 2010.

[34] F. Fanfani, C. Rossitto, A. Fagotti, P. Rosati, V. Gallotta, and G. Scambia, "Laparoscopic myomectomy at 25 weeks of pregnancy: case report," *Journal of Minimally Invasive Gynecology*, vol. 17, no. 1, pp. 91–93, 2010.

[35] A. S. Adeyemi, S. E. Akinola, and A. I. Isawumi, "Antepartum myomectomy with a live term delivery—a case report," *Nigerian Journal of Clinical Practice*, vol. 10, no. 4, pp. 346–348, 2007.

[36] J. E. N. Okonkwo and G. O. Udigwe, "Myomectomy in pregnancy," *Journal of Obstetrics and Gynaecology*, vol. 27, no. 6, pp. 628–630, 2007.

[37] L. Dracea and D. Codreanu, "Vaginal birth after extensive myomectomy during pregnancy in a 39-year-old nulliparous woman," *Journal of Obstetrics and Gynaecology*, vol. 26, no. 4, pp. 374–375, 2006.

[38] L. Melgrati, A. Damiani, G. Franzoni, M. Marziali, and F. Sesti, "Isobaric (gasless) laparoscopic myomectomy during pregnancy," *Journal of Minimally Invasive Gynecology*, vol. 12, no. 4, pp. 379–381, 2005.

[39] L. Sentilhes, F. Sergent, E. Verspyck, A. Gravier, H. Roman, and L. Marpeau, "Laparoscopic myomectomy during pregnancy resulting in septic necrosis of the myometrium," *BJOG: An International Journal of Obstetrics and Gynaecology*, vol. 110, no. 9, pp. 876–878, 2003.

[40] J. Donnez, C. Pirard, M. Smets, R. Polet, C. Feger, and J. Squifflet, "Unusual growth of a myoma during pregnancy," *Fertility and Sterility*, vol. 78, no. 3, pp. 632–633, 2002.

[41] H. Williamson, "Enucleation during the seventh lunar month of pregnancy of a uterine fibro-myoma," *Proceedings of the Royal Society of Medicine*, vol. 1, pp. 73–78, 1908.

[42] J. Stewart, "Enucleation of fibro-myoma of uterus during pregnancy," *British Medical Journal*, vol. 1, no. 2358, pp. 548–549, 1906.

[43] A. C. Wittich, E. R. Salminen, M. K. Yancey, and G. R. Markenson, "Myomectomy during early pregnancy," *Military Medicine*, vol. 165, no. 2, pp. 162–164, 2000.

[44] M. Majid, G. Q. Khan, and L. M. Wei, "Inevitable myomectomy in pregnancy," *Journal of Obstetrics and Gynaecology*, vol. 17, no. 4, pp. 377–378, 1997.

[45] A. C. Algara, A. G. Rodríguez, A. C. Vázquez et al., "Laparoscopic approach for fibroid removal at 18 weeks of pregnancy," *Surgical Technology International*, vol. 27, pp. 195–197, 2015.

[46] C. Lockyer, "Multiple myomectomy in the sixth month of pregnancy; labour at term," *Proceedings of the Royal Society of Medicine*, vol. 7, pp. 221–225, 1914.

[47] C. A. von Hoffmann, "Abdominal myomectomy during pregnancy," *California State Journal of Medicine*, vol. 9, no. 5, pp. 197–200, 1911.

[48] H. R. Andrews, "Myomectomy during pregnancy," *Proceedings of the Royal Society of Medicine*, vol. 3, pp. 164–166, 1910.

[49] WC. Swayne, "Abdominal myomectomy during pregnancy," *Proceedings of the Royal Society of Medicine*, vol. 1, pp. 129–132, 1908.

[50] A. Doran, "Myomectomy during pregnancy and labour at term in an elderly primipara: with notes on similar cases," *British Medical Journal*, vol. 2, no. 2395, pp. 1446–1447, 1906.

[51] H. M. Evans, "A case of myomectomy for subperitoneal myoma complicating pregnancy," *British Medical Journal*, vol. 2, no. 2033, p. 1673, 1899.

[52] C. Exacoustòs and P. Rosati, "Ultrasound diagnosis of uterine myomas and complications in pregnancy," *Obstetrics and Gynecology*, vol. 82, no. 1, pp. 97–101, 1993.

[53] C. A. Burton, D. A. Grimes, and C. M. March, "Surgical management of leiomyomata during pregnancy," *Obstetrics and Gynecology*, vol. 74, no. 5, pp. 707–709, 1989.

[54] R. Rella, E. Bonfadini Bossi, and D. Fagnani, "Myomectomy in pregnancy. Description of an interesting clinical case," *Minerva Ginecologica*, vol. 32, no. 4, pp. 267–269, 1980.

[55] M. A. Pelosi, M. A. Pelosi III, and S. Giblin, "Laparoscopic removal of a 1500-g symptomatic myoma during the second trimester of pregnancy," *American Association of Gynecologic Laparoscopists*, vol. 2, no. 4, pp. 457–462, 1995.

[56] A. Pelissier-Komorek, J. Hamm, S. Bonneau, E. Derniaux, C. Hoeffel-Fornes, and O. Graesslin, "Myoma and pregnancy: when medical treatment is not sufficient," *Journal de Gynecologie Obstetrique et Biologie de la Reproduction*, vol. 41, no. 3, pp. 307–310, 2012.

[57] G. Mollica, L. Pittini, E. Minganti, G. Perri, and F. Pansini, "Elective uterine myomectomy in pregnant women," *Clinical and Experimental Obstetrics and Gynecology*, vol. 23, no. 3, pp. 168–172, 1996.

[58] G. Febo, M. Tessarolo, L. Leo, S. Arduino, T. Wierdis, and L. Lanza, "Surgical management of leiomyomata in pregnancy," *Clinical and Experimental Obstetrics and Gynecology*, vol. 24, no. 2, pp. 76–78, 1997.

[59] M. Bonito, L. Gulemì, R. Basili, and D. Roselli, "Myomectomy during the first and second trimester of pregnancy," *Clinical and Experimental Obstetrics and Gynecology*, vol. 34, no. 3, pp. 149–150, 2007.

[60] E. E. Vázquez Camacho, E. Cabrera Carranco, and R. G. Sánchez Herrera, "Pedunculated twisted myoma and pregnancy. Case report," *Ginecologia y Obstetricia de Mexico*, vol. 77, no. 9, pp. 441–444, 2009.

[61] A. P. Makar, E. A. Schatteman, I. B. Vergote, and E. Desmedt, "Myomectomy during pregnancy: uncommon case report," *Acta Chirurgica Belgica*, vol. 89, no. 4, pp. 212–214, 1989.

[62] R. Horno Liria, "Myomectomy and pregnancy," *Rev Esp Obstet Ginecol*, vol. 19, pp. 214–218, 1962.

[63] M. C. Alanis, A. Mitra, and N. Koklanaris, "Preoperative magnetic resonance imaging and antepartum myomectomy of a giant pedunculated leiomyoma," *Obstetrics and Gynecology*, vol. 111, no. 2, part 2, pp. 577–579, 2008.

[64] G. Ardizzone, "Clinical and statistical considerations of 27 cases of myomectomy in pregnancy," *Rivista di Ostetricia e Ginecologia*, vol. 10, no. 12, pp. 848–860, 1955.

[65] M. Cozzi, "Myomectomy in pregnancy," *Quaderni di Clinica Ostetrica e Ginecologica*, vol. 22, no. 3, pp. 171–180, 1967.

[66] Y. Rochet, M. Cognat, D. Dargent, and E. Pollosson, "On myomectomy during pregnance (apropos of 14 observations)," *Bulletin de la Fèdèration des Sociètès de Gynècologie et Dòbstètrique de Langue Francaise*, vol. 16, pp. 462–463, 1964.

[67] F. Sciannameo, G. Madami, C. Madami et al., "Torsion of uterine fibroma associated with inguinal incarcerated hernia in pregnancy. Case report," *Minerva Ginecologica*, vol. 48, no. 11, pp. 501–504, 1996.

23

Absent Ductus Venosus Associated with Partial Liver Defect

Kenji Horie,[1] **Hironori Takahashi** ⓘ,[1] **Daisuke Matsubara,**[2] **Koichi Kataoka,**[2] **Rieko Furukawa,**[3] **Yosuke Baba** ⓘ,[1] **Akihide Ohkuchi** ⓘ,[1] **and Shigeki Matsubara** ⓘ[1]

[1]Department of Obstetrics and Gynecology, Jichi Medical University, Japan
[2]Department of Pediatrics, Jichi Medical University, Japan
[3]Department of Radiology, Jichi Medical University, Japan

Correspondence should be addressed to Hironori Takahashi; hironori@jichi.ac.jp

Academic Editor: Giovanni Monni

Absent ductus venosus (ADV) is a rare vascular anomaly. We describe a fetus/neonate with ADV with a partial liver defect. A 41-year-old woman was referred to our institute because of fetal cardiomegaly detected by routine prenatal ultrasound, which revealed absence of ductus venosus with an umbilical vein directly draining into the right atrium, consistent with extrahepatic drainage type of ADV. She vaginally gave birth to a 3,096-gram male infant at 38 weeks of gestation. Detailed ultrasound examination revealed a defect of the hepatic rectangular leaf at half a month postnatally. He showed normal development at 1.5 years of age with the liver abnormality and a Morgagni hernia. Liver morphological abnormality should also be considered as a complication of ADV.

1. Introduction

Absent ductus venous (ADV) occurs in 1/2,500 singleton pregnancies at a median gestation of 12^{+5} (range 11^{+0} to 13^{+6}) weeks [1]. This condition frequently accompanies various congenital abnormalities including cardiac anomaly, which may adversely influence the prognosis [2]. In ADV, the umbilical vein (UV) drains to the fetal systemic venous circulation through an intra- or extrahepatic route. This abnormal drainage often causes cardiac volume overload, leading to heart failure. The drainage type (intra- or extrahepatic) was reported to affect the prognosis of fetuses/infants with ADV [3].

Here, we describe a fetus/neonate prenatally diagnosed with the extrahepatic drainage type of ADV with a partial liver defect. This is, to our knowledge, the first report on ADV with this congenital abnormality.

2. Case Report

At the 30th gestational week, a 41-year-old (gravida 2, para 1 [normal vaginal delivery]) woman with no remarkable medical/family histories was referred to us because of fetal cardiomegaly detected on routine prenatal ultrasound. Fetal ultrasound revealed the absence of ductus venosus (DV) with the UV directly draining into the right atrium (Figure 1(a)), consistent with the extrahepatic drainage type of ADV. The cardiothoracic area ratio was 36.5%, within the normal range of <40% (Figure 1(b)) and heart valve regurgitation was absent. No cardiac structural abnormalities were detected, and cardiac functional parameters were normal. The parents did not desire fetal karyotyping, and, thus, amniocentesis was not performed. Direct UV flow into the systemic venous circulation (the right atrium) usually causes volume overload of the right heart, and thereby right heart failure, whose signs were carefully monitored, but they were not observed.

At 38^{+3} weeks, she showed the spontaneous onset of labor and vaginally gave birth to a 3,096-gram male infant (Apgar score 7/8 [1/5 min]). Neonatal cardiac ultrasound revealed mild aortic valve regurgitation and a slightly decreased ejection fraction, which were transient and disappeared on day 7. Detailed ultrasound examination revealed a defect of the hepatic rectangular leaf (S4: one of the largest liver leaves) at half a month postnatally. No findings indicative of liver dysfunction were observed throughout his course. Computed tomography at 1 year of age revealed atypical liver rotation with a Morgagni hernia in the liver (Figure 2). He showed normal development at 1.5 years of age.

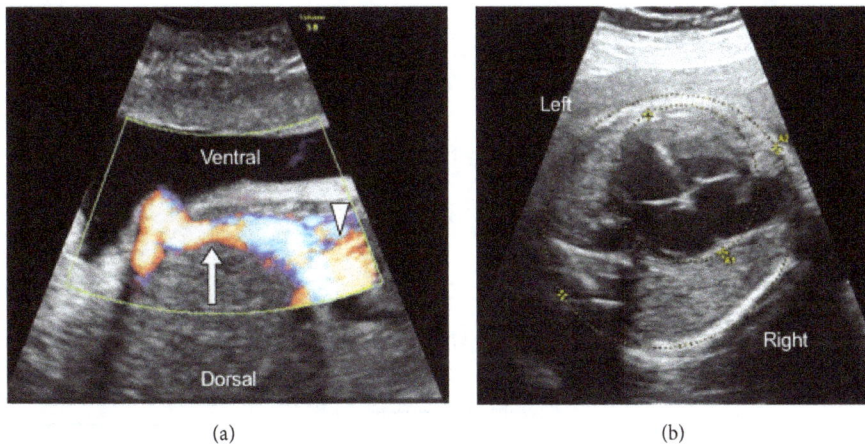

(a)   (b)

FIGURE 1: Prenatal ultrasound findings of a patient with absent ductus venosus. (a) The umbilical vein (arrow) directly flows into the right atrium (arrowhead). (b) The cardiothoracic area ratio was 36.5%.

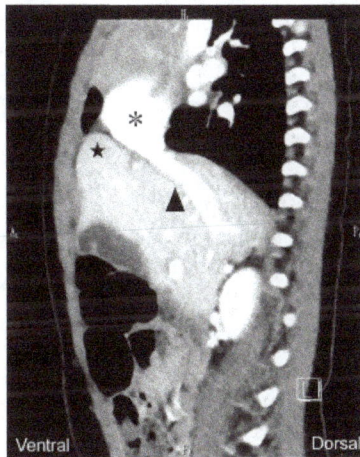

FIGURE 2: Abdominal computed tomography at 1 year of age. A Morgagni hernia (black star) can be seen, and the right atrium (asterisk) and inferior vena cava (arrowhead) are displaced on the ventral side.

3. Discussion

This is, to our knowledge, the first report of a patient with ADV accompanied by a partial liver defect. Detailed imaging analyses revealed this rare liver abnormality.

ADV is often complicated by various congenital abnormalities, associated or unassociated with chromosomal abnormalities. Congenital cardiac abnormalities are the most common, including ventricular septal defect, valve abnormalities, double outlet right ventricle, or coarctation of the aorta [2]. Various chromosomal abnormalities are also frequently observed in ADV. ADV without congenital/chromosomal abnormalities, namely, "isolated" ADV, accounts for 35-59% of all ADV [2–4]. Isolated ADV, compared with that complicated by congenital/chromosomal abnormalities, is usually associated with a better prognosis [4]. Since cardiac or chromosomal abnormality is a predominant complication and may be the main determinant of the prognosis, physicians may focus their attention on them, being less suspicious of other organ abnormalities. Here, we demonstrated that liver abnormality can coexist with ADV.

We believe that the partial liver defect is not a mere coincidence in the presence of ADV. This is because the liver and DV development are closely related. In the early developmental stage, there were two UVs, the right and left UVs, which run on the right and left sides of the liver (Figure 3(a)), with the right one disappearing during normal fetal development, and the left one eventually becoming DV, conveying oxygenated blood to the liver and inferior vena cava (Figure 3(b)). If there is some abnormality in this development/regression of the two-umbilical vein system, ADV occurs, in which oxygenated blood supply to the liver may decrease (Figure 3(c)). This insufficient blood supply to the liver (liver hypooxygenation) may cause malfunction/malsecretion of various differentiation-related substances including growth factors, cytokines, and proteins (e.g., Foxa1) [5]. As such, ADV may be closely related to liver development, and a partial liver defect may occur in association with ADV. Thus, we believe that the present liver abnormality may not be a coincidence but may be associated with ADV.

Persistent right UV and possibly its associated ADV with the partial liver defect may well explain the present patient's pathophysiology/etiology. However, patients with the persistence of right UV frequently have normal DV and some researchers considered this as statuses of normal anatomical variants [6]. A recent study revealed that 75% (9/12) of patients with the persistence of right UV were uneventful during delivery and postpartum period [7]. Thus, of patients with persistent right UV, some show normal DV without abnormalities (including liver abnormality) whereas others (the present case) show ADV and liver abnormalities. At present, we do not know the reason for this discrepancy. Possibly, various developmental factors (the time of derangement of normal regression of two UV system, its acuteness/abruptness, and its degree) may be associated with this. Further studies are necessary to clarify this issue.

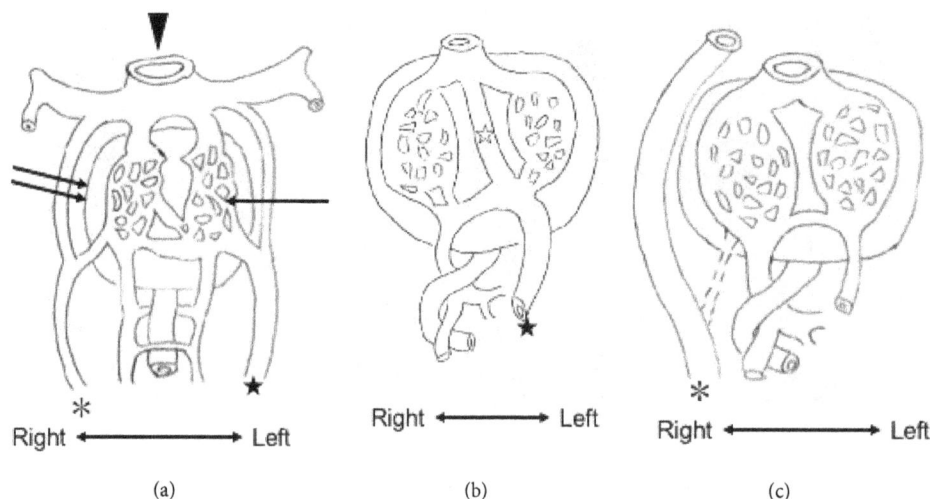

FIGURE 3: Proposed model of development in a patient with absent ductus venosus. (a) Normal fetal abdominal development at 5 weeks of gestation. Situs (arrowhead), hepatoblast (double arrows), liver sinusoid (arrow), left umbilical vein (black star), and right umbilical vein (asterisk) were indicated. (b) Normal development at 8 weeks of gestation. The right umbilical vein had regressed. Ductus venosus (DV) (white star) formed following development of the left umbilical vein (black star). (c) Abdominal development in a patient with extrahepatic absent ductus venosus at 8 weeks of gestation. The right umbilical vein (asterisk) persists and, thus, the flow of the left umbilical vein has decreased. Consequently, DV has not formed.

Putting aside this discussion, previous reports emphasized cardiac anomaly and little attention may have been paid to liver anomaly, there may have been some liver defects associated with ADV, but these remained unrecognized and unreported [2, 3]. Our patient also had a Morgagni hernia. This is an anterior right-sided defect of the diaphragm. A recent report described a Morgagni hernia concomitantly seen in a patient with ADV [8]. Considering the position of the hernia (anterior, right-sided), the hernia also may be associated with ADV.

Concerning its drainage route, ADV is divided into 2 types: intra- and extrahepatic drainage types, with the latter being in the present case. In the former intrahepatic type, the UV flow enters the liver, whereas in the latter extrahepatic type, it bypasses the liver and directly enters the inferior vena cava or right atrium. Extrahepatic ADV was correlated with a significantly poorer prognosis than intrahepatic ADV [3], which was also demonstrated by a recent review based on the largest study population to date [2]: nonsurvivors were more frequent in those with extra- than intrahepatic ADV. In extrahepatic ADV, large-volume flow directly enters the systemic circulation (the inferior vena cava or right atrium), which may lead to cardiac volume overload, causing heart failure [3, 9, 10]. Some part or all of the portal system will develop in a case with ADV. Its neighboring structure may vary with the type of ADV. The extrahepatic drainage may be more closely related to the liver defect.

We report a patient with the extrahepatic drainage type of ADV with a partial liver defect. Although it remains unclear whether this liver abnormality will affect this patient in later life, physicians should perform periodic ultrasound examination of patients with ADV. Liver morphological abnormality should also be considered as a complication of ADV, although whether its prenatal/postnatal diagnosis may affect the treatment strategy is unclear. Data accumulation is needed to determine the clinical significance of this liver abnormality associated with ADV.

Consent

Informed consent was obtained.

Authors' Contributions

Kenji Horie and Hironori Takahashi are equally contributed.

References

[1] I. Staboulidou, S. Pereira, J. De Jesus Cruz, A. Syngelaki, and K. H. Nicolaides, "Prevalence and outcome of absence of ductus venosus at 11 +0 to 13 +6 weeks," *Fetal Diagnosis and Therapy*, vol. 30, no. 1, pp. 35–40, 2011.

[2] A. Moaddab, G. Tonni, and G. Grisolia, "Predicting outcome in 259 fetuses with agenesis of ductus venosus: a multicenter experience and systematic review of the literature," *The Journal of Maternal-Fetal and Neonatal Medicine*, vol. 29, no. 22, pp. 3606–3614, 2016.

[3] C. Berg, D. Kamil, A. Geipel et al., "Absence of ductus venosus: importance of umbilical venous drainage site," *Ultrasound in Obstetrics & Gynecology*, vol. 28, no. 3, pp. 275–281, 2006.

[4] O. Shen, D. V. Valsky, B. Messing, S. M. Cohen, M. Lipschuetz, and S. Yagel, "Shunt diameter in agenesis of the ductus venosus

with extrahepatic portosystemic shunt impacts on prognosis," *Ultrasound in Obstetrics & Gynecology*, vol. 37, no. 2, pp. 184–190, 2011.

[5] C. S. Lee, J. R. Friedman, J. T. Fulmer, and K. H. Kaestner, "The initiation of liver development is dependent on Foxa transcription factors," *Nature*, vol. 435, no. 7044, pp. 944–947, 2005.

[6] R. Martinez, F. Gamez, C. Bravo et al., "Perinatal outcome after ultrasound prenatal diagnosis of persistent right umbilical vein," *European Journal of Obstetrics & Gynecology and Reproductive Biology*, vol. 168, no. 1, pp. 36–39, 2013.

[7] A. Krzyżanowski, D. Swatowski, T. Gęca et al., "Prenatal diagnosis of persistent right umbilical vein - Incidence and clinical impact. A prospective study," *Australian and New Zealand Journal of Obstetrics and Gynaecology*.

[8] P. C. Chen, J. C. Swanson, P. Masand, J. R. Rodriguez, and C. M. Mery, "Diaphragmatic Hernia Associated With Absent Ductus Venosus and Anomalous Connection of an Obliterated Umbilical Vein to the Coronary Sinus," *World Journal for Pediatric and Congenital Heart Surgery*, p. 2150135117710920, 2017.

[9] E. T. Jaeggi, J.-C. Fouron, L. K. Hornberger et al., "Agenesis of the ductus venosus that is associated with extrahepatic umbilical vein drainage: Prenatal features and clinical outcome," *American Journal of Obstetrics & Gynecology*, vol. 187, no. 4, pp. 1031–1037, 2002.

[10] R. J. Acherman, R. C. Rollins, W. J. Castillo, and W. N. Evans, "Stenosis of alternative umbilical venous pathways in absence of the ductus venosus," *Journal of Ultrasound in Medicine*, vol. 29, no. 8, pp. 1227–1231, 2010.

24

A Discussion of High-Risk HPV in a 6-Year-Old Female Survivor of Child Sexual Abuse

Connie D. Cao,[1] **Lena Merjanian,**[2] **Joelle Pierre,**[3] **and Adrian Balica**[2]

[1]*Rutgers Robert Wood Johnson Medical School, Rutgers University, New Brunswick, NJ, USA*
[2]*Department of Obstetrics, Gynecology, and Reproductive Sciences, Rutgers Robert Wood Johnson Medical School, Rutgers University, New Brunswick, NJ, USA*
[3]*Department of Surgery, Rutgers Robert Wood Johnson Medical School, Rutgers University, New Brunswick, NJ, USA*

Correspondence should be addressed to Lena Merjanian; merjanle@rutgers.edu

Academic Editor: Massimo Origoni

Background. Human papilloma viruses (HPVs) cause a variety of clinical manifestations in children including skin warts, laryngeal papillomas, and condyloma acuminatum. Whereas the mode of transmission is well understood and management of HPV infection is clearly defined by guidelines in adults, less is known about the mode of transmission, natural history of disease, and appropriate management of high-risk anogenital HPV infections in children. *Case.* The patient is a previously healthy 6-year-old female who presented with multiple vaginal lesions causing pain and discomfort and was diagnosed with HPV 18 positive CIN I. *Summary and Conclusion.* Children infected with high-risk HPV subtypes remain a vulnerable patient population, and there is minimal literature on the natural history of disease and effects of overtreatment. Based on a literature review, conservative management, HPV vaccination, and consideration of the cervical cancer screening guidelines for adolescent females are an appropriate treatment course until more studies are reported on cervical cancer screening in survivors of child sexual abuse.

1. Introduction

Human papilloma viruses (HPVs) are a family of small double-stranded DNA viruses, of which 30–40 genotypes infect the genital tract. The virus infects epithelial cells through abrasion of the skin or mucosa and can exist as a latent infection [1]. Low-risk types 6 and 11 are common causes of condyloma acuminatum. High-risk mucosal HPV types 16 and 18 have been implicated in the development of cervical, vulvar, penile, and pharyngeal malignancies. In children, there are several possible modes of transmission including perinatal vertical transmission, autoinoculation from nongenital cutaneous warts to the genitalia, and heteroinoculation from one individual to another; however, the observation of anogenital warts in children should trigger an evaluation for sexual abuse [1].

Little is known about the natural progression of high-risk HPV infection in children. It has been suggested that young children may be monitored for malignancy in a similar manner to adolescent females [1, 2]. Previous studies have demonstrated that adolescent and young women who test HPV positive with abnormal cervical cytologies can be managed with close follow-up and conservative management. Here, we discuss a pediatric patient who presented with vaginal lesions causing urinary discomfort following confirmed sexual abuse. The patient ultimately tested positive for HPV 18 and was diagnosed with CIN I.

2. Case Report

The patient is a premenarchal, 6-year-old female who presented to the emergency department (ED) with her mother because of mild discomfort with urination and "pimples" causing pain in the vaginal area. The patient was previously healthy and denied increased urinary frequency or urgency, vaginal bleeding, vaginal discharge, malaise, and fever. The patient and her mother denied inappropriate contact or touching. On physical examination, the patient was comfortable, smiling, and playful. The external pelvic examination was notable for multiple raised lesions on the labia minora

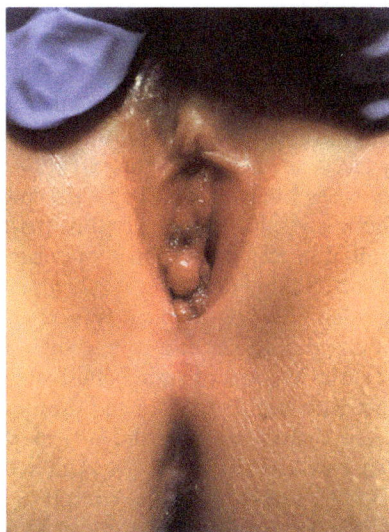

FIGURE 1: Photograph of the condylomas prior to excision.

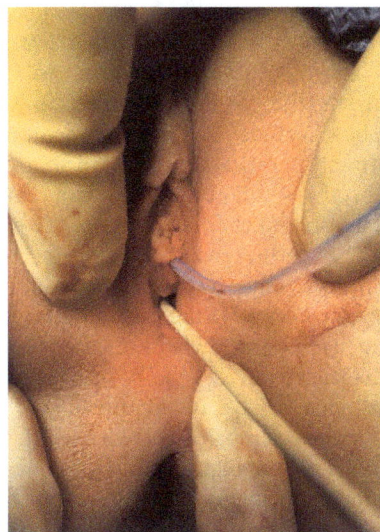

FIGURE 2: Photograph of the genital area after excision, with visualization of the urethra and vaginal introitus.

and erythema of the external genitalia. No vesicles or vaginal discharge were observed. At the ED, a clinical diagnosis of genital warts was made.

Social Work and the Department of Child Protection and Permanency were contacted. The patient and her mother were referred to a state-designated child protection center that provides crisis intervention and child abuse assessments. At the state-designated child protection center, a team of trained professionals conducted an evaluation and was able to ascertain a history of abuse from the patient by an adult, male family member living in the household. The center conducted a thorough physical examination and infection screening.

Two months after initial presentation and evaluation at the child protection center, the patient's symptoms worsened secondary to an increase in the size of the lesion. The patient was able to urinate but unable to sleep at night secondary to pain and irritation caused by rubbing. On examination, the patient had warts in the vestibule that carpeted the space between the labia minora and fourchette, obliterated the vaginal introitus, and appeared to obscure the urethra.

The patient then underwent an exam under anesthesia (EUA) and excision of vaginal lesions, as seen in Figure 1, in the lithotomy position by pediatric surgery and the gynecological team. Direct visualization of the area, without use of a hysteroscope, did not reveal any gross internal vaginal lesions. A sterile urinary catheter was placed. The condylomas were removed using smooth pickups and Metzenbaum scissors with careful visualization of the urethra, as in Figure 2. First, a 2 cm area of condyloma at the inferior portion of the vaginal introitus was removed. A second 2-3 cm lesion around the urethral meatus and third small lesion of the right labia minor were excised. Hemostasis was achieved with pressure and Surgiflo at the excision sites. A Vaginal ThinPrep Pap Test was performed and resulted in HPV 18 positive and low grade squamous intraepithelial lesion (LSIL) including cellular changes associated with HPV and cervical intraepithelial neoplasia I (CIN I). The surgical pathology

consisted of red-tan, glistening, soft tissue that measured $1.2 \times 1 \times 0.4$ cm when aggregated and was determined to be condyloma acuminatum. The patient was awakened from anesthesia and brought to the recovery room in stable condition.

At the postoperative follow-up visit, the mother and patient reported a smooth recovery with minimal pain. Exam of the surgical site in the supine frog-leg position showed that it was well healed with minimal residual disease. The patient was instructed to follow up with gynecology every 6 months and with pediatric surgery as needed. Given this patient falls outside CDC guidelines for vaccination and her pathology results, we plan to recommend HPV vaccination at the patient's next visit [3, 4].

3. Summary and Conclusion

The detection of a sexually transmitted infection (STI) in a child should raise suspicion for sexual abuse. Genital or anal condyloma acuminatum appearing for the first time in a child older than 5 years is likely to be the result of sexual transmission [5]. There is minimal safety and efficacy data on the medical treatment options for condyloma acuminatum in children younger than 12 years of age [6]. A retrospective chart-review study concluded that approximately half of the cases of anogenital warts in children spontaneously resolve [6]. As a result, nonintervention is a reasonable initial management approach for asymptomatic condylomas. Treatment options for symptomatic anogenital warts in children include local excision, laser-based ablation, cryotherapy, chemical ablation with trichloroacetic acid, podofilox gel, and imiquimod 5% cream [1]. For this patient, local excision was reasonable as the genital warts were large enough to cause symptoms. Since recurrence is possible with any treatment modality, long-term follow-up for children with anogenital warts is recommended.

While little is known about the epidemiology of HPV in children, one study demonstrated that 16% (5/31 girls) of child sex abuse victims are infected with HPV [2]. Factors associated with genital HPV infection as a result of child sexual abuse include female gender, genital warts, and increasing certainty of sexual abuse [7]. Currently, there have been no prospective studies conducted on a group of HPV-infected sexually abused children to assess the effects of age and immaturity of the reproductive tract on the course of HPV infection. As a result, researchers have proposed using studies of adolescents who voluntarily initiate sexual activity at the age of menarche as a guide to disease progression and appropriate management [2].

HPV infections behave differently in adolescent and young women when compared to older adult women [8]. Two explanations for the high rate of HPV infection in the adolescent population include the propensity for multiple sexual partners and physiology of the adolescent cervix. Hormonal changes during puberty cause cervical epithelial changes including metaplasia and the formation of a transformation zone, where squamous epithelial cells replace cervical columnar epithelial cells. Specifically, a rapid rate of squamous metaplasia was found to be a risk factor for the development of LSIL in HPV positive young women [9]. Additionally, less protective cervical mucous and larger size of the cervical ectropion during early adolescence increase the biological vulnerability of young women to genital HPV infection [10]. It has also been suggested that earlier sexual activity accelerates the process of cervical maturation [8].

The Papanicolaou (Pap) test is a screening tool for cervical cancer and has reduced the mortality rates of cervical cancer in the United States [11]. The Bethesda system standardizes reporting of cervical and vaginal cytology diagnoses by categorizing abnormal cytologies into four categories: atypical squamous cells (ASC), LSIL, high-grade squamous intraepithelial lesions (HSIL), and atypical glandular cells (AGC). With the Bethesda reporting in hand, clinicians apply the American Society of Colposcopy and Cervical Pathology algorithm for the management of abnormal Pap smears [12]. Current guidelines recommend beginning cervical cancer screening starting at the age of 21 every 3 years and HPV DNA cotesting starting at the age of 30 every 5 years [13].

These guidelines were based on studies of HPV in young women, which can provide insight regarding the management of this 6-year-old female since the natural progression of HPV in victims of child sexual abuse is not known. Although adolescent and young women have higher rates of HPV infection than older adult women, they are also more likely to clear the infection. One study noted that 65–75% of adolescent and young women were found to test negative for HPV DNA by 30 months. The same study suggested chronic HPV infection might be correlated with oncogenic, high-risk HPV viral types, indicating that high-risk viral types may more effectively evade the immune system [14]. Additionally, only 3% of young women with LSIL progressed to precancerous lesions [15]. Similarly, a different study indicated that 75% of the youngest adolescents (<16 years old) with CIN 2 had regressed within 2 years of follow-up [16]. Thus, conservative management is appropriate initial

management in adolescent girls and young women with LSIL and commonly transient HPV infection [17].

Victims of child sex abuse are an especially vulnerable population for several reasons. Often, as in this case, the sexual abuse begins prior to the age at which HPV vaccinations are routinely given; the FDA has approved HPV vaccination starting at the age of 9 in females. This patient endured sexual abuse at a young age, placing a longer time period between the time of initial infection with HPV and onset of routine cervical cancer screening at the age of 21 [4]. Moreover, a consequence of child sex abuse often is increased high-risk behavior associated with cervical cancer such as sex work and substance use. Victims of sexual abuse are more likely to lose contact with health services and drop out from the education system than women who did not experience abuse. An Australian case-control study has identified unwanted sexual experiences involving genital contact as a potential prognostic factor for invasive cervical cancer by 25 years of age [3]. Even though the efficacy of the HPV vaccine decreases from 100% to 44% in those already exposed to HPV genotypes, it is imperative that the HPV vaccine is administered to victims of child sexual abuse soon after the abuse is reported [3, 4].

This case of a 6-year-old female victim of child sexual abuse infected with high-risk HPV highlights a vulnerable patient population where there is minimal understanding of the natural course of HPV infection and appropriate management. Further study is needed to ascertain the optimal management and appropriate time to perform a Pap smear [18]. In this case, the need to follow-up with the patient should be balanced with the anxiety and effect of psychosexual morbidity associated with increased cervical screening and colposcopy at such a young age [19]. Although young females are more likely to clear HPV infections than adults, a history of sexual abuse contributes additional risk factors for cervical cancer. Based on the review of the literature on HPV infection in adolescents and young women, we recommend close patient follow-up with gynecology and pediatric surgery for an exam of the external genitalia, with EUA and excision of condyloma as needed. We will consider starting cervical cancer screening at an earlier age of 18 years in such patients and HPV vaccination prior to the age of nine [3, 4].

Acknowledgments

The authors thank the parent of the patient for providing informed consent to share this case.

References

[1] S. H. Sinal and C. R. Woods, "Human papillomavirus infections of the genital and respiratory tracts in young children," *Seminars in Pediatric Infectious Diseases*, vol. 16, no. 4, pp. 306–316, 2005.

[2] C. Stevens-Simon, D. Nelligan, P. Breese, C. Jenny, and J. M. Douglas Jr., "The prevalence of genital human papillomavirus infections in abused and nonabused preadolescent girls," *Pediatrics*, vol. 106, no. 4, pp. 645–649, 2000.

[3] Y. L. Jayasinghe, V. Sasongko, R. W. Lim et al., "The association between unwanted sexual experiences and early-onset cervical cancer and precancer by age 25: a case-control study," *Journal of Women's Health (Larchmt)*, 2016.

[4] S. M. Garland, A. K. Subasinghe, Y. L. Jayasinghe et al., "HPV vaccination for victims of childhood sexual abuse," *The Lancet*, vol. 386, no. 10007, pp. 1919-1920, 2015.

[5] J. A. Adams, N. D. Kellogg, K. J. Farst et al., "Updated guidelines for the medical assessment and care of children who may have been sexually abused," *Journal of Pediatric and Adolescent Gynecology*, vol. 29, no. 2, pp. 81–87, 2016.

[6] A. L. Allen and E. C. Siegfried, "The natural history of condyloma in children," *Journal of the American Academy of Dermatology*, vol. 39, no. 6, pp. 951–955, 1998.

[7] E. R. Unger, N. N. Fajman, E. M. Maloney et al., "Anogenital human papillomavirus in sexually abused and nonabused children: A multicenter study," *Pediatrics*, vol. 128, no. 3, pp. e658–e665, 2011.

[8] A. B. Moscicki, "Impact of HPV infection in adolescent populations," *Journal of Adolescent Health*, vol. 37, no. 6, supplement, pp. S3–S9, 2005.

[9] A.-B. Moscicki, V. Grubbs Burt, S. Kanowitz, T. Darragh, and S. Shiboski, "The significance of squamous metaplasia in the development of low grade squamous intraepithelial lesions in young women," *Cancer*, vol. 85, no. 5, pp. 1139–1144, 1999.

[10] M. L. Shew, J. D. Fortenberry, P. Miles, and A. J. Amortegui, "Interval between menarche and first sexual intercourse, related to risk of human papillomavirus infection," *The Journal of Pediatrics*, vol. 125, no. 4, pp. 661–666, 1994.

[11] K. Moore, A. Cofer, L. Elliot, G. Lanneau, J. Walker, and M. A. Gold, "Adolescent cervical dysplasia: histologic evaluation, treatment, and outcomes," *American Journal of Obstetrics & Gynecology*, vol. 197, no. 2, pp. e141–e146, 2007.

[12] D. Saslow, D. Solomon, H. W. Lawson et al., "American Cancer Society, American Society for Colposcopy and Cervical Pathology, and American Society for Clinical Pathology screening guidelines for the prevention and early detection of cervical cancer," *American Journal of Clinical Pathology*, vol. 137, no. 4, pp. 516–542, 2012.

[13] Committee on Practice B-G, "Practice bulletin no. 168: cervical cancer screening and prevention," *Obstetrics & Gynecology*, vol. 128, no. 4, pp. e111–e130, 2016.

[14] A. B. Moscicki, S. Shiboski, J. Broering et al., "The natural history of human papillomavirus infection as measured by repeated DNA testing in adolescent and young women," *Journal of Pediatrics*, vol. 132, no. 2, pp. 277–284, 1998.

[15] A.-B. Moscicki, S. Shiboski, N. K. Hills et al., "Regression of low-grade squamous intra-epithelial lesions in young women," *The Lancet*, vol. 364, no. 9446, pp. 1678–1683, 2004.

[16] K. Fuchs, S. Weitzen, L. Wu, M. G. Phipps, and L. A. Boardman, "Management of cervical intraepithelial neoplasia 2 in adolescent and young women," *Journal of Pediatric and Adolescent Gynecology*, vol. 20, no. 5, pp. 269–274, 2007.

[17] G. Y. F. Ho, R. Bierman, L. Beardsley, C. J. Chang, and R. D. Burk, "Natural history of cervicovaginal papillomavirus infection in young women," *The New England Journal of Medicine*, vol. 338, no. 7, pp. 423–428, 1998.

[18] D. Marcoux, K. Nadeau, C. McCuaig, J. Powell, and L. L. Oligny, "Pediatric anogenital warts: a 7-year review of children referred to a tertiary-care hospital in Montreal, Canada," *Pediatric Dermatology*, vol. 23, no. 3, pp. 199–207, 2006.

[19] A. Szarewski and P. Sasieni, "Cervical screening in adolescents—at least do no harm," *The Lancet*, vol. 364, no. 9446, pp. 1642–1644, 2004.

25

Placenta Accreta following Hysteroscopic Lysis of Adhesions Caused by Asherman's Syndrome: A Case Report and Literature Review

Yuko Sonan (ID),[1] **Shigeru Aoki,**[1] **Kimiko Enomoto,**[1] **Kazuo Seki,**[1] **and Etsuko Miyagi**[2]

[1]*Perinatal Maternity and Neonatal Center of Yokohama City University Medical Center, Yokohama, Japan*
[2]*Department of Obstetrics and Gynecology, Yokohama City University Hospital, Yokohama, Japan*

Correspondence should be addressed to Yuko Sonan; aiu525@yahoo.co.jp

Academic Editor: Julio Rosa-e-Silva

Asherman's syndrome is defined as partial or complete obstruction of the uterine cavity primarily caused by intrauterine procedures and infections. Hysteroscopic adhesiolysis is commonly used to treat Asherman's syndrome. Although the frequency of placenta accreta is known to increase with pregnancy after hysteroscopic adhesiolysis, precise data remain unknown. We report a case of placenta accreta following hysteroscopic lysis of adhesions caused by Asherman's syndrome and IVF treatment and review the literature on placenta accreta following hysteroscopic adhesiolysis. It is necessary to consider placenta accreta as a complication of pregnancies after hysteroscopic adhesiolysis for Asherman's syndrome, particularly in those conceived using IVF.

1. Introduction

Asherman's syndrome is defined as partial or complete obstruction of the uterine cavity due to damage to the basal layer of the endometrium [1, 2] and is primarily caused by intrauterine procedures and infections often associated with miscarriage or curettage for postpartum placental retention [1].

Hysteroscopic adhesiolysis is commonly used to treat Asherman's syndrome. Although the frequency of placenta accreta is known to increase with pregnancy after hysteroscopic adhesiolysis, precise data remain unknown.

Here, we report a case of placenta accreta following hysteroscopic lysis of adhesions caused by Asherman's syndrome and IVF treatment and review the literature on placenta accreta following hysteroscopic adhesiolysis.

2. Case Presentation

The patient was a 40-year-old primiparous woman. She was diagnosed with submucosal fibroids by her previous gynecologist 5 years prior, based on chief complaints of atypical genital bleeding and hypermenorrhea. She underwent hysteroscopic myomectomy for one 1 cm sized and one 3 cm sized submucosal fibroid located between 2 and 3 o'clock in the uterine fundus. Asherman's syndrome was suspected after the patient exhibited secondary hypomenorrhea 10 months after surgery. Therefore, hysterosalpingography and magnetic resonance imaging (MRI) were performed. Intrauterine adhesions were suspected based on hysterosalpingography findings, while uterine cavity narrowing was identified using MRI. Hysteroscopy revealed filmy adhesions consistent with myomatous tissue at the excision site, and the patient was diagnosed with Asherman's syndrome.

Eight months after diagnosis, the patient underwent hysteroscopic adhesiolysis. The filmy adhesions observed on the left side of the fundus were easily separated with Hegar cervical dilators, and an intrauterine device was inserted after dilation. The patient was diagnosed with stage I Asherman's syndrome defined by European Society for Hysteroscopy classification of intrauterine adhesions, and menstrual flow returned to normal after the operation.

While the patient had a strong desire to bear children, her inability to conceive for 7 years led her to pursue in vitro fertilization (IVF). After having a miscarriage at 7 weeks

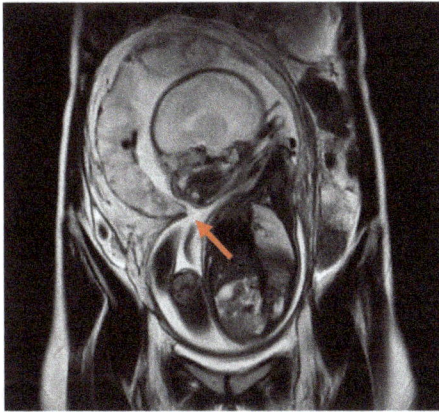

FIGURE 1: Semicircular stenosis, thought to influence adhesions in the uterus, was confirmed, and amniotic membrane sheets (tissues with a free edge visualized within the amniotic cavity) were identified (arrow).

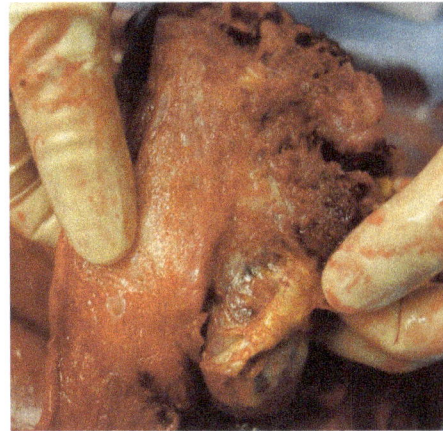

FIGURE 3: Resected uterus: placenta is present from the fundus to the posterior uterine wall. The placenta adheres diffusely to the myometrium, and partial thinning is visible at the fundus.

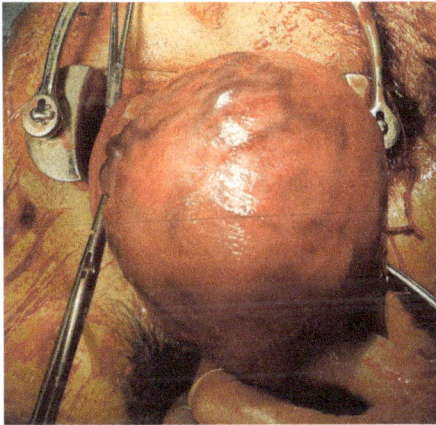

FIGURE 2: Intraoperative finding: blood vessels on the uterine surface at the placental implantation site are engorged.

of gestation, she underwent cervical dilatation and uterine curettage.

Six months after the miscarriage, the patient became pregnant again through IVF and was referred to our hospital at 7 weeks of gestation. At 19 weeks of gestation, tissues with a free edge were visualized within the amniotic cavity using obstetric ultrasound and were determined to be amniotic sheets on MRI at 31 weeks of gestation (Figure 1). The course of pregnancy was uneventful thereafter, and an elective cesarean section was performed at 38 weeks and 2 days of gestation because of a breech presentation.

The placenta adhered to the uterine wall after childbirth and could not be easily separated manually. The blood vessels on the uterine surface at the placental implantation site were engorged (Figure 2), leading us to diagnose the patient with placenta increta. The placenta remained firmly adherent to the uterine wall, and although there was almost no bleeding from the uterine cavity, cesarean hysterectomy was performed after informed consent was obtained from the patient. In the abdominal cavity, 4 cm subserosal uterine

fibroids were observed on the left side of the fundus, and adhesions thought to be caused by endometriosis were found in the right adnexa, posterior uterus, and anterior rectum. The operative time was 101 minutes, while the total blood loss was 1,584 ml (including amniotic fluid). Blood transfusion was not required. Macroscopic examination of the uterus after extraction showed the presence of placenta from the fundus to the posterior wall, diffusely adherent to the myometrium (Figure 3), along with partial thinning of the fundus.

Placenta increta was confirmed based on postpartum histological findings of placental villi invading the myometrium, without an interposed decidual plate.

The postoperative course was uneventful, and the patient was discharged in good health on the 7th postpartum day.

3. Discussion

This case highlights two points: placenta accreta must be considered as a potential complication in pregnancies after hysteroscopic adhesiolysis for Asherman's syndrome, and IVF may further increase the risk of placenta accreta.

First, we should be aware of the possibility of placental implantation disorders, placenta accrete in particular in pregnancies following hysteroscopic adhesiolysis. This patient underwent hysteroscopic adhesiolysis for intrauterine adhesions. Although approximately 90% of intrauterine adhesions are associated with intrauterine curettage in pregnant women, they can also occur in a nongravid uterus as a result of procedures like myomectomy and curettage that damage the endometrium [13]. Intrauterine adhesions are among the main long-term complications associated with hysteroscopic myomectomy [14], and Al-Inany [13] reported that multiple myomectomies are more likely to cause intrauterine adhesions than a single myomectomy. The amniotic sheets observed in this case may have been related to the intrauterine adhesions resulting from hysteroscopic myomectomy and the D&C performed because of a miscarriage.

TABLE 1: Pregnancies after hysteroscopic adhesiolysis.

Study	Delivery following hysteroscopic adhesiolysis, n	Adherent placenta, n (%)	Placenta accreta, n (%)	Postpartum hemorrhage, n (%)
Chen et al. (2017) [1]	140	6 (4.3)	3 (2.1)	11 (7.9)
Fernandez et al. (2006) [2]	21	0	3 (14.3)	3 (14.3)
Roy et al. (2010) [3]	32	3 (9.4)	1 (3.1)	5 (12.5)
Yu et al. (2008) [4]	25	3 (12.0)	2 (8.0)	-
Zikopoulos et al. (2004) [5]	20	0	2 (10.0)	-
Capella-Allouc et al. (1999) [6]	9	0	2 (22.2)	-
Bhandari et al. (2015) [7]	10	1 (10.0)	0	1 (10.0)
Liu et al. (2014) [8]	49	1 (2.0)	2 (4.1)	2 (4.1)
Katz et al. (1996) [9]	59	0	0	0
Friedman et al. (1986) [10]	23	1 (8.7)	1 (8.7)	-
Valle and Sciarra (1988) [11]	114	-	1 (0.88)	-
Feng et al. (1999) [12]	145	1 (0.7)	0	-
Total	647	16 (2.5)	17 (2.6)	22 (3.4)

Table 1 shows the results of a literature review performed by searching MEDLINE for pregnancy outcomes following hysteroscopic adhesiolysis for Asherman's syndrome [1–12]. Although the reported frequency of subsequent placenta accreta varies, a review of 12 studies published between 1986 and 2016 showed that 647 of such pregnancies ended in live birth. Of these, 17 women were diagnosed with placenta accreta, at a rate of 2.6% (17/647). Additionally, many, but not all, cases described adherent placenta and retained placenta without concomitant placenta accreta. Xiao et al. [15] reported that 64/201 cases (31.8%) had retained placenta, adherent placenta, or placenta accreta, and postpartum hemorrhage (PPH) occurred in 127/221 (63.2%) cases, suggesting that not only placenta accreta but also PPH must be considered in pregnancies after hysteroscopic adhesiolysis.

Second, IVF may increase the risk of placenta accreta. The incidence of placenta accreta is significantly higher in IVF pregnancies than in spontaneous pregnancies [16]. Esh-Broder et al. [16] reported that the rate of placenta accreta in spontaneous pregnancies was 12/752 (1.2/1000), while that in IVF pregnancies was 30/24,441 (16/1,000). The higher rate of placenta accreta in IVF pregnancies may be due to the change in endometrial environment and morphological and structural changes to the endometrium due to the IVF treatment protocol (stimulation protocol) [16].

Intrauterine adhesions (IUA) severity is associated with greater reduction in fertility [1, 3, 17], thereby increasing the likelihood that affected patients will need to undergo IVF to have a successful pregnancy. The extent of endometrial loss increases with IUA severity, which likely confers a greater risk of placenta accreta. For this reason, doctors should be aware that IVF pregnancy following hysteroscopic adhesiolysis involves a greater risk of placenta accreta.

4. Conclusion

Placenta accreta should be considered as a complication of pregnancies after hysteroscopic adhesiolysis for Asherman's syndrome, particularly in those conceived using IVF.

Authors' Contributions

Yuko Sonan and Shigeru Aoki contributed to the study design and finalization of the manuscript. Kimiko Enomoto and Kazuo Seki wrote the first draft of the manuscript. Etsuko Miyagi provided the study design and supervised the study.

References

[1] L. Chen, H. Zhang, Q. Wang et al., "Reproductive Outcomes in Patients With Intrauterine Adhesions Following Hysteroscopic Adhesiolysis: Experience From the Largest Women's Hospital in China," *Journal of Minimally Invasive Gynecology*, vol. 24, no. 2, pp. 299–304, 2017.

[2] H. Fernandez, F. Al-Najjar, A. Chauveaud-Lambling, R. Frydman, and A. Gervaise, "Fertility after treatment of Asherman's syndrome stage 3 and 4," *Journal of Minimally Invasive Gynecology*, vol. 13, no. 5, pp. 398–402, 2006.

[3] K. K. Roy, J. Baruah, J. B. Sharma, S. Kumar, G. Kachawa, and N. Singh, "Reproductive outcome following hysteroscopic adhesiolysis in patients with infertility due to Asherman's syndrome," *Archives of Gynecology and Obstetrics*, vol. 281, no. 2, pp. 355–361, 2010.

[4] D. Yu, T. C. Li, E. Xia, X. Huang, Y. Liu, and X. Peng, "Factors affecting reproductive outcome of hysteroscopic adhesiolysis

for Asherman's syndrome," *Fertility and Sterility*, vol. 89, no. 3, pp. 715–722, 2008.

[5] K. A. Zikopoulos, E. M. Kolibianakis, P. Platteau et al., "Live delivery rates in subfertile women with Asherman's syndrome after hysteroscopic adhesiolysis using the resectoscope or the Versapoint system," *Reproductive BioMedicine Online*, vol. 8, no. 6, pp. 720–725, 2004.

[6] S. Capella-Allouc, F. Morsad, C. Rongières-Bertrand, S. Taylor, and H. Fernandez, "Hysteroscopic treatment of severe Asherman's syndrome and subsequent fertility," *Human Reproduction*, vol. 14, no. 5, pp. 1230–1233, 1999.

[7] S. Bhandari, P. Bhave, I. Ganguly, A. Baxi, and P. Agarwal, "Reproductive outcome of patients with Asherman's syndrome: A SAIMS experience," *Journal of Reproduction and Infertility*, vol. 16, no. 4, pp. 229–235, 2015.

[8] X. Liu, H. Duan, and Y. Wang, "Clinical characteristics and reproductive outcome following hysteroscopic adhesiolysis of patients with intrauterine adhesion–a retrospective study," *Clinical and Experimental Obstetrics and Gynecology*, vol. 41, pp. 144–148, 2014.

[9] Z. Katz, A. Ben-Arie, S. Lurie, M. Manor, and V. Insler, "Reproductive outcome following hysteroscopic adhesiolysis in Asherman's syndrome," *International Journal of Fertility and Menopausal Studies*, vol. 41, no. 5, pp. 462–465, 1996.

[10] A. Friedman, J. Defazio, and A. Decherney, "Severe obstetric complications after aggressive treatment of asherman syndrome," *Obstetrics & Gynecology*, vol. 67, no. 6, pp. 864–867, 1986.

[11] R. F. Valle and J. J. Sciarra, "Intrauterine adhesions: hysteroscopic diagnosis, classification, treatment, and reproductive outcome," *American Journal of Obstetrics & Gynecology*, vol. 158, no. 6I, pp. 1459–1470, 1988.

[12] Z. C. Feng, B. Yang, J. Shao, and S. Liu, "Diagnostic and therapeutic hysteroscopy for traumatic intrauterine adhesions after induced abortions: clinical analysis of 365 cases," *Gynaecological Endoscopy*, vol. 8, no. 2, pp. 95–98, 1999.

[13] H. Al-Inany, "Intrauterine adhesions: an update," *Acta Obstetricia et Gynecologica Scandinavica*, vol. 80, no. 11, pp. 986–993, 2001.

[14] O. Taskin, S. Sadik, A. Onoglu et al., "Role of endometrial suppression on the frequency of intrauterine adhesions after resectoscopic surgery," *The Journal of Minimally Invasive Gynecology*, vol. 7, no. 3, pp. 351–354, 2000.

[15] S. Xiao, Y. Wan, M. Xue et al., "Etiology, treatment, and reproductive prognosis of women with moderate-to-severe intrauterine adhesions," *International Journal of Gynecology and Obstetrics*, vol. 125, no. 2, pp. 121–124, 2014.

[16] E. Esh-Broder, I. Ariel, N. Abas-Bashir, Y. Bdolah, and D. H. Celnikier, "Placenta accreta is associated with IVF pregnancies: A retrospective chart review," *BJOG: An International Journal of Obstetrics & Gynaecology*, vol. 118, no. 9, pp. 1084–1089, 2011.

[17] J. Zhao, Q. Chen, D. Cai, Z. Duan, X. Li, and X. Xue, "Dominant factors affecting reproductive outcomes of fertility-desiring young women with intrauterine adhesions," *Archives of Gynecology and Obstetrics*, vol. 295, no. 4, pp. 923–927, 2017.

26

Placental Chorangiosis: Increased Risk for Cesarean Section

Shariska S. Petersen,[1] **Raminder Khangura,**[1] **Dmitry Davydov,**[2]
Ziying Zhang,[3] **and Roopina Sangha**[1,2]

[1]*Department of Women's Health Services, Henry Ford Hospital, Detroit, MI 48202, USA*
[2]*Wayne State University School of Medicine, Detroit, MI 48202, USA*
[3]*Department of Pathology, Cytopathology Laboratory, Henry Ford Hospital, Detroit, MI 48202, USA*

Correspondence should be addressed to Shariska S. Petersen; speters8@hfhs.org

Academic Editor: Svein Rasmussen

We describe a patient with Class C diabetes who presented for nonstress testing at 36 weeks and 4 days of gestation with nonreassuring fetal heart tones (NRFHT) and oligohydramnios. Upon delivery, thrombosis of the umbilical cord was grossly noted. Pathological analysis of the placenta revealed chorangiosis, vascular congestion, and 40% occlusion of the umbilical vein. Chorangiosis is a vascular change of the placenta that involves the terminal chorionic villi. It has been proposed to result from longstanding, low-grade hypoxia in the placental tissue and has been associated with such conditions such as diabetes, intrauterine growth restriction (IUGR), and hypertensive conditions in pregnancy. To characterize chorangiosis and its associated obstetric outcomes we identified 61 cases of "chorangiosis" on placental pathology at Henry Ford Hospital from 2010 to 2015. Five of these cases were omitted due to lack of complete records. Among the 56 cases, the cesarean section rate was 51%, indicated in most cases for nonreassuring fetal status. Thus, we suggest that chorangiosis, a marker of chronic hypoxia, is associated with increased rates of cesarean sections for nonreassuring fetal status because of long standing hypoxia coupled with the stress of labor.

1. Introduction

Chorangiosis refers to the marked increase in the number of vascular channels in noninfarcted, nonischemic area of the placenta. The classic definition is more than 10 capillaries in more than 10 villi in several areas of placenta [1]. It is an uncommon finding that is widely described as a compensatory response to chronic hypoxia [1]; however, it is associated with common conditions including diabetes, hypertension, and tobacco use [2]. Using placental tissue oxygen index values, Suzuki et al. have shown an association between oxygen saturation of maternal blood in intervillous spaces and development of chorangiosis [2]. They postulate that low efficiency of oxygen transfer from maternal to fetal circulation facilitates vascular remodeling in adaptation to low oxygen supply, resulting in chorangiosis [2].

Umbilical vein thrombus is a rare occurrence and most occurrences are complications of cord compression and circulatory stasis [3]. Maternal diabetes as well as umbilical cord abnormalities including excessively long umbilical cords, true

knots, and excessively twisted umbilical cords have also been associated with umbilical cord thrombus [3, 4]. Dussaux et al. report on a case of umbilical cord thrombus noted antenatally by power Doppler which resulted in intrauterine fetal death [5]. Thus, the finding of both umbilical cord thrombus and chorangiosis in a recent case prompted a review of our recent experience at Henry Ford Hospital.

2. Case Report

A 38-year-old *gravida 7 para 5015* patient with Class C diabetes and singleton pregnancy presented at 36 + 4/7 weeks of gestation for scheduled nonstress testing with the additional report of decreased fetal movement for the last day. The patient's blood glucose logs indicated sufficient glucose control and her hemoglobin A1c one month prior to presentation was 7.1%. Fetal growth was greater than the 98th percentile with an estimated fetal weight of 3616 grams and an amniotic fluid index of 22.1 cm nineteen days prior to presentation at 33 weeks and 6 days of gestation.

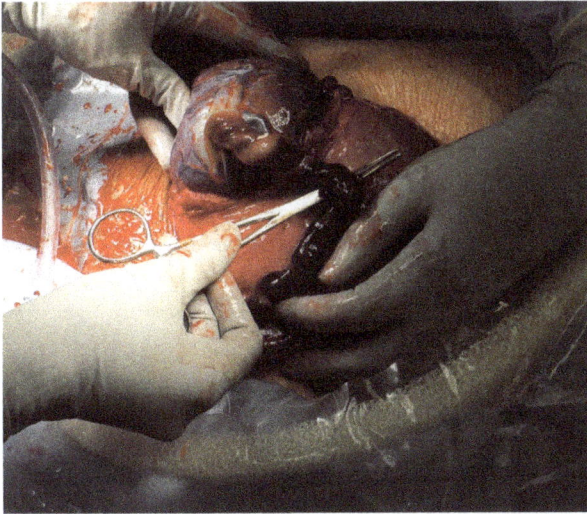

FIGURE 1: Gross umbilical cord at time of delivery.

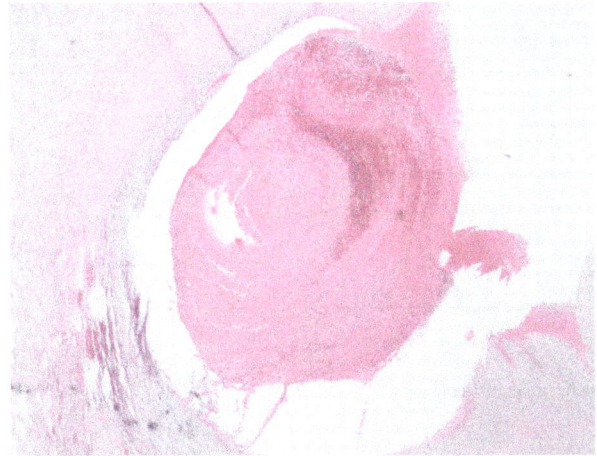

FIGURE 2: Cross section of umbilical vein with 40% thrombus occluding the vessel.

Fetal umbilical Doppler studies were not indicated and patient was monitored with twice weekly nonstress tests, which were within normal limits. She was a nonsmoker and had an overweight BMI of 28.47 kg/m^2. On presentation, bedside ultrasonography identified amniotic fluid level of 4.75 cm and the fetal heart rate tracing indicated irregular contractions with recurrent late-pattern decelerations from a baseline of *150* with moderate variability to 90 beats per minute lasting about one minute. Due to nonreassuring fetal status with oligohydramnios, delivery was affected by repeat low transverse cesarean section. At delivery, the umbilical cord was dusky and thrombus was palpable (*Figure 1*). The male infant weighed 4015 g. Resuscitation was rapid with Apgar scores 8 and 9 at 1 and 5 minutes, and other than transient hypoglycemia, the neonatal course was uneventful. The maternal postpartum course was also uncomplicated.

The placenta weighed 501 grams and the disc grossly appeared normal; however, the entire length of the cord appeared dark and mottled, showing signs of thrombosis. The pathological report described a three-vessel umbilical cord with subocclusive thrombosis of the umbilical vein, narrowing the vascular lumen by 40% (*Figure 2*). The fetal membranes were unremarkable. There were vascular congestion of the chorionic plate and a small 10 mm diameter area of subchorionic hemorrhage. Due to greater than the 10 capillaries per high power field of the chorionic villi, chorangiosis was identified (*Figure 3*).

3. Chart Review Methods

Approval for the chart review was obtained from the Institutional Review Board at Henry Ford Hospital. Patient medical record numbers were identified from the Pathology Department case index file from 2010 to 2015. Sixty-one cases of "chorangiosis" were identified by five staff cytopathologists: 5 cases were excluded due to incomplete medical record information. A descriptive analysis of the remaining 56 cases was completed using data from the integrated electronic health

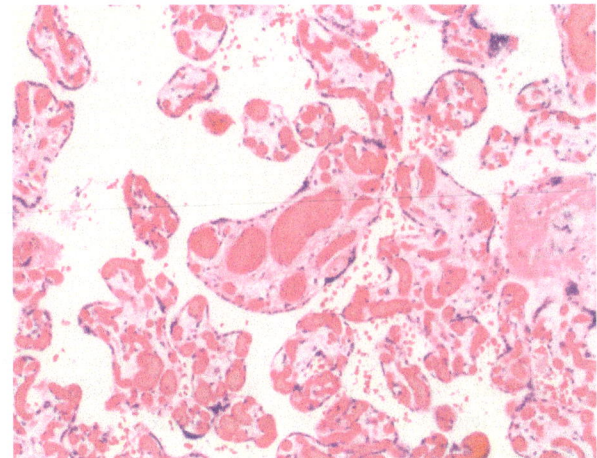

FIGURE 3: Chorionic villi with evidence of chorangiosis; more than 10 capillaries in at least 10 terminal villi in low-power fields (10x).

record within the Henry Ford Health System. We determined maternal age, BMI prior to twenty weeks of gestation, smoking status, maternal health conditions including presence of hypertensive conditions and diabetes, antenatal fetal issues including intrauterine growth restriction, gestational age at delivery, mode of delivery, indication for cesarean delivery (if performed), Apgar score, and neonatal weight through retrospective chart review.

4. Results

The demographic profile of the 56 cases with complete information is summarized in Table 1. The profile is reflective of the patients serviced by Henry Ford Hospital: obesity is a growing problem in southeast Michigan and tobacco use amongst low-income young women is a continuing national issue. As a referral hospital, we have a rich population with chronic diseases in pregnancy and patients in their late reproductive years. The obstetric outcomes are summarized

TABLE 1: Demographic profile and antenatal characteristics.

		Patients (N = 56)	Percentage of total (%)
Age	<18 years old	1	1.8
	18–34 years old	44	78.6
	≥35 years old	11	19.6
Race	Black	17	30.4
	White	30	53.6
	Latina	5	8.9
	Unknown	4	7.1
Body mass index (kg/m^2)	<18.5	1	1.8
	18.5–24.9	17	30.4
	25.0–29.9	13	23.2
	>30	25	44.6
	Unknown	1	1.8
Tobacco use	Current	5	8.9
	Former	37	66.1
	Never	12	21.4
	Unknown	2	3.6
Gestation	Singleton	47	83.9
	Twins	9	16.1
Parity	Primiparous	24	42.9
	Multiparous	32	57.1
Comorbid conditions	Hypertension	9	16.1
	Diabetes	6	10.7
	Intrauterine growth restriction	6	10.7

in Table 2. The rate of cesarean section was noted to be 51.8% with the most common indication being nonreassuring fetal heart rate. Majority of neonates were delivered at term with the average gestational age of 37.5 weeks.

While the neonatal outcomes summarized in Table 3 are largely reassuring, the occurrence of 11% of patients with growth restriction, one with intrauterine fetal demise, and one neonatal death, support the idea that chorangiosis is a pathologic entity rather than an incidental observation. Chorangiosis was only associated with umbilical cord thrombus of one placenta in this study.

5. Discussion

The etiology and clinical associations of chorangiosis are not well understood; however, this finding is associated with fetal, maternal, and placental disorders including preeclampsia, diabetes, hypertension, major congenital anomalies, air pollution, and smoking [6] and has been correlated with fetal morbidity and mortality rates as high as 42% [1]. In our recent experience, the pregnancy outcomes are much improved over those suggested by Altshuler in 1984. The average placental/birth weight ratio for this cohort, 0.17, is considered normal in studies that correlate high placenta/birth weight ratio to adverse perinatal outcomes [7, 8]. Adverse events in our review, such as neonatal death at 22 weeks of gestation, are explainable by prematurity without need to invoke chronic hypoxia.

The rate of cesarean section in this cohort was 51.8%, which was much higher than the institution rate of 29% of 15,431 deliveries during this timeframe. The most common indication for cesarean section in this cohort was fetal heart rate abnormalities. Chorangiosis was only associated with cord thrombus in the sentinel case, suggesting that the two events are separate. This is supported by a study that found no correlation between fetal vessel thrombosis and chorangiosis in twin placentas [9]. Furthermore, chorangiosis has been associated with multiple umbilical cord complications but not a single complication [4] such as umbilical cord thrombus as seen on our sentinel case. We suspect that the umbilical cord thrombus was likely related to the patient's diabetes, since infants of diabetic mothers have increased α 2-antiplasmin and decreased fibrinolysin activity resulting in higher risk of thrombus formation [5]. We postulate that the umbilical vein thrombus was recently formed, coinciding with the decreased fetal movement the patient experienced and that the chorangiosis was resultant of a long standing hypoxia.

Over two-thirds of our cohort reported being former or current smokers suggesting that chorangiosis might be a compensatory mechanism for maternal hypoxia as suggested by Akbulut et al. In addition, the rate of maternal obesity, 45%, is also exaggerated in this group. This increased rate of obesity and smoking may suggest an association between obesity, smoking, and decreased efficiency of oxygen transfer to the fetal circulation resulting in chorangiosis. In our cohort, chorangiosis did not have the reported strong association

Table 2: Obstetrical outcomes.

		All patients N = 56	Percentage of total (%)
Gestational age at delivery	<37 completed weeks	10	17.8
	>37 weeks	46	82.1
Mode of delivery	Vaginal	27	48.2
	Cesarean delivery	29	51.8
Cesarean delivery indication	Fetal heart rate abnormality	10	17.9
	Malpresentation	6	10.7
	Labor abnormality	3	5.4
	Prior cesarean delivery	7	12.5
	Other[1]	2	3.6

[1]One patient had cesarean delivery for active HSV lesion and the other for history of a 4th-degree perineal laceration.

Table 3: Neonatal outcomes.

	All neonates N = 65	All singletons N = 47	Twin gestation N = 18
Mean Apgar score at 1 minute	7.3	7.0	8.0
Mean Apgar score at 5 minutes	8.6	8.5	8.9
Mean gestational age (completed weeks)	37.5	37.9	36.4
Mean birth weight (grams)	2996.4	3189.1	2493.2
Mean placental weight (grams)	504	525.7	447.8
Placental/birth weight ratio	0.17	0.16	0.18
Born alive	63	45	18
Neonatal death	1	1	0
Intrauterine fetal demise	1	1	0

with hypertensive disorders, diabetes, or preterm deliveries. However, we are limited by the inability to compare the incidence of these comorbidities to patients with normal placentas. At our institution, placentas are sent to pathology only if there is a pregnancy/delivery complication or a clinical observation such as the cord thrombosis in the sentinel case. Thus, we do not have "normal placenta" controls, nor can we estimate the prevalence of chorangiosis in our population. An editorial by Schwartz suggests that the existence of chorangiosis in many infants with hypoxia will remain unknown because the placenta has often been discarded [10].

We have shown that cesarean delivery is enriched in patients with placental chorangiosis; however, chorangiosis is not the direct cause. Chorangiosis is a placental marker of antepartum low-grade chronic hypoxia; thus, clinical correlation of entities that may contribute to hypoxia is suggested. Our review has identified smoking history and obesity to be associated with placental chorangiosis. Obesity has been long associated with increased cesarean section rates [11]. We postulate that obesity and smoking may contribute to low-grade hypoxia resulting in chorangiosis, and this chronic hypoxic state when coupled with the stress of labor can result in nonreassuring fetal status and increased rates of cesarean delivery.

Disclosure

This research did not receive any specific grant from funding agencies in the public, commercial, or not-for-profit sectors.

References

[1] G. Altshuler, "Chorangiosis: an important placental sign of neonatal morbidity and mortality," Archives of Pathology & Laboratory Medicine, vol. 108, no. 1, pp. 71–74, 1984.

[2] K. Suzuki, H. Itoh, S. Kimura et al., "Chorangiosis and placental oxygenation," Congenital Anomalies, vol. 49, no. 2, pp. 71–76, 2009.

[3] M. A. Fritz and C. R. Christopher, "Umbilical vein thrombosis and maternal diabetes mellitus," Journal of Reproductive Medicine, vol. 26, no. 6, pp. 320–324, 1981.

[4] J. S. Chan and R. N. Baergen, "Gross umbilical cord complications are associated with placental lesions of circulatory stasis and fetal hypoxia," Pediatric and Developmental Pathology, vol. 15, no. 6, pp. 487–494, 2012.

[5] C. Dussaux, O. Picone, G. Chambon et al., "Umbilical vein thrombosis: to deliver or not to deliver at the time of diagnosis?" Clinical Case Reports, vol. 2, no. 6, pp. 271–273, 2014.

[6] M. Akbulut, H. C. Sorkun, F. Bir, A. Eralp, and E. Duzcan, "Chorangiosis: The potential role of smoking and air pollution," *Pathology Research and Practice*, vol. 205, no. 2, pp. 75–81, 2009.

[7] F. Shehata, I. Levin, A. Shrim et al., "Placenta/birthweight ratio and perinatal outcome: a retrospective cohort analysis," *BJOG: An International Journal of Obstetrics and Gynaecology*, vol. 118, no. 6, pp. 741–747, 2011.

[8] K. M. Strand, G. L. Andersen, C. Haavaldsen, T. Vik, and A. Eskild, "Association of placental weight with cerebral palsy: population-based cohort study in Norway," *BJOG: An International Journal of Obstetrics and Gynaecology*, vol. 123, no. 13, pp. 2131–2138, 2015.

[9] M. P. Chan, J. L. Hecht, and S. E. Kane, "Incidence and clinico-pathologic correlation of fetal vessel thrombosis in mono- and dichorionic twin placentas," *Journal of Perinatology*, vol. 30, no. 10, pp. 660–664, 2010.

[10] D. A. Schwartz, "Chorangiosis and its precursors: underdiagnosed placental indicators of chronic fetal hypoxia," *Obstetrical and Gynecological Survey*, vol. 56, no. 9, pp. 523–525, 2001.

[11] J. C. Dempsey, Z. Ashiny, C. F. Qiu, R. S. Miller, T. K. Sorensen, and M. A. Williams, "Maternal pre-pregnancy overweight status and obesity as risk factors for cesarean delivery," *The Journal of Maternal-Fetal & Neonatal Medicine*, vol. 17, no. 3, pp. 179–185, 2005.

27

Pregnancy after Prosthetic Aortic Valve Replacement: How Do We Monitor Prosthetic Valvular Function during Pregnancy?

Nicole Sahasrabudhe ⓘ,[1] Nickolas Teigen,[1] Diana S. Wolfe,[1] and Cynthia Taub[2]

[1]*Department of Obstetrics and Gynecology, Albert Einstein College of Medicine, Bronx, NY, USA*
[2]*Department of Cardiology, Albert Einstein College of Medicine, Bronx, NY, USA*

Correspondence should be addressed to Nicole Sahasrabudhe; nneto@montefiore.org

Academic Editor: Mehmet A. Osmanağaoğlu

Background. With modern medicine, many women after structural heart repair are deciding to experience pregnancy. There is a need for further study to identify normal echocardiographic parameters to better assess prosthetic valvular function in pregnancy. In addition, a multidisciplinary approach is essential in managing pregnant patients with complex cardiac conditions. *Case.* A 22-year-old nulliparous woman with an aortic valve replacement 18 months prior to her pregnancy presented to prenatal care at 20-week gestation. During her prenatal care, serial echocardiography showed a significant increase in the mean gradient across the prosthetic aortic valve. Multidisciplinary management and a serial echocardiography played an integral role in her care that resulted in a successful spontaneous vaginal delivery without complications. *Conclusion.* Further characterization of the normal echocardiographic parameters in pregnant patients with prosthetic valves is critical to optimize prenatal care for this patient population. This case report is novel in that serial echocardiograms were obtained throughout prenatal care, which showed significant changes across the prosthetic aortic valve. *Teaching Points.* (1) Further study is needed to identify normal echocardiographic parameters to best assess prosthetic valvular function in pregnancy. (2) Multidisciplinary management is encouraged to optimize prenatal care for women with prosthetic aortic valve replacements.

1. Introduction

Normal pregnancy induces major hemodynamic changes that require significant cardiac adaptations [1]. Increases in heart rate and plasma volume are associated with a dramatic increase in cardiac output [2]. In addition, there is a decrease in afterload due to a decrease in systemic vascular resistance during pregnancy. With modern medical and surgical techniques, many women with congenital heart disease or acquired cardiac disease are now finding themselves with improved survival and quality of life after surgical repair and are choosing to experience pregnancy.

Currently, one of the most common types of heart disease encountered during pregnancy is congenital heart disease after structural heart repair [3]. Studies have shown that hemodynamic changes of pregnancy increase the risk of cardiac complications for patients with valvular repair or replacements. In 2014, the American Heart Association and American College of Cardiology guidelines for the management of patients with valvular heart disease acknowledged that, due to an increase in cardiac output that occurs during pregnancy, the mean pressure gradient across all prostheses will increase throughout gestation [4]. The guidelines encourage the use of other hemodynamic parameters such as dimensionless index to determine the function of the aortic prosthesis. However, it does not clarify what normal echocardiographic parameters are to compensate for these hemodynamic changes in pregnancy. The European Society guidelines highlight the importance of anticoagulation during pregnancy but provide no clear guidelines as to how to monitor prosthetic valvular function in pregnancy [5].

Literature regarding management and prenatal outcomes of patients with prosthetic valves is scarce [6]. Literature on echocardiographic changes in pregnant patients with prosthetic valves is even more limited [7]. In our case report, we present a woman with a bioprosthetic aortic valve with a successful pregnancy course through the management of our MFM-Cardiology Joint program.

2. Case

A 20-year-old female presented to the emergency department with chest pain, dyspnea, fever, and chills for 3 weeks. She was an active intravenous heroin abuser at the time and had been attempting to wean herself off heroin. During her evaluation, her blood cultures were notable for *Streptococcus mitis*. The diagnosis of bacterial endocarditis with severe aortic valve vegetation was made after a transthoracic echocardiography was performed. The patient was started on intravenous antibiotics on the day of admission and a cardiothoracic surgery consultation was made. On hospital day number 2, the patient was taken to the operating room for a bovine pericardial patch repair of a fistula and aortic valve replacement with a 21 mm bioprosthetic valve. The patient remained hospitalized for 36 days and was discharged to a drug rehabilitation program once she was medically cleared.

When the patient presented to cardiology for followup 1.5 years after her aortic valve replacement, the patient was 22 years old and 20 weeks pregnant with a recorded body mass index of 29 kg/m². The patient had been enrolled in a methadone maintenance program and had not used intravenous heroin for 6 months. She was promptly referred to our maternal-fetal medicine and cardiology joint program, a multidisciplinary collaboration created to manage pregnant women with preexisting or acquired cardiac conditions. An echocardiogram was performed during her first prenatal care visit showing a heart rate of 61 bpm, peak velocity of 360.5 m/s, peak gradient across valve of 52 mmHg, mean gradient across valve of 28.9 mmHg, and dimensionless index 0.36.

Joint prenatal care and cardiology clinic visits were scheduled, during which routine prenatal care and cardiology evaluations were performed. The patient was placed on 81 mg of aspirin for the duration of her pregnancy to decrease her risk of thrombosis. Echocardiogram was repeated at 32 weeks and 37 weeks of gestation. At 32-week gestation, the echocardiogram showed a heart rate of 69 bpm, peak velocity of 386.9 m/s, peak gradient across valve 59.9 mmHg, mean gradient across valve 36.1 mmHg, and dimensionless index 0.43. At 37-week gestation, heart rate was 76, peak velocity of 339.3 m/s, peak gradient across valve 46.1 mmHg, mean gradient across valve 22.6 mmHg, and dimensionless index 0.45. The patient was asymptomatic and denied any cardiac symptoms.

A multidisciplinary meeting included subspecialists of cardiology, maternal-fetal medicine, anesthesiology, criticalcare, and labor and delivery nursing to create a delivery plan. A consensus was reached that a vaginal delivery would be safe for this patient without an assisted second stage, unless obstetrically indicated. A plan was made for telemetry monitoring immediately postpartum given higher risk of arrhythmia at that time.

The patient presented to the labor and delivery triage unit at 40-week 0-day gestation complaining of contractions and was found to be in spontaneous labor. As discussed during our multidisciplinary meeting, the patient received endocarditis prophylaxis and underwent expectant management of her labor. The patient did not require an assisted second stage of delivery and proceeded to have a spontaneous vaginal delivery. Within 10 hours of admission, she delivered a healthy male infant with Apgar scores of 9 at 1 min and 9 at 5 min, weighing 3770 grams with estimated blood loss of 350 ml. Her postpartum care was uneventful. Her echocardiography on postpartum day 1 showed a heart rate of 63 bpm, peak velocity of 325.8 m/s, peak gradient across valve 42.5 mmHg, mean gradient across valve 25.3 mmHg, and dimensionless index 0.36. The patient was discharged on postpartum day 3 without any complications. At her 6-week postpartum visit, the patient received an intrauterine device (IUD) for contraception.

3. Discussion

The assessment and management of prosthetic heart valves during pregnancy pose several clinical challenges. Data on prosthetic aortic valve function in pregnancy is limited and high transaortic gradients observed during pregnancy may be concerning. Therefore, it is imperative that a multidisciplinary approach be used to optimize pregnancy outcomes.

Pregnancies in women with prosthetic heart valves have been associated with an increased incidence of adverse outcomes. Lawley et al., in a meta-analysis of 11 studies capturing 499 pregnancies among women with heart valve prosthesis, pooled estimate of maternal mortality was 1.2/100 pregnancies, for mechanical valves subgroup 1.8/100 and bioprosthetic subgroup 0.7/100, overall pregnancy loss 20.8/100 pregnancies, perinatal mortality 5.0/100 births, and thromboembolism 9.3/100 pregnancies [8]. Despite these risks, the hemodynamic adaptations of pregnancy may be well tolerated in women with bioprosthetic valves as long as the valve is functioning normally, and there is no other significant cardiac disease. However, there still is limited data to illustrate optimal monitoring guidelines for pregnant patients with prosthetic heart valves. Additionally, the normal echocardiographic parameters for these prosthetic heart valves to accommodate the hemodynamic changes of pregnancy are not well understood.

Data on hemodynamic adaptations in pregnancy in women with structural heart disease are scarce and have not been described in a longitudinal manner [9]. The 2014 American Heart Association and American College of Cardiology Guidelines for patients with valvular heart disease acknowledge that the mean pressure gradients across all prostheses will increase throughout gestation secondary to an increase in cardiac output [4]. The guidelines also encourage the use of other hemodynamic parameters such as dimensionless index to determine the function of the aortic prosthesis. The European Society guidelines also highlight the importance of anticoagulation during pregnancy for these patients but no clear recommendations exist for monitoring prosthetic valvular function in pregnancy such as interval echocardiogram and normal echocardiographic parameters with the changes in pregnancy [5].

TABLE 1: Serial echocardiogram measurements through gestation.

Gestational age	Heart rate (bpm)	Peak velocity (cm/sec)	Peak gradient across valve (mmHg)	Mean gradient across valve (mmHg)	Pulse wave velocity time integral (m)	Dimensionless index
			Echocardiographic parameters			
Prepregnancy	63	274.2	30.1	18.4		
20 weeks	61	360.5	52	28.9	31.2	0.36
32 weeks	69	386.9	59.9	36.1	35.7	0.43
37 weeks	76	339.3	46.1	22.6	29.2	0.45
Postpartum day 1	63	325.8	42.5	25.3	26.7	0.36

However, there is no concrete guideline as to how obstetricians and cardiologists can optimally manage these patients other than getting a baseline and repeat echocardiograms if the patient becomes symptomatic. There has been little published regarding normal and abnormal echocardiography parameters in pregnant patients with prosthetic valves. Normal and abnormal echocardiographic parameters have been described for nonpregnant patients with prosthetic aortic valves, but there is limited data as to the changes in these parameters due to hemodynamic changes of pregnancy [10].

In our patient, there was a significant increase in the mean gradient across the prosthetic aortic valve until around 32 weeks to 36.1 mmHg (Table 1), which could be interpreted as significant aortic prosthetic valve stenosis in nonpregnant patients. But it is difficult to interpret the data as such, given that we do not have enough information to identify stenosis in the pregnant population. Hemodynamic changes of pregnancy with a substantial increase in cardiac output were likely responsible for this change, especially since our patient did not experience signs and symptoms of aortic stenosis. Throughout her pregnancy, we observed a gradual increase in the mean gradient across the bioprosthetic aortic valve until around 32 weeks and subsequent stabilization during the rest of third trimester and return to baseline soon after the delivery (Figure 1). The same trend is observed for cardiac output throughout her pregnancy (Figure 2).

Lesniak-Sobelga and colleagues studied pregnancy outcomes of 259 women with cardiac disease, of which 54 patients had aortic valve disease [6]. This study reports that, in women with severe aortic stenosis, pregnancy can lead to sudden clinical deterioration. Results of echocardiographic examinations revealed an increase in aortic gradients throughout gestation. However, these were patients with native valve dysfunctions.

Heuvelman et al. described pregnancy outcomes of 40 women after successful aortic valve replacements [7]. There were increased maternal cardiac and obstetrical complications such as heart failure, arrhythmia, valve thrombosis, preeclampsia, and preterm delivery. The authors recommend careful monitoring of these high risk patients but there are no concrete guidelines as to how that can be accomplished.

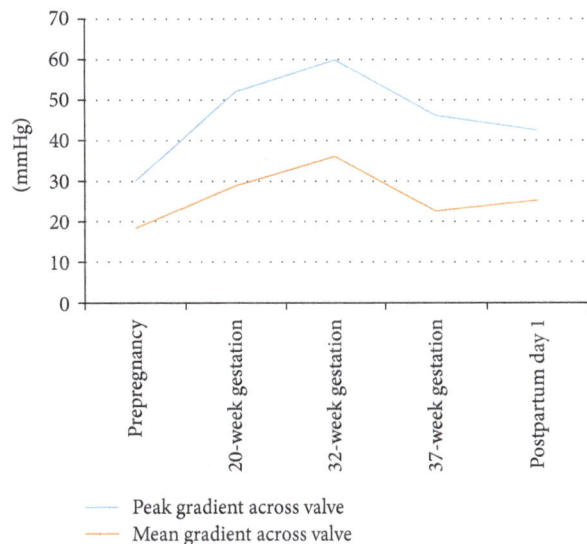

FIGURE 1: Serial echocardiographic measurements of the mean and peak prosthetic aortic valve gradients over time.

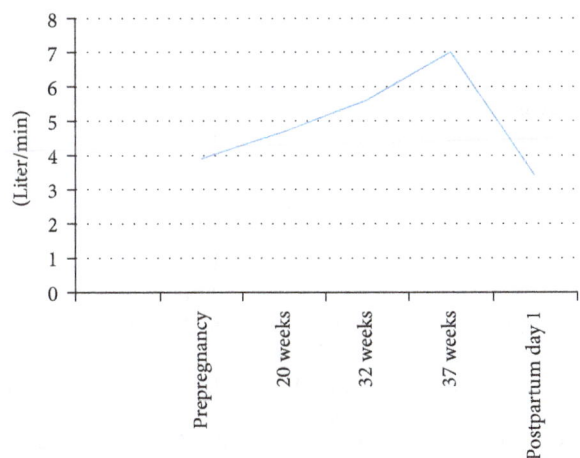

FIGURE 2: Changes in cardiac output during prepregnancy, antepartum, and postpartum periods.

Limited data suggests that, for patients with bioprosthetic valves, pregnancy may accelerate structural valve degeneration [10]. The team caring for a pregnant woman with history of aortic valve replacement or any valvular dysfunction should be prepared for possible maternal cardiac decompensation. Creating a multidisciplinary delivery plan with maternal-fetal medicine, cardiology, anesthesia, and labor and delivery nursing plays a critical role in successful perinatal outcomes.

This case describes the use of multidisciplinary planning and serial echocardiography throughout pregnancy as a way to monitor and improve perinatal outcomes. In the past, pregnant patients with aortic valve disease posed a great risk of maternal mortality and morbidity. Now with modern medicine, these patients are undergoing successful aortic valve replacements with improved quality of life and are choosing to experience pregnancy. However, there is limited information on how to best assess and evaluate pregnant patients with prosthetic valves. This case report is novel in that serial echocardiograms were obtained throughout prenatal care, which showed significant changes across the prosthetic aortic valve. The significance of these changes is not well understood. Therefore, there is a need for further data in obtaining serial echocardiograms on pregnant patients with prosthetic valves to delineate what normal echocardiographic parameters are in order to assess their cardiac risk during pregnancy. Because the physiologic changes of pregnancy can have an impact on prosthetic valvular function, we recognize that it is crucial to develop clear echocardiographic parameters to stratify their risk of cardiac complications.

Our case also illustrates that patients with serious medical comorbidities such as our patient with aortic valve replacement may greatly benefit from a multidisciplinary team approach to optimize their medical care.

References

[1] J. J. Duvekot, E. C. Cheriex, F. A. A. Pieters, P. P. C. A. Menheere, and L. L. H. Peeters, "Early pregnancy changes in hemodynamics and volume homeostasis are consecutive adjustments triggered by a primary fall in systemic vascular tone," *American Journal of Obstetrics & Gynecology*, vol. 169, no. 6, pp. 1382–1392, 1993.

[2] J. J. Duvekot and L. L. H. Peeters, "Maternal cardiovascular hemodynamic adaptation to pregnancy," *Obstetrical & Gynecological Survey*, vol. 49, suuplement 12, pp. S1–S14, 1994.

[3] K. J. Lindley, S. N. Conner, and A. G. Cahill, "Adult congenital heart disease in pregnancy," *Obstetrical & Gynecological Survey*, vol. 70, no. 6, pp. 397–407, 2015.

[4] R. A. Nishimura, C. M. Otto, R. O. Bonow et al., "2014 AHA/ACC guideline for the management of patients with valvular heart disease: a report of the American College of Cardiology/American Heart Association Task Force on Practice Guidelines," *Journal of the American College of Cardiology*, vol. 63, no. 22, pp. e57–e185, 2014.

[5] European Society of Gynecology (ESG), Association for European Paediatric Cariology (AEPC), German Society for Gender Medicine (DGesGM) et al., "ESC guidelines on the management of cardiovascular diseases during pregnancy: the task force on the management of cardiovascular diseases during pregnancy of the European Society of Cardiology (ESC)," *European Heart Journal*, vol. 24, no. 32, pp. 3147–3197, 2011.

[6] A. Leśniak-Sobelga, W. Tracz, M. Kostkiewicz, P. Podolec, and M. Pasowicz, "Clinical and echocardiographic assessment of pregnant women with valvular heart diseases - Maternal and fetal outcome," *International Journal of Cardiology*, vol. 94, no. 1, pp. 15–23, 2004.

[7] H. J. Heuvelman, B. Arabkhani, J. M. J. Cornette et al., "Pregnancy outcomes in women with aortic valve substitutes," *American Journal of Cardiology*, vol. 111, no. 3, pp. 382–387, 2013.

[8] C. M. Lawley, S. J. Lain, C. S. Algert, J. B. Ford, G. A. Figtree, and C. L. Roberts, "Prosthetic heart valves in pregnancy, outcomes for women and their babies: A systematic review and meta-analysis," *BJOG: An International Journal of Obstetrics & Gynaecology*, vol. 122, no. 11, pp. 1446–1455, 2015.

[9] J. Cornette, T. P. E. Ruys, A. Rossi et al., "Hemodynamic adaptation to pregnancy in women with structural heart disease," *International Journal of Cardiology*, vol. 168, no. 2, pp. 825–831, 2013.

[10] B. R. Badduke, W. R. E. Jamieson, R. T. Miyagishima et al., "Pregnancy and childbearing in a population with biologic valvular prostheses," *The Journal of Thoracic and Cardiovascular Surgery*, vol. 102, no. 2, pp. 179–186, 1991.

28

A Case of Placenta Percreta Managed with Sequential Embolisation Procedures

Shannon Armstrong-Kempter [ID],[1,2] Supuni Kapurubandara,[1,3,4] Brian Trudinger,[3] Noel Young,[2,5] and Naim Arrage[1,4]

[1]Department of Women's and Newborn Health, Westmead Hospital, Westmead, NSW 2145, Australia
[2]Western Sydney University, Campbelltown, NSW 2560, Australia
[3]University of Sydney, Camperdown, NSW 2006, Australia
[4]Sydney West Advanced Pelvic Surgery Unit, NSW, Australia
[5]Department of Radiology, Westmead Hospital, Westmead, NSW 2145, Australia

Correspondence should be addressed to Shannon Armstrong-Kempter; smj.armstrong@gmail.com

Academic Editor: Akihide Ohkuchi

Background. The incidence of morbidly adherent placenta, including placenta percreta, has increased significantly over recent years due to rising caesarean section rates. Historically, abnormally invasive placenta has been managed with caesarean hysterectomy; however nonsurgical interventions such as uterine artery embolisation (UAE) are emerging as safe alternative management techniques. UAE can be utilised to decrease placental perfusion and encourage placental resorption, thereby reducing the risk of haemorrhage and other morbidities. *Case.* We describe one of the very few reported cases of placenta percreta which was successfully treated primarily with sequential artery embolisation. Our patient underwent four embolisation procedures over a period of 248 days, with no major morbidity or complications. *Conclusion.* Repeat UAE may be a beneficial primary management modality in cases of placenta percreta with bladder involvement.

1. Introduction

Placenta percreta is a serious obstetric complication where the placental villi penetrate through the myometrium into the uterine serosa and possibly adjacent organs. There are three degrees of morbidly adherent placenta (MAP): placenta accreta, increta, and percreta. Placenta percreta is the most severe but least common form of this condition, accounting for 7% of abnormally implanted placentas; however it is associated with a significantly higher maternal morbidity than the other varieties [1, 2]. The incidence of morbidly adherent placenta, including placenta percreta, has increased significantly over recent years, which has been attributed to increasing rates of caesarean delivery, although the mechanism remains speculative [3]. The most appropriate management for this life threatening condition is debated. We report a case that presented at the end of the first trimester with successful

conservative management and detailed angiographic and ultrasound imaging.

2. Case Presentation

A 38-year-old female, G7P3 (three previous lower segment caesarian sections and 3 prior surgical terminations), presented to our hospital with a massive haemorrhage after surgical termination of pregnancy. The gestational age estimate was 14 weeks based on biparietal diameter on bedside ultrasound performed preoperatively at a private clinic. No formal ultrasound had been performed during her current pregnancy. A dilation of cervix and suction curettage were performed. Significant haemorrhage occurred with the loss exceeding 1000 ml. Syntocinon was administered intramuscularly and a Foley catheter was inserted into the uterus for

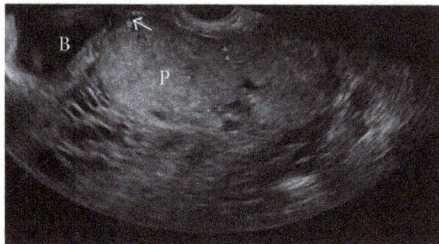

FIGURE 1: Retained placental tissue (P), 55 mm in diameter. Minimal myometrium noted between bladder (B) and placental tissue (arrowed).

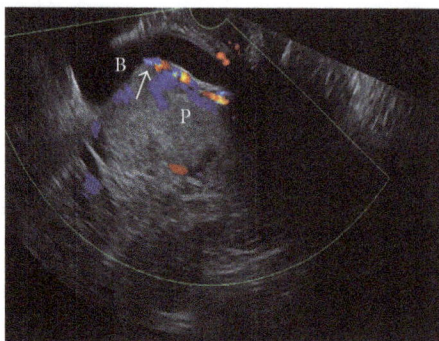

FIGURE 2: Large dilated vessels (arrowed) in the placental bed (P), possibly extending into bladder (B).

tamponade. The patient was transferred from the clinic to a tertiary hospital.

Upon arrival the patient was stable and there was no evidence of ongoing active blood loss. The patient was managed conservatively overnight after admission. A formal ultrasound scan performed the next day demonstrated retained placental tissue (with vascularity) at the site of previous caesarean scar, suggestive of a morbidly adherent placenta (see Figures 1 and 2).

Given the stability of the patient, she was offered the option of hysterectomy, placental resection, conservative management with arterial embolisation, or expectant management. The patient preferred to avoid a hysterectomy so as to preserve fertility as well as any other form of surgical intervention given the risk of significant surgical morbidity. A multidisciplinary discussion involving the treating team, urogynaecology, maternal-fetal medicine, and interventional radiology took place and together with the patient it was decided to proceed with arterial embolisation while leaving the placenta in situ. Given the lack of robust evidence with respect to embolisation and subsequent follow-up, it was decided that embolisation with very close outpatient monitoring would be the safest management option for this patient (see Table 1).

3. Discussion

The most appropriate management of placenta percreta with bladder involvement remains somewhat unclear. While a range of management options are presented in the literature, there is a lack of good quality data to indicate which management option is preferable, largely due to the paucity of such cases. These can be broadly categorised into hysterectomy with placenta in situ, placental resection, and conservative management modalities with or without a planned interval hysterectomy.

Conservative management, where the placenta is left in situ, can include expectant management, methotrexate administration, uterine artery embolisation (UAE), or a combination of these modalities. Conservative management offers the main advantages of minimising the risk of haemorrhage and other significant surgical morbidities at the time of delivery, as well as preserving fertility. One review ($n = 407$) found that 85.7% of women conceived following conservative treatment in all forms of morbidly adherent placenta (MAP); however in cases of placenta percreta specifically only 10% (1/10) had a subsequent pregnancy [4, 5]. It is also important to consider the significant recurrence risk of MAP, which has been reported to be as high as 29% [4]. Serious complications such as secondary haemorrhage, sepsis, and the need for emergency hysterectomy may occur with conservative management, and have been reported up to many months after delivery; thus this approach requires close surveillance.

In one of the largest case series of conservatively managed placenta percreta ($n = 119$), 61% of patients experienced at least one postoperative complication, compared to 12% in placental resection and caesarean hysterectomy groups [6]. The most common complications were emergency hysterectomy (50%) (even up to 9 months after caesarean section), haemorrhage (44%), sepsis (25%), and bladder injury (17%) [6]. Management with methotrexate has been described in some small case series and reports, with results ranging from successful placental resorption without complications [7–10] to significant complications including coagulopathy, haemorrhage, and need for secondary hysterectomy or placental removal [11–14]. Uterine artery embolisation has been used to manage placenta percreta primarily and in cases of postpartum haemorrhage; however a significant proportion of these (18–62%) may still require hysterectomy [5, 15–17]. For cases managed successfully with expectant management alone, reports of complete resorption range from 8 months to 3 years postpartum [18, 19]. It has been suggested by a number of case reports and series that leaving the placenta in situ at the time of delivery with a planned interval hysterectomy at a later date may be a safe management option, as there may be markedly decreased vascularity, allowing for technically easier hysterectomy with a reduced rate of peri- and postoperative complications [20–23]. However, this requires extensive planning and multidisciplinary input and there is insufficient consistent evidence to suggest an appropriate timeline before which a definitive interval hysterectomy should be offered. The unpredictability of complications with conservative management and associated morbidity necessitate taking a cautious, individualised approach with each case given the lack of robust evidence.

Local placental resection has also been presented as a conservative surgical alternative in cases of placenta percreta with bladder involvement; however there have been mixed

TABLE 1: A timeline summary of the management of this patient.

Days after surgical uterine evacuation	Events and Images
Day 22	(i) Ultrasound showed persistent retained placental tissue with significant vascularity and extension into bladder with no overlying myometrium, suggestive of placenta percreta with bladder involvement (See Figure 3) (ii) Multidisciplinary discussion between gynaecologist, urogynaecologist, maternal fetal medicine specialist, and patient (iii) The options of management discussed included expectant management, abdominal hysterectomy, or uterine artery embolisation (iv) Uterine artery embolisation was decided
Day 33	(i) Initial angiogram showed very large, tortuous, abnormal uterine arteries, particularly on the left side; thus it was decided to proceed with initial embolisation with the view that multiple procedures would be required to adequately devascularise the retained placental tissue (ii) This decision was based on attempting to minimise undue ischemia and pain to the patient, and therein any hospital admissions, as well as minimising the radiation exposure to this young patient by spreading the embolisation over multiple session (iii) Left sided arterial embolisation performed via microcatheter, using Boston Scientific Helical pushable metal coils (4 mm + 6 mm) and Boston scientific contour embolisation particles (250–350 microns) (See Figures 4, 5, and 6)
Day 36	(i) Ultrasound showed persistence of retained placental tissue with significant vascularity
Day 54	(i) Pelvic angiogram showed persistent uterine vascular abnormality with some regression since the initial embolisation procedure (ii) Further embolisation of two arterial branches of the left internal iliac artery (iii) Regression of persistent PV bleeding and return of regular menses
Day 57	(i) Serum beta HCG 7
Day 107	(i) Angiogram showed further improvement of the uterine vascular abnormality (ii) Further embolisation of a branch of the right internal iliac artery
Day 177	(i) Pelvic angiogram showed a single abnormal feeding vessel to the vascular anomaly off the right internal iliac artery, which was successfully embolised (ii) No further abnormal vessels, including intraperitoneal feeding vessels, were identified (See Figure 7)
Day 241	(i) Ultrasound showed persistent uterine mass (16 × 15 × 10 mm); however this was avascular and significantly reduced in size as compared to earlier ultrasound images (See Figure 8)
Day 248	(i) Hysteroscopy was performed which showed no evidence of residual placental tissue over the anterior uterine wall. Endometrium overlying possible remnant placental tissues could not be ruled out. A uterine septum was identified which was divided with scissors (See Figure 9)
Day 283	(i) Patient was well, continuing to have regular menstrual periods with no abnormal bleeding

results depending on the resection method utilised. In one prospective study (n = 68), local resection was performed via retrovesical and parametrial dissection with subsequent repair of the anterior wall defect, with 26% of patients requiring secondary hysterectomy, the majority due to extensive uterine destruction, and two cases of inadvertent ureteric ligation [24]. In a retrospective review of local resection (n = 17), there were no reported cases of urological complications and only two cases of haemorrhage, neither requiring hysterectomy [6]. One small cohort study (n = 19) has proposed a method of local resection involving myometrial excision leaving the area of placental involvement of the bladder intact and uterine artery balloon occlusion, which

has shown a reduced rate of postpartum haemorrhage, secondary hysterectomy, and duration of hospital stay when compared to leaving the placenta in situ [25, 26]. A systematic review found that partial resection resulted in a subsequent pregnancy in 19/26 (73%) cases of morbidly adherent placenta [5].

Caesarean hysterectomy has historically been the treatment of choice for abnormally invasive placenta, where the placenta along with the uterus is removed at the time of delivery. This minimises the risk of long term complications, such as sepsis, haemorrhage, and need for emergency hysterectomy. However, there is considerable morbidity associated with this procedure, with significant intraoperative and

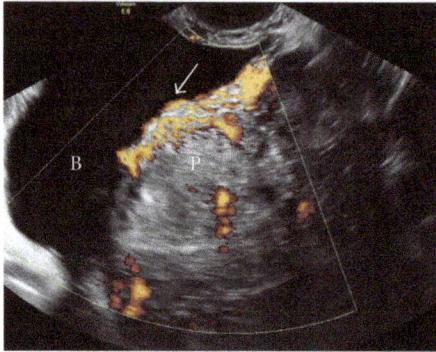

FIGURE 3: Ongoing evidence of adherent placenta (P) with likely bladder (B) invasion (arrowed) and dilated vesical and uterine vessels.

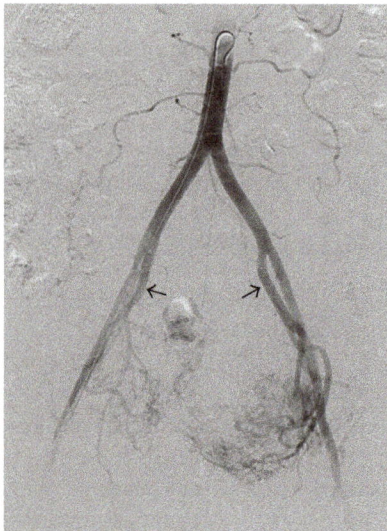

FIGURE 4: Pelvic angiogram—early arterial phase. Both internal iliac arteries (arrowed) show extensive abnormal arterial supply to the uterus, more evident on the left.

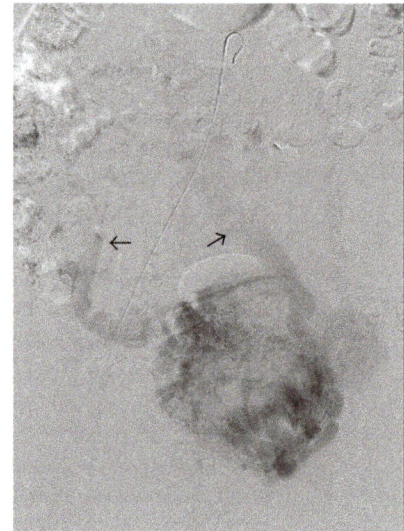

FIGURE 5: Pelvic angiogram—late venous phase. Early venous drainage to internal iliac veins (arrowed).

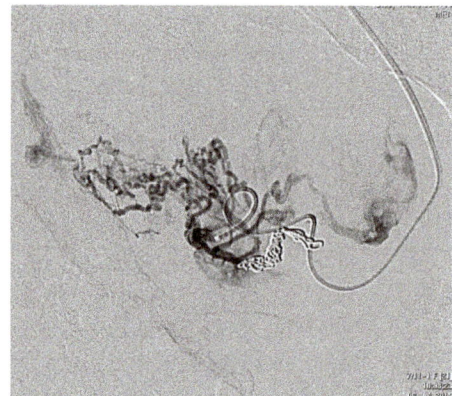

FIGURE 6: Microcatheter metal coil embolisation of the abnormal left internal iliac arteries.

postoperatively complications, including maternal death (up to 5%) [27]. Urology involvement preoperatively has been shown to reduce the rates of urological complications [28]. A large retrospective review (n = 66) found that 30% of cases managed with caesarean hysterectomy resulted in some form of complication, with 17% suffering a bladder injury and 7.6% postoperative haemorrhage [6]. Conversely, one prospective case series (n = 58) had only 6.9% of patients enduring a bladder injury and 1.7% requiring reoperation due to haemorrhage; however, almost one-third (29.3%) received more than 4 units of red blood cells [29]. There have been a number of case reports presenting modified caesarean hysterectomy methods, with techniques such as intentional cystotomy and resection of the affected bladder wall with subsequent bladder repair [30], subtotal hysterectomy with invasive portion of placenta left in situ [31], and retrograde caesarean hysterectomy [32]. These methods have been proposed in an attempt to minimise urological complications and intraoperative blood loss; however they lack sufficient

supporting evidence and do not seem to result in a significant reduction of morbidity. Caesarean hysterectomy in conjunction with arterial embolisation and/or arterial balloon occlusion has been shown to reduce intraoperative blood loss and transfusion requirements when compared to caesarean hysterectomy alone [6, 33, 34].

This is one of the first reported cases of serial embolisation for the primary management of placenta percreta. While there have been other case reports of sequential arterial embolisation, to our knowledge, this is the first report of so many embolisation procedures, utilised as the only management method [8, 35]. Given the fact that our patient did not have a progressing pregnancy and that she had completed her family but was eager for uterine conservation and also very compliant, we were able to try this uterine sparing method. In a retrospective review including nine cases managed with primary arterial embolisation, 78% (7/9) did not experience major morbidity, with only two requiring hysterectomy [36] and resorption of placental tissue has been

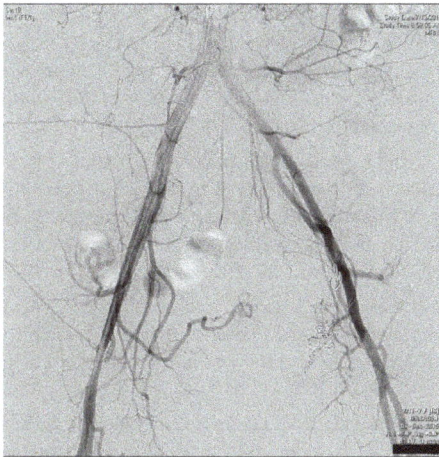

FIGURE 7: Pelvic angiogram following serial embolisation shows no persisting abnormal uterine vessels.

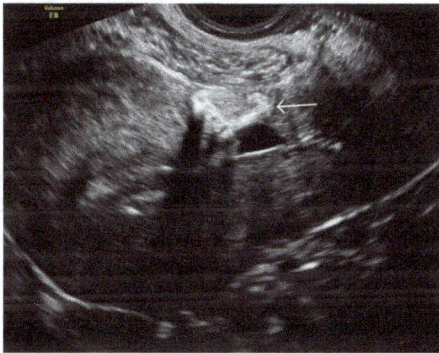

FIGURE 8: Avascular echogenic mass ($16 \times 15 \times 10$ mm) at the site of caesarean scar (arrowed).

reported after 4–6 months with no complications [16, 37–39]. However, there may be significant adverse outcomes associated with this management option, including secondary PPH, DIC, and emergency hysterectomy [36, 40, 41]. There may also be adverse outcomes resulting directly from arterial embolisation, including postembolisation syndrome, uterine scarring, endometrial atrophy, and secondary amenorrhoea [42, 43]. One systematic review found that arterial embolisation resulted in a subsequent menstruation in 6/10 (60%) but subsequent pregnancy was not reported in any (0/7) cases, which is significantly lower than other forms of conservative management or partial resection and may be associated with significant increased risk [5]. Our patient had a successful outcome, given we were able to conserve the uterus and achieve regression of placental tissue without encountering any significant morbidity during the process. There was a significant risk of life threatening haemorrhage as with any case of conservatively managed placenta percreta. This risk was further increased given the extensive blood supply to the retained placental tissue identified in initial angiogram, which took four embolisation procedures to adequately devascularise. The treatment took nine months and required extensive monitoring and intervention; however this is within

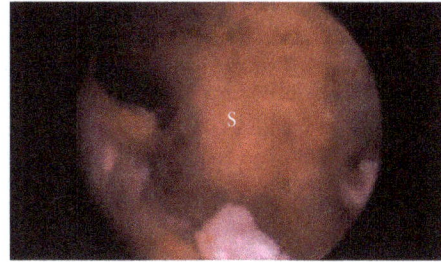

FIGURE 9: Uterine septum (S). Otherwise normal uterine cavity.

the range of 4–12 months as reported by other similar case studies in the literature [5, 8, 35, 37, 38].

4. Conclusion

While the incidence of morbidly adherent placenta, including placenta percreta, is sure to increase in the years to come, there is a lack of robust evidence regarding the most appropriate management; thus management must be individualised. We present a case of a successfully managed placenta percreta with serial arterial embolisation procedures over a period of nine months, which resulted in placental regression and uterine preservation without significant morbidity.

Consent

The patient described in this case has provided written consent for its publication.

Acknowledgments

The authors would like to thank Priscilla Bonura, Westmead Hospital Maternal Fetal Medicine Unit, for performing the ultrasound examinations.

References

[1] S. Wu, M. Kocherginsky, and J. U. Hibbard, "Abnormal placentation: twenty-year analysis," *American Journal of Obstetrics & Gynecology*, vol. 192, no. 5, pp. 1458–1461, 2005.

[2] J. M. Palacios-Jaraquemada, "Caesarean section in cases of placenta praevia and accreta," *Best Practice & Research Clinical Obstetrics & Gynaecology*, vol. 27, no. 2, pp. 221–232, 2013.

[3] K. Guleria, B. Gupta, S. Agarwal, A. Suneja, N. Vaid, and S. Jain, "Abnormally invasive placenta: Changing trends in diagnosis and management," *Acta Obstetricia et Gynecologica Scandinavica*, vol. 92, no. 4, pp. 461–464, 2013.

[4] K. M. Cunningham, A. Anwar, and S. W. Lindow, "The recurrence risk of placenta accreta following uterine conserving management," *Journal of Neonatal-Perinatal Medicine*, vol. 8, no. 4, pp. 293–296, 2016.

[5] C. N. Steins Bisschop, T. P. Schaap, T. E. Vogelvang, and P. C. Scholten, "Invasive placentation and uterus preserving treatment modalities: A systematic review," *Archives of Gynecology and Obstetrics*, vol. 284, no. 2, pp. 491–502, 2011.

[6] C. Clausen, L. Lönn, and J. Langhoff-Roos, "Management of placenta percreta: A review of published cases," *Acta Obstetricia et Gynecologica Scandinavica*, vol. 93, no. 2, pp. 138–143, 2014.

[7] Y.-H. Yee, F.-T. Kung, P.-C. Yu, T.-Y. Hsu, and Y.-F. Cheng, "Successful conservative management of placenta previa totalis and extensive percreta," *Taiwanese Journal of Obstetrics and Gynecology*, vol. 47, no. 4, pp. 431–434, 2008.

[8] D. M. Sherer, C. Gorelick, A. Zigalo, S. Sclafani, H. L. Zinn, and O. Abulafia, "Placenta previa percreta managed conservatively with methotrexate and multiple bilateral uterine artery embolizations," *Ultrasound in Obstetrics & Gynecology*, vol. 30, no. 2, pp. 227-228, 2007.

[9] N. Heiskanen, J. Kröger, S. Kainulainen, and S. Heinonen, "Placenta percreta: Methotrexate treatment and MRI findings," *American Journal of Perinatology*, vol. 25, no. 2, pp. 91-92, 2008.

[10] N. Akdemir, A. S. Cevrioğlu, S. Özden, Y. Gündüz, and G. Ilhan, "Successful treatment of Placenta Percreta through a combinatorial treatment involving a Bakri Balloon and Methotrexate - a case report," *Ginekologia Polska*, vol. 86, no. 8, pp. 631–634, 2015.

[11] T. Çirpan, C. Y. Sanhal, S. Yücebilgin, and S. Özşener, "Conservative management of placenta previa percreta by leaving placental tissue in situ with arterial ligation and adjuvant methotrexate therapy," *Journal of the Turkish German Gynecology Association*, vol. 12, no. 2, pp. 127–129, 2011.

[12] A. M. E. Hays, K. C. Worley, and S. R. Roberts, "Conservative management of placenta percreta: Experiences in two cases," *Obstetrics & Gynecology*, vol. 112, no. 2, pp. 425-426, 2008.

[13] L. E. Silver, C. J. Hobel, L. Lagasse, J. W. Luttrull, and L. D. Platt, "Placenta previa percreta with bladder involvement: New considerations and review of the literature," *Ultrasound in Obstetrics & Gynecology*, vol. 9, no. 2, pp. 131–138, 1997.

[14] H.-P. Dinkel, P. Dürig, P. Schnatterbeck, and J. Triller, "Percutaneous treatment of placenta percreta using coil embolization," *Journal of Endovascular Therapy*, vol. 10, no. 1, pp. 158–162, 2003.

[15] M. Teixidor Viñas, E. Chandraharan, M. V. Moneta, and A. M. Belli, "The role of interventional radiology in reducing haemorrhage and hysterectomy following caesarean section for morbidly adherent placenta," *Clinical Radiology*, vol. 69, no. 8, pp. e345–e351, 2014.

[16] P. Soyer, O. Morel, Y. Fargeaudou et al., "Value of pelvic embolization in the management of severe postpartum hemorrhage due to placenta accreta, increta or percreta," *European Journal of Radiology*, vol. 80, no. 3, pp. 729–735, 2011.

[17] J. Zeng, Y. L. Shi, J. Y. Luo, S. Zhou, and M. Y. Luo, "Complications and related determinants in 13669 pregnant women," *Journal of Central South University (Medical Sciences)*, vol. 38, no. 11, pp. 1092–1098, 2013.

[18] S. Pather, S. Strockyj, A. Richards, N. Campbell, B. de Vries, and R. Ogle, "Maternal outcome after conservative management of placenta percreta at caesarean section: a report of three cases and a review of the literature," *Australian and New Zealand Journal of Obstetrics and Gynaecology*, vol. 54, no. 1, pp. 84–87, 2014.

[19] M. Sawada, S. Matsuzaki, K. Mimura, K. Kumasawa, M. Endo, and T. Kimura, "Successful conservative management of placenta percreta: Investigation by serial magnetic resonance imaging of the clinical course and a literature review," *Journal of Obstetrics and Gynaecology Research*, vol. 42, no. 12, pp. 1858–1863, 2016.

[20] M. E. Ochalski, A. Broach, and T. Lee, "Laparoscopic Management of Placenta Percreta," *Journal of Minimally Invasive Gynecology*, vol. 17, no. 1, pp. 128–130, 2010.

[21] S. B. L. Teo, D. Kanagalingam, H.-K. Tan, and L.-K. Tan, "Massive postpartum haemorrhage after uterus-conserving surgery in placenta percreta: The danger of the partial placenta percreta," *BJOG: An International Journal of Obstetrics & Gynaecology*, vol. 115, no. 6, pp. 789–792, 2008.

[22] E. Fay, B. Norquist, J. Jolley, and M. Hardesty, "Conservative Management of Invasive Placentation: Two Cases with Different Surgical Approaches," *American Journal of Perinatology Reports*, vol. 06, no. 02, pp. e212–e215, 2016.

[23] P. S. Lee, R. Bakelaar, C. Brennan Fitpatrick, S. C. Ellestad, L. J. Havrilesky, and A. A. Secord, "Medical and surgical treatment of Placenta percreta to optimize bladder preservation," *Obstetrics & Gynecology*, vol. 112, no. 2, pp. 421–424, 2008.

[24] J. M. Palacios Jaraquemada, M. Pesaresi, J. C. Nassif, and S. Hermosid, "Anterior placenta percreta: Surgical approach, hemostasis and uterine repair," *Acta Obstetricia et Gynecologica Scandinavica*, vol. 83, no. 8, pp. 738–744, 2004.

[25] M. Teixidor Viñas, A. Belli, S. Arulkumaran, and E. Chandraharan, "Prevention of postpartum haemorrhage and hysterectomy in patients with Morbidly Adherent Placenta: A cohort study comparing outcomes before and after introduction of the Triple-P procedure," *Ultrasound in Obstetrics & Gynecology*, 2014.

[26] E. Chandraharan, "Should the Triple-P procedure be used as an alternative to peripartum hysterectomy in the surgical treatment of placenta percreta?" *Women's Health Journal (WHJ)*, vol. 8, no. 4, pp. 351–353, 2012.

[27] R. Washecka and A. Behling, "Urologic complications of placenta percreta invading the urinary bladder: a case report and review of the literature." *Hawaii Medical Journal*, vol. 61, no. 4, pp. 66–69, 2002.

[28] M. K. Ng, G. S. Jack, D. M. Bolton, and N. Lawrentschuk, "Placenta Percreta With Urinary Tract Involvement: The Case for a Multidisciplinary Approach," *Urology*, vol. 74, no. 4, pp. 778–782, 2009.

[29] A. Camuzcuoglu, M. Vural, N. G. Hilali et al., "Surgical management of 58 patients with placenta praevia percreta," *Wiener Klinische Wochenschrift*, vol. 128, no. 9-10, pp. 360–366, 2016.

[30] S. Matsubara, A. Ohkuchi, M. Yashi et al., "Opening the bladder for cesarean hysterectomy for placenta previa percreta with bladder invasion," *Journal of Obstetrics and Gynaecology Research*, vol. 35, no. 2, pp. 359–363, 2009.

[31] R. Faranesh, R. Shabtai, S. Eliezer, and S. Raed, "Suggested approach for management of placenta percreta invading the urinary bladder," *Obstetrics & Gynecology*, vol. 110, no. 2, pp. 512–515, 2007.

[32] S. Matsuzaki, K. Yoshino, K. Kumasawa et al., "Placenta percreta managed by transverse uterine fundal incision with retrograde cesarean hysterectomy: a novel surgical approach," *Clinical Case Reports*, vol. 2, no. 6, pp. 260–264, 2014.

[33] S. Sumigama, A. Itakura, T. Ota et al., "Placenta previa increta/percreta in Japan: A retrospective study of ultrasound findings, management and clinical course," *Journal of Obstetrics and Gynaecology Research*, vol. 33, no. 5, pp. 606–611, 2007.

[34] G. Cali, F. Forlani, L. Giambanco et al., "Prophylactic use of intravascular balloon catheters in women with placenta accreta,

increta and percreta," *European Journal of Obstetrics & Gynecology and Reproductive Biology*, vol. 179, pp. 36–41, 2014.

[35] A. El-Messidi, C. Morissette, W. Faught, and L. Oppenheimer, "Application of 3-D Angiography in the Management of Placenta Percreta Treated with Repeat Uterine Artery Embolization," *Journal of Obstetrics and Gynaecology Canada*, vol. 32, no. 8, pp. 775–779, 2010.

[36] S. Timmermans, A. C. van Hof, and J. J. Duvekot, "Conservative management of abnormally invasive placentation," *Obstetrical & Gynecological Survey* , vol. 62, no. 8, pp. 529–539, 2007.

[37] D. Clément, G. Kayem, and D. Cabrol, "Conservative treatment of placenta percreta: A safe alternative," *European Journal of Obstetrics & Gynecology and Reproductive Biology*, vol. 114, no. 1, pp. 108-109, 2004.

[38] F. Alkazaleh, M. Geary, J. Kingdom, J. R. Kachura, and R. Windrim, "Elective Non-Removal of the Placenta and Prophylactic Uterine Artery Embolization Postpartum as a Diagnostic Imaging Approach for the Management of Placenta Percreta: A Case Report," *Journal of Obstetrics and Gynaecology Canada*, vol. 26, no. 8, pp. 743–746, 2004.

[39] Y. Y. Cheng, J. I. Hwang, S. W. Hung et al., "Angiographic Embolization for Emergent and Prophylactic Management of Obstetric Hemorrhage: A Four-Year Experience," *Journal of the Chinese Medical Association*, vol. 66, no. 12, pp. 727–734, 2003.

[40] G. Luo, S. C. Perni, C. Jean-Pierre, R. N. Baergen, and M. Predanic, "Failure of conservative management of placenta previa-percreta," *Journal of Perinatal Medicine*, vol. 33, no. 6, pp. 564–568, 2005.

[41] M. Y. Chung, Y. K. Y. Cheng, S. C. H. Yu, D. S. Sahota, and T. Y. Leung, "Nonremoval of an abnormally invasive placenta at cesarean section with postoperative uterine artery embolization," *Acta Obstetricia et Gynecologica Scandinavica*, vol. 92, no. 11, pp. 1250-1255, 2013.

[42] A. N. Diop, P. Chabrot, A. Bertrand et al., "Placenta accreta: Management with uterine artery embolization in 17 cases," *Journal of Vascular and Interventional Radiology*, vol. 21, no. 5, pp. 644–648, 2010.

[43] M. Alanis, B. S. Hurst, P. B. Marshburn, and M. L. Matthews, "Conservative management of placenta increta with selective arterial embolization preserves future fertility and results in a favorable outcome in subsequent pregnancies," *Fertility and Sterility*, vol. 86, no. 5, pp. 1514–e7, 2006.

29

Severe Maternal Morbidity Associated with Systemic Lupus Erythematosus Flare in the Second Trimester of Pregnancy

Matthew J. Blitz ⓘ and Adiel Fleischer

Division of Maternal-Fetal Medicine, Department of Obstetrics and Gynecology, Long Island Jewish Medical Center, Donald and Barbara Zucker School of Medicine at Hofstra/Northwell, New Hyde Park, NY, USA

Correspondence should be addressed to Matthew J. Blitz; mblitz@northwell.edu

Academic Editor: Seung-Yup Ku

Pregnancy in women with systemic lupus erythematosus (SLE) is associated with an increased risk of adverse maternal and fetal outcomes. Here, we present a case of severe maternal morbidity in a 23-year-old primigravida with SLE and secondary Sjögren's syndrome who experienced a life-threatening multisystem flare at 17 weeks of gestational age. She presented to the emergency department complaining of cough with hemoptysis and shortness of breath. She developed hypoxic respiratory failure and was admitted to the intensive care unit. Bronchoscopy confirmed diffuse alveolar hemorrhage. Physical exam and laboratory evaluation were consistent with an active SLE flare, pancytopenia, and new-onset lupus nephritis. After counseling regarding disease severity, poor prognosis, and recommendation for therapy with cytotoxic agents, she agreed to interruption of pregnancy which was achieved by medical induction. Her course was further complicated by thrombotic microangiopathy and generalized tonic-clonic seizures attributable to posterior reversible encephalopathy syndrome versus neuropsychiatric SLE. This case represents one of the most extreme manifestations of lupus disease activity associated with pregnancy that has been reported in the literature and emphasizes the importance of preconception evaluation and counseling and a multidisciplinary management approach in cases with a complex and evolving clinical course.

1. Introduction

Systemic lupus erythematosus (SLE) is a chronic autoimmune disease that predominantly affects women of childbearing age. Pregnancy in women with SLE is associated with an increased risk of adverse maternal and fetal outcomes. Here, we present a case of severe maternal morbidity in a young woman with SLE and secondary Sjögren's syndrome who experienced a life-threatening multisystem flare which required a prolonged stay in the intensive care unit and interruption of pregnancy in the second trimester. Although many cases of life-threatening and even fatal maternal complications of SLE have been described in the literature, there are few reported cases in which such a large number of different organ systems are affected, as we describe here. With such an uncertain and complex disease course, clinical management can be very challenging, necessitating a multidisciplinary approach to care.

2. Case Presentation

A 23-year-old primigravida at 17 weeks of gestational age presented to the emergency department complaining of worsening cough with intermittent hemoptysis, shortness of breath, and chest pain which had been present for several weeks and exacerbated by light physical activity. Her past medical history was significant for SLE with secondary Sjögren's syndrome diagnosed 6 years before based on findings of arthritis, malar rash, positive antinuclear antibodies (ANA), elevated anti-double-stranded DNA (anti-dsDNA), and the presence of anti-Ro/SSA antibodies. She had no prior surgery and was not taking any medications. She reported no SLE flares in the past few years and had discontinued hydroxychloroquine (HCQ) approximately one year earlier. Her obstetrician referred her for a maternal-fetal medicine consultation in early pregnancy, at which time she acknowledged that she was no longer under the care of

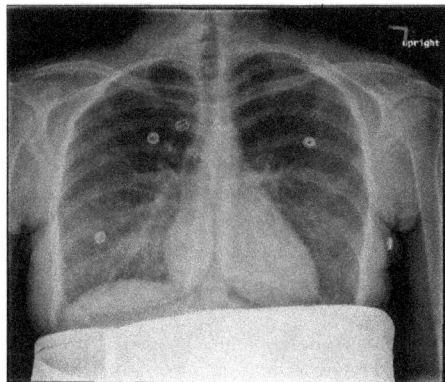

FIGURE 1: Chest radiograph on the day of admission noted indistinct increased markings and a patchy opacity in the right lower lung.

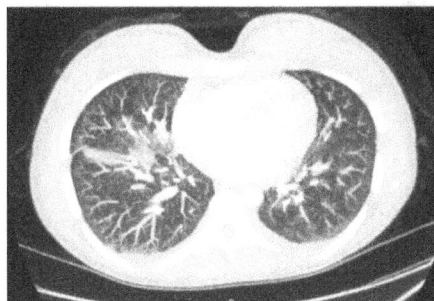

FIGURE 2: Chest computed tomography angiography (CTA) on the day of admission noting patchy infiltrate in the right middle and lower lung lobes and small bilateral pleural effusions.

a rheumatologist. She did not receive any risk assessment or counseling prior to conception. Two months prior to pregnancy, her serum creatinine was 0.74 mg/dL and her systolic and diastolic blood pressures ranged from 100 to 120 mm Hg and from 70 to 80 mm Hg, respectively. Of note, she was treated with antibiotics for pneumonia three times in the past 14 months and was known to have a recent negative purified protein derivative (PPD) skin test.

Upon arrival to the hospital, she was awake and alert and in no apparent distress. Her heart rate was 116 beats per minute. She was afebrile and normotensive with a respiratory rate of 16 breaths per minute and an oxygen saturation of 100% on room air. Abdominal exam noted a gravid, nontender uterus. Her respiratory effort appeared normal and her lungs were clear to auscultation. A subtle malar rash and diffuse, white ulcerative plaques were visualized on the buccal mucosa and palate. Bilateral lower extremity pitting edema was noted. The physical exam was otherwise unremarkable. Abdominal ultrasound demonstrated an intrauterine pregnancy with a fetal heart rate of 150 beats per minute. Laboratory evaluation was significant for a hemoglobin and hematocrit of 6.1 g/dL and 18.5%, respectively. The white blood cell (WBC) count was 3,300/uL and the platelet count was 101,000/uL. Serum creatinine was 1.04 mg/dL and urine protein/creatinine ratio was 4.7. A 24-hour urine collection contained over 3 grams of protein. Antiphospholipid antibody testing was performed. On hospital day (HD) 1, anticardiolipin IgG and IgM were 24 GPL and 8 MPL, respectively, and repeat testing on HD2 yielded 34 GPL and 11 MPL, respectively (medium or high titer typically defined as >40 GPL or MPL). Anti-beta2-glycoprotein I antibody screen was negative. Lupus anticoagulant assays, which included dilute Russell viper venom time (dRVVT) and silica clotting time (SCT), were negative. An electrocardiogram (EKG) showed sinus tachycardia. Chest radiography featured indistinct increased markings and a patchy opacity in the right lower lung (Figure 1). Chest computed tomography angiography (CTA) found no evidence of pulmonary embolism but did reveal a patchy infiltrate in the right middle and lower lobes with small bilateral pleural effusions and enlarged hilar lymph nodes

(Figure 2). After initial evaluation by the obstetrical and emergency medicine teams, consultations were requested with pulmonology, infectious disease, rheumatology, hematology, and nephrology to assist in further management. The decision was made to admit the patient for treatment of suspected community-acquired pneumonia (CAP), new-onset nephrotic syndrome likely secondary to lupus nephritis, and an active SLE flare associated with pancytopenia, malar rash, oral ulcers, and lymphadenopathy.

The patient was started on intravenous ceftriaxone and azithromycin for CAP and HCQ and pulse methylprednisolone for the SLE flare. Thromboprophylaxis was initiated with enoxaparin. She received a transfusion of two units of packed red blood cells (PRBCs) for severe anemia described as normocytic and direct coombs test positive. Indirect bilirubin and lactate dehydrogenase (LDH) were increased, serum haptoglobin was decreased, and a peripheral smear showed a few schistocytes and some spherocytes; these findings were most consistent with autoimmune hemolytic anemia. Overall, her pancytopenia was thought to be multifactorial. In the coming days, there was evidence of continued hemolysis despite steroid administration with a persistently elevated LDH and low serum haptoglobin (<20 mg/dL), as well as repeat peripheral smears demonstrating numerous schistocytes. Of note, a repeat direct coombs test was negative. Collectively, these findings were concerning for other (nonimmune) causes of hemolysis such as microangiopathic hemolytic anemia (MAHA) or thrombotic thrombocytopenic purpura (TTP). A normal ADAMTS13 activity level subsequently ruled out the latter.

On HD5, the patient was started on supplemental oxygen via nasal cannula after it was noted that her oxygen saturation on room air decreased to below 90%. Over the next few days her oxygen requirements gradually increased to 6 L/min. Pulmonary edema was suspected based on diffuse b-lines on lung ultrasound and repeat chest radiograph noting increased bilateral pleural effusions. All intravenous fluids were discontinued, and furosemide was administered. Improvement in lower extremity edema and good urine output were noted. However, she continued to experience shortness of breath with oxygen saturation as low as 80% on supplemental

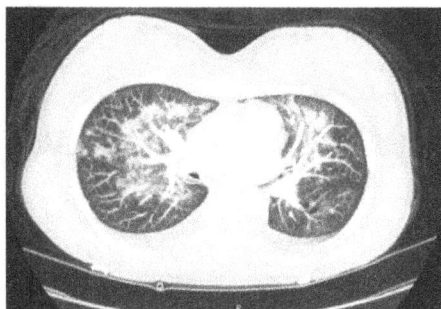

FIGURE 3: Repeat chest computed tomography angiography (CTA) on hospital day 5 featuring progressive ground-glass opacities bilaterally, which, in the setting of continued hemoptysis, was concerning for diffuse alveolar hemorrhage.

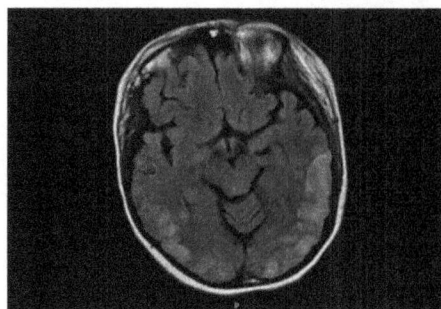

FIGURE 4: Brain magnetic resonance imaging (MRI) demonstrated symmetrical bilateral hyperintensities on T2-weighted imaging and fluid-attenuated inversion recovery (FLAIR) sequences consistent with cerebrocortical edema.

oxygen. A repeat chest CTA noted progressive ground-glass opacities bilaterally (Figure 3), which, in the setting of continued hemoptysis, increased concern for diffuse alveolar hemorrhage (DAH). On HD8 she was transferred to the intensive care unit for worsening hypoxia despite diuresis, antibiotic therapy, and steroids. Therapeutic plasma exchange (TPE) was performed with a plan for 4 additional sessions. Fiberoptic bronchoscopy with sequential bronchoalveolar lavage (BAL) demonstrated grossly hemorrhagic fluid consistent with DAH.

Given the severity of maternal disease, poor prognosis for the fetus, and recommendation for more aggressive therapy, the patient was counseled for termination of pregnancy. The patient understood that the risk of early-onset preeclampsia and extreme preterm delivery was high even if her pulmonary and renal status were to improve significantly. She was induced and delivered vaginally on HD10. Cyclophosphamide, an alkylating agent associated with gonadal toxicity and teratogenicity, was administered after a suboptimal response to steroids and TPE.

In the first few days after delivery, her blood pressures were persistently elevated (≥140/90 mm Hg) but generally below severe range (160/110 mm Hg). A repeat 24-hour urine collection on HD 14 was found to have a total protein of more than 17 grams. Serum creatinine increased to 1.02 mg/dL. On HD22, a kidney biopsy was performed, which revealed lupus nephritis, diffuse global proliferative type, class IV-G (A), and an active thrombotic microangiopathy (TMA) in several arterioles and glomerular vascular poles. The patient was discharged home on HD25 on prednisone and HCQ for lupus, losartan for hypertension, and furosemide for edema associated with nephrotic syndrome. She was also to continue cyclophosphamide infusions outpatient.

Less than two weeks after discharge, the patient was readmitted with symptomatic anemia and progressive lower extremity edema. She was also noted to have worsening hypertension (systolic blood pressure 160–200 mm Hg), acute kidney injury (creatinine 1.7 → 2.5 mg/dL), and worsening thrombocytopenia (platelet count 81,000 → 52,000/uL). Serum LDH increased to 1,028 U/L. These findings were suspicious for an SLE flare-induced TMA exacerbation versus atypical hemolytic uremic syndrome (aHUS). Pulse dose

steroids were again administered. Nicardipine infusion was started for blood pressure optimization. Approximately one hour after a transfusion of PRBCs was started, the patient was found to have altered mental status. She then experienced a series of generalized tonic-clonic seizures in quick succession without recovery between episodes. This was followed by a postictal state. Lorazepam and levetiracetam were administered. She was intubated and mechanically ventilated for airway protection and transferred to the ICU for status epilepticus. Urgent brain MRI demonstrated symmetrical bilateral hyperintensities on T2-weighted imaging and fluid-attenuated inversion recovery (FLAIR) sequences consistent with cerebrocortical edema (Figure 4); there was no evidence of acute infarct or hemorrhage. Neurology was consulted. Posterior reversible encephalopathy syndrome (PRES) and neuropsychiatric SLE (NPSLE) were highest in the differential diagnosis. Eclampsia was thought less likely at more than 3 weeks postpartum, after delivery of a 17-week fetus. After an inadequate hematologic response to pulse dose steroids, eculizumab, a monoclonal antibody and complement inhibitor, was started. Over the next few days, the platelet count and LDH began improving, suggesting a response to this treatment. The patient received a total of 5 units of PRBCs and 3 doses of eculizumab and was successfully extubated on HD5 after readmission. Repeat antiphospholipid antibody testing was performed. Anticardiolipin IgG and IgM decreased to 4 GPL and 3 MPL, respectively. Anti-beta2-glycoprotein I antibody screen and lupus anticoagulant functional assays remained negative. She was discharged home on HD13 on labetalol and amlodipine for blood pressure control, HCQ and prednisone for lupus, levetiracetam for seizure prophylaxis, and cefuroxime for meningitis prophylaxis given that eculizumab increases susceptibility to Neisseria infection.

Over the next several months, she experienced continued seizure activity and frequent headaches which required intermittent hospitalization.

3. Discussion

It is well established that pregnant women with SLE have an increased risk of adverse maternal and fetal outcomes, including, among others, preeclampsia, venous thromboembolism, infection, unplanned cesarean delivery, fetal growth restriction, preterm birth, and fetal loss [1]. In addition, maternal mortality may be 20-fold higher in women with SLE [2]. Active disease and lupus nephritis are nearly always present in such cases, and the two major causes of death are complications from lupus disease activity and opportunistic infection [3].

Based on the numerous risks associated with pregnancy, it is recommended that women with SLE have a preconception evaluation and multidisciplinary management with maternal-fetal medicine and rheumatology during pregnancy. Active SLE at the time of conception is a predictor of adverse outcomes; it is suggested that the disease be quiescent for six months prior to attempting pregnancy [4]. Laboratory testing should, at a minimum, include antiphospholipid antibodies (lupus anticoagulant, IgG and IgM anticardiolipin antibodies, IgG and IgM anti-beta2-glycoprotein I antibodies), anti-Ro/SSA and anti-La/SSB antibodies, and an assessment of renal function (creatinine, spot urine protein/creatinine ratio). Women who have anti-Ro/SSA and anti-La/SSB antibodies should have intensive fetal surveillance for heart block with weekly pulsed-Doppler fetal echocardiography (to measure the mechanical PR interval) starting at 16–18 weeks and continuing through 26–28 weeks of pregnancy. Ideally, all women with SLE should be on HCQ and low-dose aspirin during pregnancy, unless otherwise contraindicated. Women who continue HCQ during pregnancy have fewer disease flares, improved outcomes, and, in mothers with anti-Ro/SSA and anti-LA/SSB antibodies, a reduced risk of fetal heart block [5]. Low-dose aspirin started at 12–16 weeks of gestation reduces the risk of preeclampsia and fetal growth restriction [6]. Discontinuation of medications used to control disease activity increases the risk of flares and associated pregnancy complications. Serial ultrasound examinations should be performed to assess fetal growth and antepartum fetal surveillance should be initiated in the third trimester.

Renal involvement is common in patients with SLE and may be suspected in the presence of proteinuria or an elevated serum creatinine. Lupus nephritis is diagnosed and classified based on histopathologic findings on renal biopsy [7]. Most patients with this condition have an immune complex-mediated glomerular disease. The most common and most severe form of lupus nephritis is class IV, defined histologically as involvement of more than 50 percent of glomeruli on light microscopy [8]. Class IV disease is further subclassified based on whether affected glomeruli are segmentally (S) or globally (G) affected and whether the inflammatory activity of the lesions is active (A), chronic (C), or both (A/C). Hypertension and nephrotic syndrome, consisting of heavy proteinuria, hypoalbuminemia, and peripheral edema, are often seen in active class IV disease and patients characteristically have low complement levels (C3) and elevated anti-dsDNA levels.

Involvement of the renal vasculature in cases of lupus nephritis is a poor prognostic sign. In thrombotic microangiopathy (TMA), damage to the endothelial cells of small arterioles and capillaries results in microvascular thrombosis.

Nearly all TMAs cause microangiopathic hemolytic anemia (MAHA) and thrombocytopenia. MAHA results from intravascular fragmentation of red blood cells, which produces schistocytes on peripheral blood smear.

Alveolar hemorrhage is a rare, life-threatening complication which occurs in approximately 0.5–3.7% of nonpregnant SLE patients [9, 10] and has also been reported during pregnancy in a limited number of case reports and case series [11–13]. This is typically associated with active class III or IV lupus nephritis and increased disease activity. Microvascular injury is thought to result from immune complex deposition in the alveolar wall with induction of apoptosis [14, 15]. The mortality rate for SLE patients with DAH may exceed 50% [9, 16]. It is important to recognize that hemoptysis is reported in less than two-thirds of such cases [17]. More frequent signs and symptoms are hypoxemia, dyspnea, cough, and fever. Thus, DAH can easily be mistaken for pneumonia or pulmonary edema [18]. In patients with lupus nephritis, clinical suspicion for DAH should be increased in the presence of acute pulmonary symptoms, new radiographic infiltrates, and a falling hematocrit, even in the absence of hemoptysis. The diagnosis is established by flexible bronchoscopy with sequential BAL. Characteristically, lavage aliquots are progressively more hemorrhagic and Prussian blue staining reveals hemosiderin-containing macrophages [19, 20]. High clinical suspicion, early diagnosis, and aggressive therapy with glucocorticoids and cyclophosphamide are the cornerstones of DAH management in patients with SLE. Ventilatory support and blood transfusion should be offered as necessary. Although it is uncertain whether it improves survival, plasma exchange therapy is frequently offered to remove circulating immune complexes from the blood, especially in cases where there is an inadequate clinical response to cyclophosphamide [21].

Posterior reversible encephalopathy syndrome (PRES), characterized by headache, visual disturbances, confusion, and seizures, is an underrecognized condition associated with SLE [22]. Pregnancy-related PRES in women *without* SLE occurs most frequently in conjunction with preeclampsia-eclampsia [23]. Disruption of the blood brain barrier secondary to endothelial dysfunction results in vasogenic edema, often in the parietooccipital regions; this produces a characteristic magnetic resonance imaging (MRI) finding of hyperintense signal in affected areas on T2-weighted imaging [24, 25]. At the time of presentation, most SLE patients diagnosed with PRES have hypertension, lupus nephritis, and active disease with multiple complications [26, 27].

Although it is one of the most prevalent complications of lupus, likely affecting the majority of patients at some time in their disease course, NPSLE is arguably the most poorly understood [28, 29]. NPSLE associated with pregnancy has been addressed in scant case reports and case series [30, 31]. Nervous system involvement can produce a complex array of neurological, psychiatric, and behavioral manifestations that increase morbidity and mortality. The American College of Rheumatology (ACR) has developed a standardized nomenclature system which defines 19 NPSLE syndromes involving the central and peripheral nervous systems [32]. Cognitive dysfunction, headaches, and psychiatric disorders are some of the most common NPSLE syndromes [29, 33]. In all cases, NPSLE is a diagnosis of exclusion; all other possible etiologies of the observed neuropsychiatric symptoms must be considered and excluded, including electrolyte abnormalities, infection, renal failure, and drug effects. In the absence of a gold standard diagnostic test, this may represent a significant clinical challenge, especially in pregnancy and the postpartum period, where pregnancy-specific conditions such as preeclampsia-eclampsia may produce the same symptoms. The pathogenesis of NPSLE is multifactorial and involves inflammatory cytokines, autoantibodies, and immune complexes that contribute to vasculopathic, cytotoxic, and autoantibody-mediated neuronal dysfunction [34]. Management remains empirical without any standardized, evidence-based approach to treatment [35].

Antiphospholipid syndrome (APS) is an autoimmune disorder characterized by vascular thromboses and/or pregnancy morbidity in the presence of persistent antiphospholipid antibodies. A small subset of patients with APS (<1%) develop multiple organ failure secondary to widespread thrombotic disease, a condition referred to as catastrophic APS (CAPS) which has a mortality rate of up to 50% [36]. A definitive diagnosis requires simultaneous involvement of 3 or more organs and histopathologic confirmation in at least one organ or tissue. In the case described here, the patient did not meet criteria for APS. She did have anticardiolipin antibodies but at titers below the threshold to meet APS laboratory criteria (>40 GPL or MPL). However, the clinical similarities with CAPS are worth noting. Although it is possible that serial laboratory evaluation during her first hospital admission would have yielded an anticardiolipin IgG titer > 40 GPL, the anticardiolipin results during her second admission demonstrate that they were not persistent and, therefore, not consistent with APS or CAPS.

Termination of pregnancy in the second trimester, prior to viability, to preserve the health of the mother in cases of severe SLE disease activity is infrequent and usually performed to facilitate more aggressive treatment. Although the physiologic changes of pregnancy, including an increase in glomerular filtration rate and renal plasma flow, may worsen preexisting renal disease, there is not sufficient evidence to suggest that interruption of pregnancy, in and of itself, has a beneficial effect on the resolution of an acute disease flare. However, it is theoretically possible that a rapid decline in pregnancy hormone levels, particularly estrogen, may be advantageous [37]. Immunosuppressive medications used to treat SLE, such as cyclophosphamide, are known to cross the placenta and have teratogenic effects. In addition, this particular medication has been associated with premature and irreversible ovarian failure. It should only be offered, after appropriate counseling, in cases where no alternative therapy is available.

In the case presented here, the patient did not have many of the known prepregnancy predictors of adverse pregnancy outcomes. Specifically, she did not have any recent disease exacerbations, antiphospholipid antibodies, thrombocytopenia, prior lupus nephritis, or prior use of antihypertensive medications [1, 38]. However, as a primigravida, she was at increased risk for flare during pregnancy [39]. In addition,

her discontinuation of HCQ prior to pregnancy, lack of preconception counseling, and lapse in rheumatologic care placed her at increased risk of pregnancy morbidity.

In summary, SLE disease flares can occur at any time during pregnancy and with unpredictable severity. All women with a diagnosis of SLE should be offered a preconception evaluation and consultation, with a goal of reducing adverse pregnancy outcomes through health education, risk assessment, and appropriate interventions. In cases with a complex and evolving clinical course, the importance of a collaborative and multidisciplinary management approach must be emphasized. Furthermore, it is essential that management occur at a tertiary referral center with experience managing critically ill high-risk obstetric patients.

References

[1] J. P. Buyon, M. Y. Kim, M. M. Guerra et al., "Predictors of pregnancy outcomes in patients with lupus: A cohort study," *Annals of Internal Medicine*, vol. 163, no. 3, pp. 153–163, 2015.

[2] M. E. Clowse, M. Jamison, E. Myers, and A. H. James, "A national study of the complications of lupus in pregnancy," *American Journal of Obstetrics & Gynecology*, vol. 199, no. 2, pp. 127.e1–127.e6, 2008.

[3] J. Ritchie, A. Smyth, C. Tower, M. Helbert, M. Venning, and V. D. Garovic, "Maternal deaths in women with lupus nephritis: A review of published evidence," *Lupus*, vol. 21, no. 5, pp. 534–541, 2012.

[4] L.-W. Kwok, L.-S. Tam, T. Y. Zhu, Y.-Y. Leung, and E. K. Li, "Predictors of maternal and fetal outcomes in pregnancies of patients with systemic lupus erythematosus," *Lupus*, vol. 20, no. 8, pp. 829–836, 2011.

[5] A. Saxena, P. M. Izmirly, B. Mendez, J. P. Buyon, and D. M. Friedman, "Prevention and treatment in utero of autoimmune-associated congenital heart block," *Cardiology in Review*, vol. 22, no. 6, pp. 263–267, 2014.

[6] S. Roberge, K. Nicolaides, S. Demers, J. Hyett, N. Chaillet, and E. Bujold, "The role of aspirin dose on the prevention of preeclampsia and fetal growth restriction: systematic review and meta-analysis," *American Journal of Obstetrics & Gynecology*, vol. 216, no. 2, pp. 110–120.e6, 2017.

[7] M. M. Schwartz, S. M. Korbet, and E. J. Lewis, "The prognosis and pathogenesis of severe lupus glomerulonephritis," *Nephrology Dialysis Transplantation*, vol. 23, no. 4, pp. 1298–1306, 2008.

[8] J. J. Weening, V. D. D'Agati, and M. M. Schwartz, "The classification of glomerulonephritis in systemic lupus erythematosus revisited," *Journal of the American Society of Nephrology*, vol. 15, no. 2, pp. 241–250, 2004.

[9] M. R. Zamora, M. L. Warner, R. Tuder, and M. I. Schwarz, "Diffuse alveolar hemorrhage and systemic lupus erythematosus: clinical presentation, histology, survival, and outcome," *Medicine*, vol. 76, no. 3, pp. 192–202, 1997.

[10] C. A. Dos Santos Andrade, T. Mendonça, F. Farinha et al., "Alveolar hemorrhage in systemic lupus erythematosus: A cohort review," *Lupus*, vol. 25, no. 1, pp. 75–80, 2016.

[11] K. Gaither, K. Halstead, and T. C. Mason, "Pulmonary alveolar hemorrhage in a pregnancy complicated by systemic lupus

erythematosus," *Journal of the National Medical Association*, vol. 97, no. 6, pp. 831–833, 2005.

[12] M. P. Keane, C. J. M. Van De Ven, J. P. Lynch III, and W. J. McCune, "Systemic lupus during pregnancy with refractory alveolar haemorrhage: Recovery following termination of pregnancy," *Lupus*, vol. 6, no. 9, pp. 730–733, 1997.

[13] M.-Y. Chang, J.-T. Fang, Y.-C. Chen, and C.-C. Huang, "Diffuse alveolar hemorrhage in systemic lupus erythematosus: a single center retrospective study in Taiwan," *Renal Failure*, vol. 24, no. 6, pp. 791–802, 2002.

[14] M. D. Hughson, Z. He, J. Henegar, and R. McMurray, "Alveolar hemorrhage and renal microangiopathy in systemic lupus erythematosus," *Arch Pathol Lab Med*, vol. 125, no. 4, pp. 475–483, 2001.

[15] J. W. Eagen, V. A. Memoli, J. L. Roberts, G. R. Matthew, M. M. Schwartz, and E. J. Lewis, "Pulmonary hemorrhage in systemic lupus erythematosus," *Medicine (United States)*, vol. 57, no. 6, pp. 545–560, 1978.

[16] S.-K. Kwok, S.-J. Moon, J. H. Ju et al., "Diffuse alveolar hemorrhage in systemic lupus erythematosus: Risk factors and clinical outcome: Results from affiliated hospitals of Catholic University of Korea," *Lupus*, vol. 20, no. 1, pp. 102–107, 2011.

[17] M. Shen, X. Zeng, X. Tian et al., "Diffuse alveolar hemorrhage in systemic lupus erythematosus: A retrospective study in China," *Lupus*, vol. 19, no. 11, pp. 1326–1330, 2010.

[18] A. S. Santos-Ocampo, B. F. Mandell, and B. J. Fessler, "Alveolar hemorrhage in systemic lupus erythematosus: Presentation and management," *CHEST*, vol. 118, no. 4, pp. 1083–1090, 2000.

[19] D. W. Golde, M. J. Cline, W. L. Drew, H. Z. Klein, and T. N. Finley, "Occult Pulmonary Haemorrhage in Leukaemia," *British Medical Journal*, vol. 2, no. 5964, pp. 166–168, 1975.

[20] A. De Lassence, J. Fleury-Feith, E. Escudier, J. Beaune, J. F. Bernaudin -, and C. Cordonnier, "Alveolar hemorrhage: Diagnostic criteria and results in 194 immunocompromised hosts," *American Journal of Respiratory and Critical Care Medicine*, vol. 151, no. 1, pp. 157–163, 1995.

[21] C. Ednalino, J. Yip, and S. E. Carsons, "Systematic review of diffuse alveolar hemorrhage in systemic lupus erythematosus: Focus on outcome and therapy," *JCR: Journal of Clinical Rheumatology*, vol. 21, no. 6, pp. 305–310, 2015.

[22] N. Gatla, N. Annapureddy, W. Sequeira, and M. Jolly, "Posterior reversible encephalopathy syndrome in systemic lupus erythematosus," *JCR: Journal of Clinical Rheumatology*, vol. 19, no. 6, pp. 334–340, 2013.

[23] Y. Wen, B. Yang, Q. Huang, and Y. Liu, "Posterior reversible encephalopathy syndrome in pregnancy: a retrospective series of 36 patients from mainland China," *Irish Journal of Medical Science*, vol. 186, no. 3, pp. 699–705, 2017.

[24] C. Lamy, C. Oppenheim, J. F. Méder, and J. L. Mas, "Neuroimaging in posterior reversible encephalopathy syndrome," *Journal of Neurogenetics*, vol. 14, no. 2, pp. 89–96, 2004.

[25] J. E. Fugate, D. O. Claassen, H. J. Cloft, D. F. Kallmes, O. S. Kozak, and A. A. Rabinstein, "Posterior reversible encephalopathy syndrome: associated clinical and radiologic findings," *Mayo Clinic Proceedings*, vol. 85, no. 5, pp. 427–432, 2010.

[26] C.-C. Lai, W.-S. Chen, and Y.-S. Chang, "Clinical features and outcomes of posterior reversible encephalopathy syndrome in patients with systemic lupus erythematosus," *Arthritis Care & Research*, vol. 65, no. 11, pp. 1766–1774, 2013.

[27] A. Budhoo and G. M. Mody, "The spectrum of posterior reversible encephalopathy in systemic lupus erythematosus," *Clinical Rheumatology*, vol. 34, no. 12, pp. 2127–2134, 2015.

[28] H. Ainiala, J. Loukkola, J. Peltola, M. Korpela, and A. Hietaharju, "The prevalence of neuropsychiatric syndromes in systemic lupus erythematosus," *Neurology*, vol. 57, no. 3, pp. 496–500, 2001.

[29] R. L. Brey, S. L. Holliday, A. R. Saklad et al., "Neuropsychiatric syndromes in lupus: prevalence using standardized definitions," *Neurology*, vol. 58, no. 8, pp. 1214–1220, 2002.

[30] G. R. De Jesus, B. C. Rodrigues, M. I. Lacerda et al., "Gestational outcomes in patients with neuropsychiatric systemic lupus erythematosus," *Lupus*, vol. 26, no. 5, pp. 537–542, 2017.

[31] S. Aoki, N. Kobayashi, A. Mochimaru, T. Takahashi, and F. Hirahara, "Seizures associated with Lupus during pregnancy," *Clinical Case Reports*, vol. 4, no. 4, pp. 366–368, 2016.

[32] "The American College of Rheumatology nomenclature and case definitions for neuropsychiatric lupus syndromes," *Arthritis & Rheumatism*, vol. 42, no. 4, pp. 599–608, 1999.

[33] E. Harboe, A. B. Tjensvoll, S. Maroni et al., "Neuropsychiatric syndromes in patients with systemic lupus erythematosus and primary Sjögren syndrome: A comparative population-based study," *Annals of the Rheumatic Diseases*, vol. 68, no. 10, pp. 1541–1546, 2009.

[34] A. Popescu and A. H. Kao, "Neuropsychiatric systemic lupus erythematosus," *Current Neuropharmacology*, vol. 9, no. 3, pp. 449–457, 2011.

[35] A. Bortoluzzi, M. Padovan, I. Farina, E. Galuppi, F. De Leonardis, and M. Govoni, "Thherapeutic strategies in severe neuropsychiatric systemic lupus erythematosus: Experience from a tertiary referral centre," *Reumatismo*, vol. 64, no. 6, pp. 350–359, 2012.

[36] S. Bucciarelli, G. Espinosa, R. Cervera et al., "Mortality in the catastrophic antiphospholipid syndrome: causes of death and prognostic factors in a series of 250 patients," *Arthritis & Rheumatology*, vol. 54, no. 8, pp. 2568–2576, 2006.

[37] R. W. McMurray and W. May, "Sex hormones and systemic lupus erythematosus: Review and meta-analysis," *Arthritis & Rheumatology*, vol. 48, no. 8, pp. 2100–2110, 2003.

[38] E. Borella, A. Lojacono, M. Gatto et al., "Predictors of maternal and fetal complications in SLE patients: a prospective study," *Immunologic Research*, vol. 60, no. 2-3, pp. 170–176, 2014.

[39] M. A. Saavedra, A. Sánchez, S. Morales, J. E. Navarro-Zarza, U. Ángeles, and L. J. Jara, "Primigravida is associated with flare in women with systemic lupus erythematosus," *Lupus*, vol. 24, no. 2, pp. 180–185, 2015.

30

A Case of Primary Uterina Lymphoma Presenting with Bleeding, Pelvic Pain, and Dysmenorrhea

Lilian Yukari Miura ⓘ,[1] **Miriam Anyury Daquin Maure**,[2] **Monica Tessmann Zomer**,[1] **Reitan Ribeiro** ⓘ,[1] **Teresa Cristina Santos Cavalcanti**,[3] and **William Kondo** ⓘ[1]

[1]*Vita Batel Hospital, Rua Alferes Angelo Sampaio, 1896 Curitiba, PR, Brazil*
[2]*Complejo Hospitalario Metropolitano, Via Simon Bolivar, Panama City, Panama*
[3]*Citolab, Rua Vicente Machado 1192 Curitiba, PR, Brazil*

Correspondence should be addressed to William Kondo; williamkondo@yahoo.com

Academic Editor: Giampiero Capobianco

Primary non-Hodgkin's lymphoma (NHL) can arise from lymphatic cells located in solid organs (extranodal) and it accounts for 25 to 35% of all NHL. Primary lymphoma on the female genital tract (PLFGT) is a rare disease, comprising 0.2 to 1.1% of all extranodal lymphomas in the female population. In this paper, the authors report an extremely rare case of a 48-year-old woman who exhibited an abnormal uterine bleeding, pelvic pain, and dysmenorrhea history. The transvaginal ultrasound showed an anteverted uterus measuring 153 cm^3 in volume, with intramural leiomyomas. She underwent a total laparoscopic hysterectomy with bilateral salpingectomy. The histologic evaluation of the specimen showed a follicular lymphoma with diffuse pattern in the endometrium. This report illustrates the difficulty in the diagnosis of primary lymphomas of the female genital tract.

1. Introduction

Primary non-Hodgkin's lymphoma (NHL) may arise from lymphatic cells located in solid organs (extranodal) and it accounts for 25 to 35% of all NHL [1–4]. Most of the sites related to this disease are in the gastrointestinal tract and the central nervous system. However, less commonly this pathology may also arise from adrenal glands, thyroid, breasts, bone, prostate, and female genital tract [5–7]. Primary lymphoma on the female genital tract (PLFGT) is a rare disease, which comprises 0.2 to 1.1% of all extranodal lymphomas in the female population [8–10].

The main histological subtypes of non-Hodgkin's lymphoma are the diffuse large B-cell lymphoma, follicular lymphoma, and Burkitt lymphoma [9–11]. Immunohistochemistry studies are important to achieve a correct diagnosis [12–14].

The ovaries are the most common site of PLFGT, followed by the uterine cervix and the uterine body, which is very rare [9, 15]. Usually, in these women the endometrial involvement is secondary to a systemic lymphoma affecting the cervix [15].

2. Case Report

A 48-year-old woman, G4 P2 C2, came to our service complaining about abnormal uterine bleeding, pelvic pain, and dysmenorrhea for the last 6 months. She was under clinical treatment for the uterine bleeding with continuous use of hormonal contraceptive (Gestodene 75 mcg + Ethinylestradiol 30 mcg). She had a past surgical history of cholecystectomy, cesarean section, abdominoplasty, and bilateral tubal ligation. The gynecological examination was unremarkable.

On bimanual examination, the uterus was mobile and had a normal size. There was no increase in the volume of the ovaries. Transvaginal ultrasound showed an anteverted uterus, measuring 153 cm^3, with a heterogeneous pattern, with intramural leiomyomas at the posterior uterine wall. Pap smear was negative for neoplasia.

She underwent a laparoscopic hysterectomy with bilateral salpingectomy for a presumed abnormal uterine bleeding and leiomyomas not responding to clinical treatment. The laparoscopic hysterectomy was performed according to the previously reported surgical technique [16]. The surgical

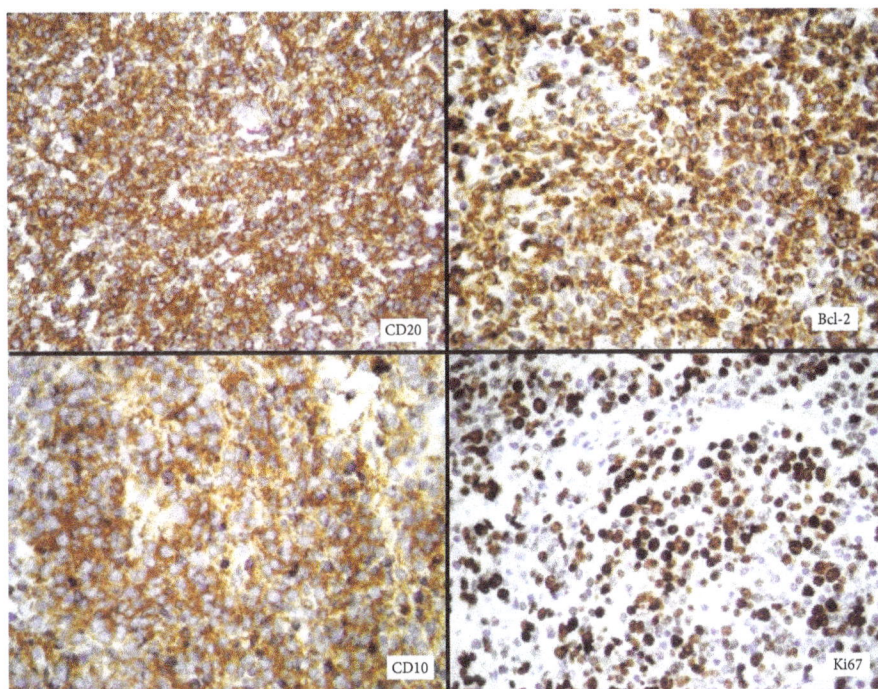

FIGURE 1: Immunohistochemistry showing positivity of the antibodies CD20, Bcl-2, and CD10 in atypical lymphocytes and Ki67 in 50% of all lymphocytes.

procedure was uneventful and lasted 90 minutes. Estimated intraoperative blood loss was 20 cc. The patient was discharged from the hospital, 24 hours after the surgery. The histological evaluation of the specimen identified a dense lymphoid infiltrated in the endometrium, with a diffuse follicular pattern. Immunohistochemical analysis showed CD20, Bcl-2, and CD10 positivity in atypical lymphocytes and Ki67 positivity in 50% of all lymphocytes, leading to a diagnosis of follicular lymphoma with diffuse pattern in the endometrium (Figure 1).

After clinical staging, the disease was diagnosed as follicular lymphoma of the endometrium stage IV, due to the involvement of the bone marrow. The patient was submitted to chemotherapy with six cycles of R-CHOP (rituximab + cyclophosphamide, hydroxydaunorubicin, oncovin, and prednisone), after surgery. Follow-up PET/CT was made sixteen months after surgery and demonstrated increased activity in the retroperitoneum, and it was decided to maintain rituximab for 2 more years.

3. Discussion

Lymphomas are malignant tumors that affect the immune system, most commonly, the lymph nodes. However, 40% of the lymphomas are extra nodal [17–20]. When the female genital tract is compromised, which represents 30 to 40% of the cases, it is usually secondary to disseminated disease [21]. Primary lymphoma involving the female genital tract is an uncommon condition, in which the ovaries and cervix are the most frequently affected sites [8–10, 15]. The involvement of extra nodal sites means the worst prognosis [22]. The prognosis usually is analyzed based on the Ann Arbor staging system

TABLE 1: Ann Arbor staging system.

Stage I	Involvement of a single lymph node region (I) or lymphatic structure (Ie)
Stage II	Involvement of 2 or more lymph node regions on same side of diaphragm (II) or with limited, contiguous extralymphatic tissue involvement (IIe)
Stage III	Both sides of the diaphragm are involved and may include spleen (IIIe) or local tissue involvement (IIIe)
Stage IV	Multiple/disseminated involvement of one or more extralymphatic organs, or isolated extralymphatic organ involvement without adjacent regional lymph node involvement, but with disease in distant site (s), or any involvement of the liver, bone marrow, pleura, or cerebrospinal fluid (i.e., bone marrow)
(A) or (B)	Designates absence/presence of "B" symptoms
(E)	Localized, solitary involvement of extra lymphatic tissue, excluding liver and bone marrow

(Table 1), size and extension of the disease, age, number of nodes affected, LDH level, and lymphoma's grade [20].

It usually occurs in women during the fifth decade of life. Nevertheless, it depends on the histological subtype; as an example, diffuse large B-cell lymphoma is more common between 35 and 45 years old, whereas follicular lymphoma is more frequent in people aged over 50, and Burkitt lymphoma affects children from five to ten years old [23].

The diagnosis is very difficult because of the rarity of this entity. In addition, there is no typical presentation of the symptoms; usually, it depends on the site where the cancer is confined [23]. Some of the symptoms of PLFGT are abnormal uterine bleeding, pelvic pain, abdominal distension, and bloating [17–19]. The "B" symptoms are not frequent in this population, unless the disease has an aggressive behavior along with a large tumor burden [24–26]. In the follicular lymphoma subtype, the clinical presentation usually has an indolent course. Survival rate is very high even without treatment, but it can exhibit a variable clinical presentation, with some patients suffering from aggressive disease [23].

Since clinical evaluation and imaging studies cannot give a definitive diagnosis, most PLFGT is initially treated as being any other common gynecologic malignancy. The definitive diagnosis is obtained after surgery during the pathological examination of the surgical specimen [8]. Immunohistochemistry plays a fundamental role in the characterization of the antibodies and in the classification of the subtypes of lymphomas [27, 28].

The main histological subtype of non-Hodgkin's lymphoma is the diffuse large B-cell lymphoma [9, 11]. The second most common is the follicular lymphoma, followed by Burkitt lymphoma [9]. Immunohistochemical studies are useful to achieve a correct diagnosis, as some low-grade lymphomas (particularly follicular lymphomas and MALT-type lymphomas) are difficult to be distinguished from benign reactive diseases such as severe chronic cervicitis or follicular cervicitis [12–14].

In this case, the patient presented no specific symptoms. She underwent a total laparoscopic hysterectomy for a presumed benign disease (leiomyoma and increased uterine bleeding). The diagnosis of follicular lymphoma with diffuse pattern coming from the endometrium was confirmed after anatomopathological and immunohistochemical evaluations.

The treatment of PLFGT consists of a multimodal approach, including the gynecologist, the clinical oncologist, and the radiation oncologist, trying to individualize each treatment. As this type of lymphoma often compromises premenopausal women, it is very important to consider the patient's fertility. Chemotherapy induces irreversible damage to the ovarian tissue, which leads to premature ovarian failure. This is an important issue that must be discussed with the patient, and the possibility of oocyte or embryo cryopreservation must be remembered in those patients who desire future childbearing [9]. Temporary ovary suppression with GnRH agonists is another alternative, to attempt to reduce the occurrence of premature ovarian failure. However, this procedure is still controversial [29]. Patients who have indication for radiotherapy treatment may be benefited from the ovarian transposition. In this procedure, the ovaries are sutured into the paracolic gutter, in order to attempt to maintain them outside the radiation field, postoperatively [30].

R-CHOP regimen is the standard treatment for follicular lymphoma and includes rituximab plus cyclophosphamide, hydroxydaunorubicin, oncovin (vincristine), and prednisone or prednisolone. The cyclophosphamide is considered a high-risk gonadotoxic drug, oncovin a medium risk [29].

In the posttreatment follow-up, tumor remission is usually evaluated by PET-CT (positron emission tomography-computed tomography) [23].

4. Conclusion

PLFGT is a rare condition. Different clinical presentations may lead to a difficult diagnosis, frequently misunderstood during the preoperative setting. Due to the scarce number of cases, there is no formal protocol for the management of PLFGT. Although rare, PLFGT should be considered in the differential diagnosis of organic diseases, leading to increased uterine bleeding and pelvic pain.

References

[1] R. Newton, J. Ferlay, V. Beral, and S. S. Devesa, "The epidemiology of non-Hodgkin's lymphoma: comparison of nodal and extra-nodal sites," *International Journal of Cancer*, vol. 72, no. 6, pp. 923–930, 1997.

[2] B. Vannata and E. Zucca, "Primary extranodal B-cell lymphoma: current concepts andtreatment strategies," *The Chinese Clinical Oncology Journal*, vol. 4, no. 1, article 10, 2015.

[3] J. J. Castillo, E. S. Winer, and A. J. Olszewski, "Sites of extranodal involvement are prognostic in patients with diffuse large B-cell lymphoma in the rituximab era: An analysis of the Surveillance, Epidemiology and End Results database," *American Journal of Hematology*, vol. 89, no. 3, pp. 310–314, 2014.

[4] J. Yun, S. J. Kim, J. A. Kim et al., "Clinical features and treatment outcomes of non-hodgkin's lymphomas involving rare extranodal sites: a single-center experience," *Acta Haematologica*, vol. 123, no. 1, pp. 48–54, 2010.

[5] G. Ryan, G. Martinelli, M. Kuper-Hommel et al., "Primary diffuse large B-cell lymphoma of the breast: prognostic factors and outcomes of a study by the international extranodal lymphoma study group," *Annals of Oncology*, vol. 19, no. 2, pp. 233–241, 2008.

[6] M. Mian, G. Gaidano, A. Conconi et al., "High response rate and improvement of long-term survival with combined treatment modalities in patients with poor-risk primary thyroid diffuse large B-cell lymphoma: an international extranodal lymphoma study group and intergruppo Italiano linfomi study," *Leukemia & Lymphoma*, vol. 52, no. 5, pp. 823–832, 2011.

[7] A. Martinez, M. Ponzoni, C. Agostinelli et al., "Primary bone marrow lymphoma: an uncommon extranodal presentation of aggressive non-hodgkin lymphomas," *The American Journal of Surgical Pathology*, vol. 36, no. 2, pp. 296–304, 2012.

[8] L. Singh, R. Madan, R. Benson, and G. K. Rath, "Primary non-hodgkins lymphoma of uterine cervix: a case report of two patients," *The Journal of Obstetrics and Gynecology of India*, vol. 66, no. 2, pp. 125–127, 2016.

[9] D. Nasioudis, P. N. Kampaktsis, M. Frey, S. S. Witkin, and K. Holcomb, "Primary lymphoma of the female genital tract: an analysis of 697 cases," *Gynecologic Oncology*, vol. 145, no. 2, pp. 305–309, 2017.

[10] J. A. Bennett, E. Oliva, V. Nardi, N. Lindeman, J. A. Ferry, and A. Louissaint, "Primary endometrial marginal zone lymphoma (MALT Lymphoma): a unique clinicopathologic entity," *The American Journal of Surgical Pathology*, vol. 40, no. 9, pp. 1217–1223, 2016.

[11] F. Kosari, Y. Daneshbod, R. Parwaresch, M. Krams, and H.-H. Wacker, "Lymphomas of the female genital tract: a study of

186 cases and review of the literature," *The American Journal of Surgical Pathology*, vol. 29, no. 11, pp. 1512–1520, 2005.

[12] N. N. Van Renterghem, P. P. De Paepe, R. R. Van den Broecke, C. Bourgain, and R. Serreyn, "Primarylymphoma of the cervix uteri: a diagnostic challenge. Report of two casesand review of the literature," *European Journal of Gynaecological Oncology*, vol. 26, pp. 36–38, 2005.

[13] A. Anagnostopoulos, N. Mouzakiti, S. Ruthven, J. Herod, and M. Kotsyfakis, "Primary cervical anduterine corpus lymphoma; a case report and literature review," *International Journal of Clinical and Experimental Medicine*, vol. 6, pp. 298–306, 2013.

[14] F. Binesh, M. Karimi zarchi, H. Vahedian, and Y. Rajabzadeh, "Primary malignant lymphoma of the uterine cervix," *BMJ Case Reports*, vol. 2012, 2012.

[15] F. C. Tahmasebi, S. Roy, J. E. Kolitz, F. Sen, J. Laser, and X. Zhang, "Primary extranodal marginal zone lymphoma of the endometrium: report of four cases and review of literature," *International Journal of Clinical and Experimental Pathology*, vol. 8, no. 3, pp. 3036–3044, 2015.

[16] W. Kondo, M. T. Zomer, A. W. Branco, L. C. Stunitz, A. J. BrancoFilho, and S. Nichele, "Surgical technique of total laparoscopic hysterectomy," *Brazilian Journal of Videoendoscopic Surgery*, vol. 3, no. 3, pp. 139–149, 2010.

[17] V. D. Mandato, R. Palermo, A. Falbo et al., "Primary diffuse large B-cell lymphoma of the uterus: case report and review," *Anticancer Reseach*, vol. 34, no. 8, pp. 4377–4390, 2014.

[18] S. Guastafierro, A. Tedeschi, C. Criscuolo et al., "Primary extranodal non-hodgkin's lymphoma of the vagina: a case report and a review of the literature," *Acta Haematologica*, vol. 128, no. 1, pp. 33–38, 2012.

[19] N. Clemente, L. Alessandrini, M. Rupolo et al., "Primary non-hodgkin's lymphoma of the vulva: a case report and literature review," *Medicine*, vol. 95, no. 10, Article ID e3041, 2016.

[20] A. Ferreira and T. M. Cunha, "Envolvimento do aparelho genital feminino por linfoma," *Acta Radiológica Portuguesa*, vol. 23, no. 91, pp. 25–32, 2011.

[21] S. Patni and I. Thompson, "Genital tract lymphoma: a rare malignancy," *Journal of Obstetrics & Gynaecology*, vol. 25, no. 3, pp. 289–291, 2005.

[22] W.-K. Lee, E. W. F. Lau, V. A. Duddalwar, A. J. Stanley, and Y. Y. Ho, "Abdominal manifestations of extranodal lymphoma: spectrum of imaging findings," *American Journal of Roentgenology*, vol. 191, no. 1, pp. 198–206, 2008.

[23] E. Pinto, S. Batista, C. Lourenço, J. Gonçalves, and G. Ramalho, "Gynecological lymphomas Linfomas ginecológicos," *ActaObstetGinecol Port*, vol. 8, no. 2, pp. 201–205, 2014.

[24] A. S. Lagoo and S. J. Robboy, "Lymphoma of the female genital tract: current status," *International Journal of Gynecological Pathology*, vol. 25, no. 1, pp. 1–21, 2006.

[25] A. K. Ahmad, P. Hui, B. Litkouhi et al., "Institutional review of primary non-Hodgkin lymphoma of the female genital tract a 33-year experience," *International Journal of Gynecological Cancer*, vol. 24, no. 7, pp. 1250–1255, 2014.

[26] E. Zucca and F. Cavalli, "Extranodal lymphomas," *Annals of Oncology*, vol. 11, no. 3, pp. 219–222, 2000.

[27] J. H. M. Heeren, A. M. Croonen, and J. M. A. Pijnenborg, "Primary extranodal marginal zone B-cell lymphoma of the female genital tract: a case report and literature review," *International Journal of Gynecological Pathology*, vol. 27, no. 2, pp. 243–246, 2008.

[28] G. Yang, J. Deisch, M. Tavares, Q. Haixia, C. Cobb, and A. S. Raza, "Primary B-cell lymphoma of the uterine cervix: presentation in Pap-test slide and cervical biopsy," *Diagnostic Cytopathology*, vol. 45, no. 3, pp. 235–238, 2017.

[29] Z. Blumenfeld, H. Zur, and E. J. Dann, "Gonadotropin-releasing hormone agonist cotreatment during chemotherapy may increase pregnancy rate in survivors," *The Oncologist*, vol. 20, no. 11, pp. 1283–1289, 2015.

[30] N. S. Moawad, E. Santamaria, A. Rhoton-Vlasak, and J. L. Lightsey, "Laparoscopic ovarian transposition before pelvic cancer treatment: ovarian function and fertility preservation," *Journal of Minimally Invasive Gynecology*, vol. 24, no. 1, pp. 28–35, 2017.

31

Group A *Streptococcus* Septic Shock after Surgical Abortion: A Case Report and Review of the Literature

Stephanie C. Tardieu and Elizabeth Schmidt

Department of Obstetrics and Gynecology, Hofstra Northwell School of Medicine, Hofstra University,
North Shore-LIJ University Hospital, 270-05 76th Avenue, New Hyde Park, NY 11040, USA

Correspondence should be addressed to Stephanie C. Tardieu; stephanie.tardieu@gmail.com

Academic Editor: Irene Hoesli

Group A *Streptococcus* (GAS) causing puerperal sepsis is a leading cause of maternal mortality worldwide. Although rare, GAS infection is a relatively significant public health concern because of its propensity to evolve rapidly into septic shock, streptococcal toxic shock syndrome, and death. We report the case of a 27-year-old patient who presented with GAS septic shock after undergoing a surgical termination of pregnancy and was treated successfully and recovered without sequelae. GAS septic shock should always be included in the differential diagnosis of any patient who develops sepsis after a surgical abortion. Patients with GAS septic shock have a rapid clinical decline and need aggressive fluid management, early initiation of broad-spectrum antibiotics, and rapid surgical intervention.

1. Introduction

Group A *Streptococcus* (GAS) infection is a leading cause of death from puerperal sepsis worldwide [1]. Prior to the antibiotic era, GAS infections were a major cause of peripartum morbidity and mortality [2]. Currently, approximately 246 cases of puerperal GAS infection are reported every year in the United States [3].

Although its incidence remains relatively rare, GAS infection is significant because of its potential to progress rapidly to septic shock, organ damage, and streptococcal toxic shock syndrome (TSS), which are associated with significant morbidity and mortality. Patients with invasive GAS infections who develop septic shock, streptococcal TSS, or necrotizing fasciitis have mortality rates of 45%, 38%, and 29%, respectively [3].

This is the first case report of invasive GAS infection after a surgical abortion. We present the clinical presentation, management, and treatment of a patient who presented with septic shock secondary to GAS infection after a first-trimester surgical termination of pregnancy.

2. Case Report

A 27-year-old gravida 6, para 3033 female was brought to the emergency room with a fever and severe lower abdominal pain that had begun 5 hours earlier. She had undergone a dilation and curettage at 6 weeks' gestation 24 hours prior to presentation at a private outpatient family planning clinic unaffiliated to our institution. Her pain was sharp and diffuse and associated with nausea, vomiting, rigors, and dyspnea. She denied rashes, vaginal bleeding, or abnormal vaginal discharge.

Upon presentation to the emergency room, the patient's vital signs were as follows: blood pressure of 130/69, heart rate of 131 beats per minute, respiratory rate of 18 breaths per minute, oxygen saturation on room air of 100%, and temperature of 38.0°C (100.4°F). Within the hour, she became hypotensive with a blood pressure of 77/54, heart rate of 111, respiratory rate of 20, and oxygen saturation of 99% on room air. Her temperature rose to 39.6°C (103.4°F), and her blood pressure dropped to 60/30 during resuscitative efforts.

The patient appeared pale and diaphoretic but was alert, awake, and oriented. Lung fields were bilaterally clear without rales, wheezes, or rhonchi. Her abdomen was soft and nondistended with diffuse tenderness to light palpation and positive rebound and guarding. Pelvic examination revealed an open cervix with copious amounts of opaque mucous discharge draining from the cervical os with no foul odor. The uterus was 6 weeks in size, and there were severe cervical motion and uterine tenderness on bimanual examination.

Initial labs were as follows: white blood cell count (WBC), $9.4 \times 10^3/mm^3$; hemoglobin, 11.9 g/dL; hematocrit, 34.1%; platelets, $257 \times 10^3/mm^3$; and lactate, 2.5 mg/dL. Creatinine, liver function tests, and coagulation profile were normal. Transvaginal ultrasound (TVUS) revealed a normal-sized uterus with the endometrial lining measuring 9.5 mm containing heterogeneous material that was negative to Doppler interrogation. A computed tomography (CT) scan of the abdomen and pelvis with contrast was negative for intra-abdominal pathology.

Her past medical history included asthma and rheumatoid arthritis, and she had a penicillin allergy producing angioedema.

In the emergency room, two intravenous lines (IVs) were started, and the patient was resuscitated with three liters of Lactated Ringer. She was started on IV ertapenem and metronidazole for presumed endometritis. A Foley catheter was inserted. Given her continued hemodynamic instability despite adequate fluid resuscitation, the decision was made to perform an emergency dilation and curettage and diagnostic laparoscopy.

Intraoperatively, no gross abnormalities of the uterus, adnexa, bowel, appendix, gall bladder, or liver were seen. Dilation and curettage produced minimal hemorrhagic tissue that was sent to pathology. The patient remained hypotensive and was treated with dopamine for vasopressor support. The intraoperative lactate level was 4.5 mg/dL.

Postoperatively, the patient was admitted to the surgical intensive care unit. Her lactate level postoperatively was 4.6 mg/dL. On postoperative day 1, she continued to report severe, diffuse abdominal pain with rebound and guarding. She was febrile with a maximum temperature of 38.8°C (102°F) and continued to require dopamine for vasopressor support. Metronidazole was discontinued and vancomycin was started. Her lactate level decreased to 1.1 mg/dL, and her WBC was $10.9 \times 10^3/mm^3$.

On postoperative day 2, the patient remained febrile with a temperature of 39.1°C (102.5°F) with decreased abdominal pain. She was weaned off vasopressor support. Her cervical cultures and blood cultures from admission were positive for group A beta-hemolytic *Streptococcus* from both tubes. Antibiotics were changed from vancomycin to clindamycin. Her WBC dropped to $4.2 \times 10^3/mm^3$.

On postoperative day 3, the patient's abdominal pain continued to improve. She had fundal tenderness without rebound or guarding. She was afebrile for 24 hours and was transferred to the inpatient gynecology floor. A second set of blood cultures drawn on postoperative day 2 were negative for GAS. She remained afebrile on postoperative day 4 and was discharged on postoperative day 5 with a peripherally inserted central catheter line and IV ertapenem to be continued for 14 days. No retained products of conception were found on pathology.

The patient provided written informed consent for the treatment and for publication of this case.

3. Discussion

Surgical abortion is a safe and reliable surgical procedure for termination of pregnancy. The overall frequency of infections following surgical abortion in the first trimester is 0.27% [4]. Case reports of invasive GAS infection in the literature include infection in the puerperal period as well as after medical abortion [5, 6]. US Centers for Disease Control data from 2005 to 2012 estimates that the incidence of puerperal invasive GAS infection is approximately 246 cases per year with a mortality rate of 10.6% [3]. However, to our knowledge, this is the first case report being published on GAS sepsis after a surgical abortion.

Puerperal GAS infections vary in presentation from mild endometritis to invasive life-threatening infections [7]. The classic presentation of puerperal GAS infection is a woman who presents within 48 hours from delivery or abortion with fever, rigor, and severe abdominal pain. Clinical findings can include purulent vaginal discharge, uterine tenderness, nausea, and vomiting [7]. A key characteristic that distinguishes GAS sepsis from other types of sepsis is the patient's rapid clinical deterioration despite appropriate resuscitative measures with fluids and broad-spectrum antibiotics [8]. The presence of hypotension, tachycardia, and leukocytosis are signs that TSS is developing, which is associated with higher mortality rates [3, 9].

Toxic shock syndrome (TSS) develops in up to 14–20% of patients with invasive GAS infection [10]. Its diagnosis carries a poor prognosis and a high mortality rate [3, 9]. Diagnosis of TSS is made when GAS is isolated from a sterile (blood, cerebrospinal fluid, pleura, peritoneal fluid, tissue biopsy, or a surgical wound) or nonsterile site (vagina, throat, sputum, or skin) in a patient with hypotension (systolic blood pressure < 90) who has at least two of the following organ dysfunctions: renal impairment (creatinine > 2 mg/Dl), coagulopathy (platelets < 100,000 mm³ or disseminated intravascular coagulopathy), liver impairment (LFTs > 2x the upper limit of normal), acute respiratory distress syndrome, generalized erythematous macular rash that may desquamate, and/or soft tissue necrosis [11].

In puerperal or postabortion GAS sepsis, necrosis of the uterus and adnexa may be present [12]. Atypical presentations include necrotizing fasciitis involving the limbs and cervix [6, 12, 13]. Cases of puerperal TSS causing myositis, rhabdomyolysis, disseminated intravascular coagulopathy, and acute respiratory distress syndrome have been reported [14]. Rare complications may include septic ovarian thrombosis and septic arthritis [15]. Early diagnosis of complications associated with invasive GAS infection is vital, as early surgical intervention by debridement or hysterectomy may be necessary. Surgical intervention with hysterectomy is crucial when signs of deeper invasion are present and necrosis is suspected [16].

TABLE 1: Diagnostic work-up for postabortion sepsis.

Blood work	CBC w/differential
	CMP
	Coagulation profile (PT/INR, aPTT, fibrinogen)
	Lactate
	Arterial blood gas
Imaging	Chest X-ray
	Transvaginal ultrasound
	CT abdomen and pelvis with contrast or MRI
Cultures	Blood cultures
	Cervical cultures
	Vaginal discharge cultures (including cultures for trichomonas, gonorrhea, chlamydia, and candida)
	Cultures of endometrial biopsy or curettage specimen
	Urine culture
Other tests	Urinalysis
Consultation	Gynecology (including family planning subspecialist if available)
	Infectious disease
	Hospital infectious control services
	Surgery (general and other subspecialists)
	Critical care

CBC: complete blood count; CMP: comprehensive metabolic panel; PT/INR: prothrombin time/international normalized ratio; aPTT: activated partial thromboplastin time; CT: computed tomography; MRI: magnetic resonance imaging.

Clinicians should have a high index of suspicion for invasive GAS infection when evaluating a patient with postabortion sepsis. Work-up should include a complete blood count with differential, renal, and liver function tests, coagulation profile (PT/INR, aPTT, and fibrinogen), lactate, and cervical and/or wound cultures at presentation (Table 1) [7]. A swab or blood culture positive for GAS is necessary for diagnosis but should not delay aggressive management with fluid resuscitation and broad-spectrum IV antibiotics [17]. Gram stain will show Gram-positive cocci in chains or in pairs. Bandemia > 10% may be present even in the absence of leukocytosis [1]. Hemoconcentration or hemolysis may also be present [1]. Arterial blood gases are important for monitoring lactate, pH, and arterial oxygenation levels. A chest X-ray should be ordered for patients with dyspnea and low oxygen saturation. Other sources of infection should also be ruled out including urinary tract infection, pyelonephritis, and endometritis. Imaging with CT, magnetic resonance imaging, or TVUS provides clinical information about the presence of an abscess and retained products of conception. However, normal imaging should not delay aggressive management.

Imaging may demonstrate an edematous uterus that is larger than expected. GAS does not usually create abscesses or produce gas. The presence of gas in the endomyometrium may point to another bacterial etiology for postabortion sepsis or septic shock such as infection with *Clostridium sordellii*. These infections typically lack a fever and produce a leukemoid reaction (WBC 50–200 × 10³/mm³) and diffuse capillary leakage [18].

Early treatment of GAS sepsis requires antibiotic therapy combined with aggressive fluid resuscitation. Once shock develops, the mortality rate approaches 45–60% [3, 9].

Infectious disease consultation should be obtained as soon as possible. IV benzylpenicillin (4 million units every 4 hours) is the first-line antibiotic. Clindamycin should be added in cases of severe sepsis and septic shock (900 mg every 8 hours). Patients with a penicillin allergy, as was the case for this patient, can be treated with a broad-spectrum cephalosporin and vancomycin (15 mg/kg every 12 hours) [19]. The length of treatment should be individualized and determined in collaboration with infectious disease specialists. Patients with positive blood cultures should be treated for at least 14 days.

Given the critical nature of invasive GAS infections, rapidly deteriorating women require treatment in an intensive care unit [20]. When TSS is present, volume deficits are large and can require up to 10 to 20 liters of fluid resuscitation per day [21]. Vasopressor therapy will usually be required. Strict monitoring of fluid intake and output is important to prevent sequelae of fluid overload. If the patient continues to deteriorate despite antibiotic therapy and adequate fluid resuscitation, it is necessary to consider deeper signs of infection such as necrosis. Surgical intervention is required when a confirmed GAS infection is present with signs of organ dysfunction [9]. In our case, diagnostic laparoscopy and dilation and curettage were performed. Necrosis and gangrene were not observed in our patient; however, there are cases of necrosis and necrotizing fasciitis of the uterus and adnexa requiring hysterectomy, adnexectomy, and debridement of necrosed tissues [12, 22]. The use of intravenous immunoglobulin in the treatment of puerperal GAS sepsis is debated; however, most favor its administration in patients with TSS to boost the patient's passive immunity [23, 24].

Given its rarity, screening of carriage for GAS is not thought to be helpful in the prevention of invasive disease.

Thus far, optimal prevention and vaccination are not yet available. GAS transmission can occur from inhalation or direct contact with droplets of saliva and nasal or vaginal secretions. It can also occur through skin-to-skin contact with those who have infected lesions. The need for rigorous personal hygiene and hand washing should be emphasized to the patient, her close contacts, and healthcare workers who are caring for her. Although rare, healthcare workers can acquire GAS infections from patients. The CDC has issued guidelines for screening and prophylaxis to prevent transmission of invasive GAS infections to household contacts and to persons involved in their healthcare [8, 25].

Healthcare workers should always wear protective equipment including gloves, masks, and gown when directly caring for the patient [8]. Patients should be placed in an isolated room with contact precautions and strict hand hygiene practices should be employed. Close contacts and healthcare workers who have a sore throat, skin infection, vaginitis, or a needle stick within the 30-day period spent treating the patient should receive screening and an evaluation by an infectious disease specialist [8]. Discussion about who requires screening and antibiotic regimens for a positive screen are beyond the scope of this paper but can be found in our referenced literature [25].

4. Conclusion

This presentation of a patient who developed postabortion GAS septic shock highlights the fact that these patients can deteriorate rapidly and require aggressive fluid management, early initiation of broad-spectrum antibiotics, and concurrent rapid surgical intervention. Although the patient in this report did not develop streptococcal TSS, she did develop septic shock with a rapid clinical decline. We believe that she would have developed TSS had she not received timely aggressive medical and surgical intervention. Early involvement of infectious disease, critical care, and surgical specialists were vital to the patient's positive outcome, highlighting the need for an interdisciplinary approach when caring for patients with GAS sepsis. GAS infection should be included in the differential diagnosis of postabortion sepsis, as it requires aggressive management and an interdisciplinary approach to avoid life-threatening septic shock, TSS, end-organ failure, and death.

References

[1] D. Maharaj, "Puerperal pyrexia: a review. Part I," *Obstetrical and Gynecological Survey*, vol. 62, no. 6, pp. 393–399, 2007.

[2] D. Charles and B. Larsen, "Streptococcal puerperal sepsis and obstetric infections: a historical perspective," *Reviews of Infectious Diseases*, vol. 8, no. 3, pp. 411–422, 1986.

[3] G. E. Nelson, T. Pondo, K.-A. Toews et al., "Epidemiology of invasive group a streptococcal infections in the United States, 2005–2012," *Clinical Infectious Diseases*, vol. 63, no. 4, pp. 478–486, 2016.

[4] U. D. Upadhyay, S. Desai, V. Zlidar et al., "Incidence of emergency department visits and complications after abortion," *Obstetrics and Gynecology*, vol. 125, no. 1, pp. 175–183, 2015.

[5] N. Gendron, C. Joubrel, S. Nedellec et al., "Group A Streptococcus endometritis following medical abortion," *Journal of Clinical Microbiology*, vol. 52, no. 7, pp. 2733–2735, 2014.

[6] J. L. Daif, M. Levie, S. Chudnoff, B. Kaiser, and S. Shahabi, "Group a streptococcus causing necrotizing fasciitis and toxic shock syndrome after medical termination of pregnancy," *Obstetrics and Gynecology*, vol. 113, no. 2, pp. 504–506, 2009.

[7] P. B. Mead and W. C. Winn, "Vaginal-rectal colonization with group A streptococci in late pregnancy," *Infectious Diseases in Obstetrics and Gynecology*, vol. 8, no. 5-6, pp. 217–219, 2000.

[8] N. Palaniappan, M. Menezes, and P. Willson, "Group A streptococcal puerperal sepsis: management and prevention," in *The Obstetrician and Gynaecologist*, vol. 14, pp. 9–16, 2012.

[9] B. H. Rimawi, D. E. Soper, and D. A. Eschenbach, "Group a streptococcal infections in obstetrics and gynecology," *Clinical Obstetrics and Gynecology*, vol. 55, no. 4, pp. 864–874, 2012.

[10] S. Shinar, Y. Fouks, S. Amit et al., "Clinical Characteristics of and Preventative Strategies for Peripartum Group A Streptococcal Infections," *Obstetrics and Gynecology*, vol. 127, no. 2, pp. 227–232, 2016.

[11] D. L. Stevens and A. E. Bryant, "Severe group A streptococcal infections in Streptococcus pyogenes," in *Basic Biology to Clinical Manifestations*, University of Oklahoma Health Sciences Center, Oklahoma, Okla, USA, 2016.

[12] D. E. Castagnola, M. K. Hoffman, J. Carlson, and C. Flynn, "Necrotizing cervical and uterine infection in the postpartum period caused by Group A Streptococcus," *Obstetrics and Gynecology*, vol. 111, no. 2, pp. 533–535, 2008.

[13] C. R. McHenry, T. Azar, A. J. Ramahi, and P. L. Collins, "Monomicrobial necrotizing fasciitis complicating pregnancy and puerperium," *Obstetrics and Gynecology*, vol. 87, no. 5, pp. 823–826, 1996.

[14] A. S. Dofferhoff and J. M. Sporken, "Puerperal toxic shock syndrome caused by Group A beta-hemolytic streptococci," *Nederlands Tijdschrift Voor Geneeskunde*, vol. 137, pp. 609–612, 1993.

[15] M. Gourlay, C. Gutierrez, A. Chong, and R. Robertson, "Group a streptococcal sepsis and ovarian vein thrombosis after an uncomplicated vaginal delivery," *Journal of the American Board of Family Practice*, vol. 14, no. 5, pp. 375–380, 2001.

[16] S. M. Hamilton, D. L. Stevens, and A. E. Bryant, "Pregnancy-related group a streptococcal infections: temporal relationships between bacterial acquisition, infection onset, clinical findings, and outcome," *Clinical Infectious Diseases*, vol. 57, no. 6, pp. 870–876, 2013.

[17] W. Schummer and C. Schummer, "Two cases of delayed diagnosis of postpartal streptococcal toxic shock syndrome," *Infectious Disease in Obstetrics and Gynecology*, vol. 10, no. 4, pp. 217–222, 2002.

[18] M. J. Aldape, A. E. Bryant, and D. L. Stevens, "Clostridium sordellii infection: epidemiology, clinical findings, and current perspectives on diagnosis and treatment," *Clinical Infectious Diseases*, vol. 43, no. 11, pp. 1436–1446, 2006.

[19] D. Stevens, A. Bisno, H. Chambers et al., "Practice guidelines for the diagnosis and management of skin and soft tissue infections: 2014 update by the Infectious Diseases Society of America," *Clinical Infectious Diseases*, vol. 59, pp. 147–159, 2014.

[20] H. M. C. Kramer, J. M. Schutte, J. J. Zwart, N. W. E. Schui-
temaker, E. A. P. Steegers, and J. Van Roosmalen, "Maternal
mortality and severe morbidity from sepsis in the Netherlands,"
Acta Obstetricia et Gynecologica Scandinavica, vol. 88, no. 6, pp.
647–653, 2009.

[21] D. L. Stevens, "Streptococcal toxic-shock syndrome: Spectrum
of disease, pathogenesis, and new concepts in treatment,"
Emerging Infectious Diseases, vol. 1, no. 3, pp. 69–78, 1995.

[22] D. L. Stevens and A. Bryant, "Pregnancy-related group A streptococcal infection," 2016, http://www.uptodate.com.

[23] M. M. Alejandria, M. A. Lansang, L. F. Dans, and J. B. Manta-
ring, "Intravenous immunoglobulin for treating sepsis and septic
shock," *The Cochrane Database of Systematic Reviews*, vol. 1,
p. CD001090, 2002.

[24] J. Darenberg, N. Ihendyane, J. Sjölin et al., "Intravenous immu-
noglobulin G therapy in streptococcal toxic shock syndrome: a
European randomized, double-blind, placebo-controlled trial,"
Clinical Infectious Diseases, vol. 37, no. 3, pp. 333–340, 2003.

[25] The Prevention of Invasive Group A Streptococcal Infections
Workshop Participants, "Prevention of invasive group A streptococcal disease among household contacts of case patients and
among postpartum and postsurgical patients: Recommendations from the Centers for Disease Control and Prevention,"
Clinical Infectious Diseases, vol. 36, no. 2, p. 243, 2003.

32

Fetal Midgut Volvulus with Meconium Peritonitis Detected on Prenatal Ultrasound

Emanuelle J. Best ⓘ,[1] **Cecelia M. O'Brien,**[1,2] **Wendy Carseldine,**[1,2] **Aniruddh Deshpande,**[3] **Rebecca Glover,**[4] **and Felicity Park**[1,2]

[1]*Maternity and Gynaecology, John Hunter Hospital, New Lambton Heights, NSW, Australia*
[2]*Maternal Fetal Medicine Unit, John Hunter Hospital, New Lambton Heights, NSW, Australia*
[3]*Department of Paediatric Surgery, John Hunter Children's Hospital, New Lambton Heights, NSW, Australia*
[4]*Neonatal Intensive Care Unit, John Hunter Children's Hospital, New Lambton Heights, NSW, Australia*

Correspondence should be addressed to Emanuelle J. Best; emanuelle.best@hnehealth.nsw.gov.au

Academic Editor: Svein Rasmussen

Background. Fetal volvulus is a rare, yet life-threatening condition that requires skilful diagnosis and management. Volvulus occurs when bowel loops become twisted and the twisting of the mesenteric artery leads to congestion, impaired venous return, and bowel necrosis. *Case Description.* We present a case of fetal ileal volvulus suspected on third trimester ultrasound, complicated by premature labour, small bowel necrosis, and meconium peritonitis. Progressive dilatation and decreased peristalsis of echogenic bowel were noted in the early part of the third trimester. Daily surveillance ultrasound was performed and spontaneous labour occurred at 32 weeks' gestation. A proactive postnatal approach guided by prenatal sonographic findings allowed prompt treatment and an urgent laparotomy was performed for an ileal volvulus with necrosis and meconium peritonitis. A segment of small bowel volvulus was resected and an end-to-end anastomosis was performed with uneventful recovery. *Discussion.* Clinically signs of fetal midgut volvulus are not pathognomonic, such as intestinal dilatation, abdominal mass, ascites, peritoneal calcifications, or polyhydramnios; thus, the diagnosis is often challenging. Complications reported in the literature include perforation and haemorrhagic ascites, which may lead to anaemia, hypovolemia, heart failure, and fetal demise. *Conclusion.* This case highlights the importance of assessing the fetal bowel as a part of routine third trimester ultrasound. The case describes the complexity of diagnosis in the fetus, important considerations along with multidisciplinary team approach to management.

1. Introduction

Fetal volvulus is a rare, yet life-threatening condition that requires skilful diagnosis and management. Volvulus occurs when bowel loops become twisted around the mesenteric artery or its branches [1]. The twisting of the mesenteric artery leads to intestinal and vascular congestion, leading to impaired venous return and bowel necrosis [2].

The diagnosis of this condition can be challenging, as the antenatal clinical presentation is often nonspecific. From the literature, clinical symptoms include decreased fetal movements, increased fundal height due to polyhydramnios, or a nonreassuring cardiotocography (CTG) [1]. Ultrasound findings that may increase suspicion of fetal midgut volvulus may include dilated bowel loops, intraabdominal calcifications, abdominal mass, polyhydramnios, gastric dilatation, and ascites. Doppler studies can demonstrate an elevated peak systolic velocity in the middle cerebral artery due to severe fetal anaemia, secondary to haemorrhagic ascites. Complications of fetal volvulus that are reported in the literature include bowel perforation, hypovolemia, heart failure, pleural and pericardial effusions, and fetal demise [2–5].

This report details the management of fetal segmental ileal volvulus diagnosed on ultrasonography in the 3rd trimester.

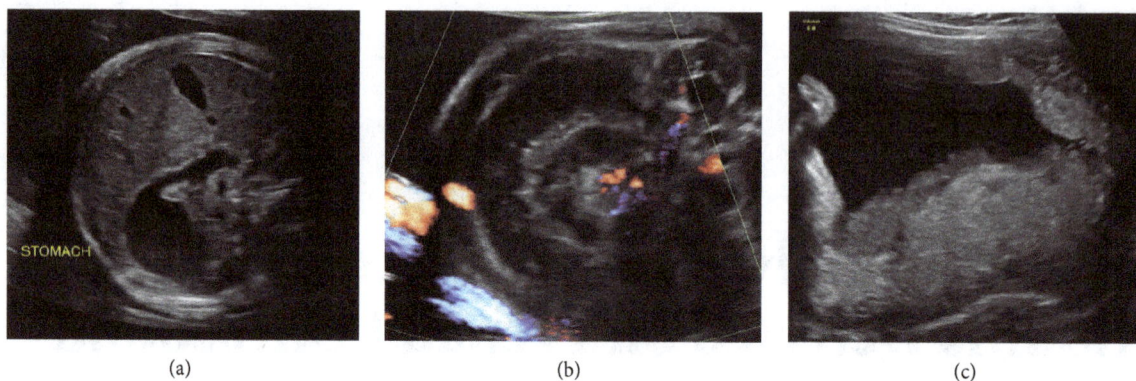

FIGURE 1: Ultrasound images of the key antenatal findings: (a) dilated appearing stomach with relatively normal duodenal diameter, not consistent with duodenal atresia; (b) concentric small bowel visible around the twisted mesenteric pedicle (whirlpool sign) and the superior mesenteric vein malpositioned on the left of the artery; and (c) dense sediment noted in the amniotic fluid, which was noted to be bile at the time of delivery.

2. Case Presentation

A 22-year-old woman, gravida 3, para 2, was referred to our tertiary centre at 31 weeks and 5 days' gestation due to a nonreassuring antenatal CTG with mild fetal tachycardia and decreased fetal movements. Initial ultrasound examination showed a moderately dilated fetal stomach, distended bowel loops, and aperistalsis (Figure 1). Doppler studies were normal, there was no evidence of fetal anaemia, and the amniotic fluid index was within normal range.

Further investigations included an amniocentesis, which demonstrated a normal fluorescence in situ hybridization (FISH) for chromosomes 21, 18, and 13 in a female fetus. A single nucleotide polymorphism (SNP) microarray showed a 0.56 Mb deletion at 16q23.3 loci of uncertain clinical significance, which was not parentally inherited. Maternal viral serology, Kleihauer, and cystic fibrosis testing were negative. Fetal echocardiogram confirmed a small pericardial effusion in an otherwise normal study.

Daily ultrasound surveillance showed persisting bowel dilatation up to 18 mm in diameter, with increasing echogenicity noted over time, with minimal peristalsis and loss of definition in the bowel wall, indicating oedema as shown in Figure 2. The coffee-bean and whirlpool signs were both evident; the latter is shown in Figures 1 and 2. At 32 weeks' gestation, corticosteroids were administered for fetal lung maturity in light of the progressive bowel dilatation and further discussions were being undertaken with continued multidisciplinary team input.

At 32 weeks and 2 days' gestation, labour began spontaneously. A live female infant was delivered vaginally with a birthweight of 2450 g (greater than 97th percentile for gestation). Apgar scores were 9^1 and 9^5 without significant requirement for resuscitation. The arterial cord gas showed a pH of 7.28 and lactate of 5.4 mmol/L, and the venous cord gas gave a pH of 7.44 and lactate of 3.8 mmol/L. The infant was admitted to the Neonatal Intensive Care Unit (NICU) at 15 minutes of age for respiratory support with continuous positive airway pressure (CPAP).

On day 1 of life, the baby remained well with no abdominal signs and a contrast swallow was performed, which did not show obvious malrotation (Figure 3(a)). The baby was kept fasted and remained under close surveillance for clinical signs or symptoms of distress. An abdominal X-ray on day 2 showed a pneumoperitoneum (Figure 3(b)). An urgent laparotomy was then performed, with findings of an ileal volvulus with meconium peritonitis (Figure 4). This required resection of the necrotic small bowel volvulus segment with a successful end-to-end anastomosis achieved.

On day 2, the infant's postoperative haemoglobin was 101 g/L and 1 unit of packed red blood cells was transfused which increased the level to 129 g/L. The postoperative course was otherwise uncomplicated with discharge home on day 7. Surgical follow-up occurred at thirteen weeks chronological age (five weeks corrected age), where the infant was found to have good scar healing and a soft nondistended abdomen. Feeding and weight gain were appropriate along with a reported normal bowel function.

On histopathological examination, the resected small intestine showed established necrosis with organisation including fibrous replacement of necrotic muscularis propria and secondary adhesions. Fibroblastic proliferation was also seen within the mesentery, which showed focal necrosis and recanalisation of mesenteric vessels. These findings are consistent with a clinical diagnosis of volvulus. The necrosis and organisation were well established at the time of resection on postnatal day 2, which is consistent with antenatal occurrence. There was no focal lesion found to explain the cause of the volvulus with no evidence of Meckel's diverticulum, tumour, or malignancy.

3. Discussion

Our case highlights the clinical benefit of prenatal sonographic findings in prompt postnatal care of fetal volvulus.

The incidence of fetal volvulus is not described in the literature; however, symptomatic neonatal intestinal rotation has been estimated at 1 in 6000 [3]. Small bowel related

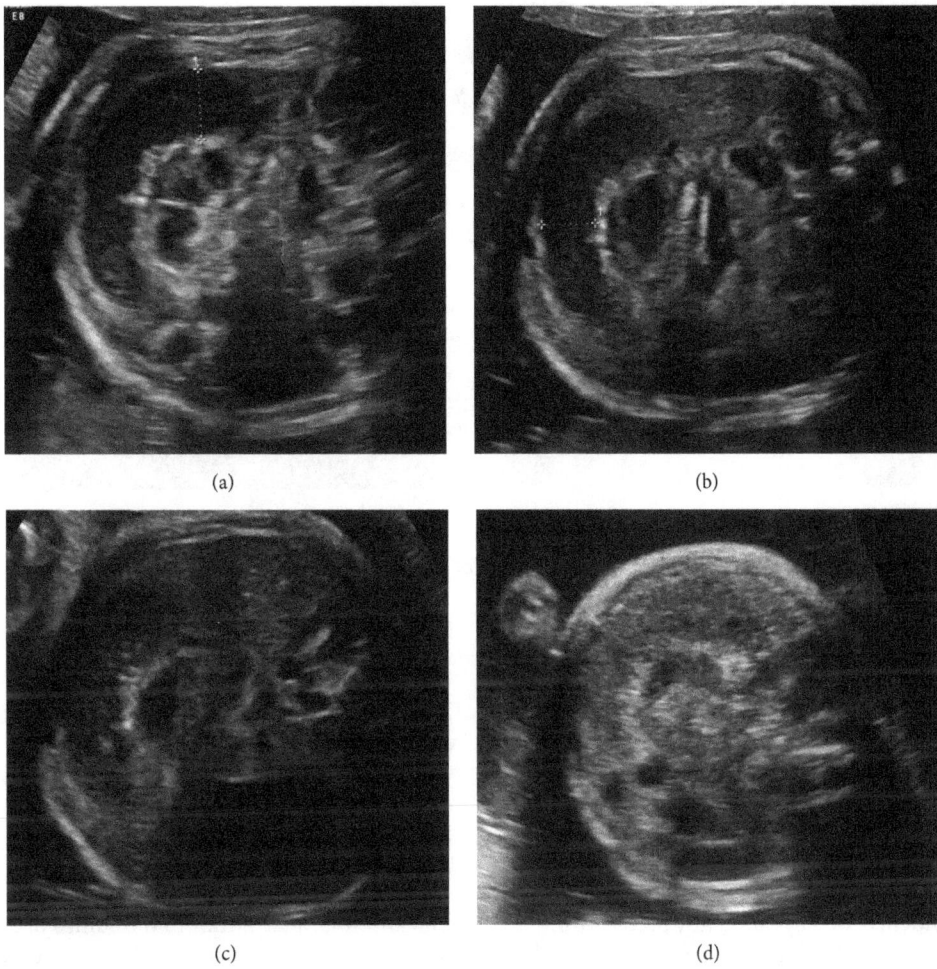

(a)

(b)

(c)

(d)

FIGURE 2: Ultrasound images showing progressive changes within the fetal bowel over time. (a) At 31^{+6} weeks, echolucent bowel contents with a diameter of 14 mm. (b) At 31^{+6} weeks, a loss of clear bowel wall border. (c) At 32 weeks, increasing echogenic particles within the bowel lumen. (d) At 32^{+1} weeks, bowel contents appear echogenic.

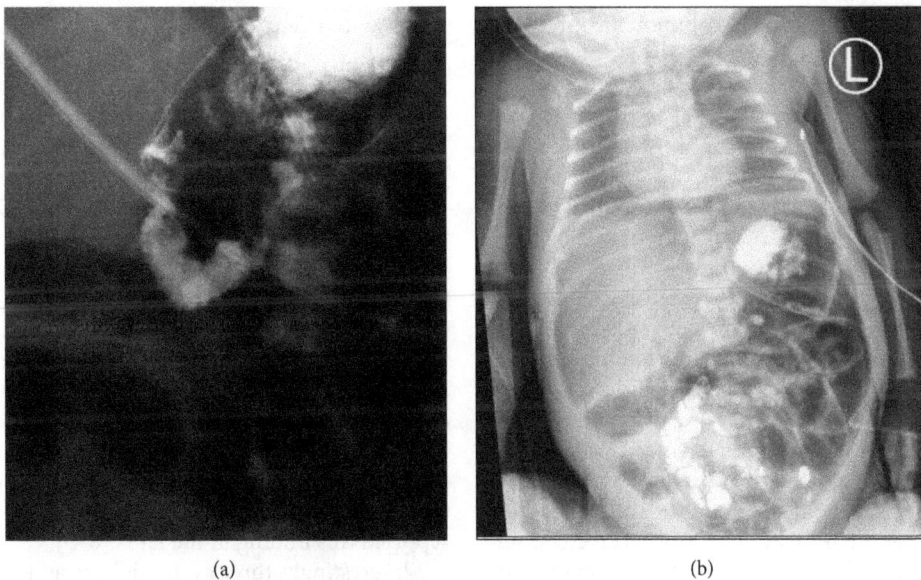

(a)

(b)

FIGURE 3: Radiographic images from day 1 and day 2 postnatally. (a) Contrast study performed on day 1 of life excluding malrotation and (b) large pneumoperitoneum evident on abdominal X-ray on day 2 of life.

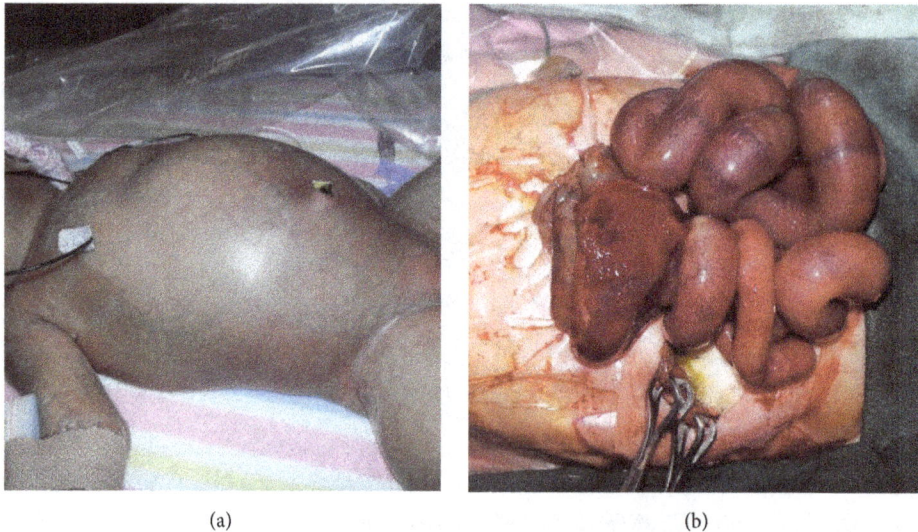

FIGURE 4: Clinical photos: (a) clinical appearance of infant on day 2 of life with erythematous, distended abdomen, and (b) in operating theatres ileal volvulus visible with a necrotic segment on the left side.

complications such as atresia, obstruction, and volvulus have a reported incidence of 1 in 1500 and 1 in 3000 [4, 5]. There are three types of volvulus presenting in the prenatal or newborn period, namely, classic type, segmental type, and volvulus without malposition. Firstly, the classic type is defined as malposition of bowel due to clockwise rotation of the small bowel and ascending colon, around the superior mesenteric artery without evidence of any anomaly predisposing to the rotation [6]. Segmental volvulus has been described as twisting of bowel loops due to an anomaly such as meconium ileus (related to cystic fibrosis), atresia, mesenteric defects, duplication or mesenteric cysts, congenital diaphragmatic hernia or abdominal wall defects, or alternatively can be classified as idiopathic [7]. Lastly, volvulus without malposition is a diagnosis of exclusion and is more common in extremely premature or low birthweight infants [6]. It is thought to be due to the insufficient fixation of the intestines due to prematurity. The latter is rare and difficult to diagnose due to the lack of consistent clinical signs, unlike the classic type.

Symptoms and signs of fetal volvulus may include decreased fetal movements, polyhydramnios, nonreassuring CTG, dilated bowel loops, gastric dilatation and ascites on diagnostic ultrasound, or ultrasound evidence of fetal anaemia (middle cerebral artery peak systolic velocity greater than or equal to 1.5 MoM) secondary to haemorrhagic ascites [1]. Complications of fetal volvulus may include bowel perforation, hypovolemia, heart failure, pleural and pericardial effusions, or fetal demise [2, 8–10].

Intestinal obstruction and haemorrhagic ascites can lead to the complication of fetal anaemia, which occurred in 4 (36%) of the 11 case reports in the literature. Three studies from Noreldeen et al., Tan et al., and Kornacki et al. all reported cases of fetal volvulus where ascites was identified on prenatal ultrasound and an elevated MCA PSV was detected, suggestive of fetal anaemia, with the diagnosis of volvulus confirmed on postnatal laparotomy [1, 10, 11].

However, in the case reported by Noreldeen et al., after an emergency caesarean was performed at 31 weeks, the fetus was found to be severely anaemic, requiring resuscitation with endotracheal intubation and a blood transfusion as well as an emergency laparotomy [1]. Steffensen et al. reported a fetal demise occurring in utero at 38 weeks of gestation due to cardiovascular failure from midgut volvulus and severe fetal anaemia, after ultrasound findings of ascites and dilated bowel loops were present from 15 weeks' gestation. The infant was later found to have intestinal atresia and arthrogryposis [2].

The most extensive retrospective case series by Sciarrone et al. was reported recently in 2016 [8]. This included eight cases of fetal volvulus and description of the ultrasound findings that led to the diagnosis [8]. In all eight cases, prominent bowel loops were visualised on prenatal ultrasound. Polyhydramnios was a notable finding in three of the eight cases and ascites was present in two cases. Chao et al. had found that the whirlpool sign, which is a spiral shaped mass made up of dilated bowel loops seen on ultrasound, is a useful indicator of fetal volvulus [12]. This prenatal ultrasound sign was present in eight of the nine cases in their 3-year prospective study and thus reported to have a sensitivity of 89% and specificity of 92%. Conversely, in the case series by Sciarrone et al. the whirlpool sign was visualised in only one of the eight cases [8]. The coffee-bean sign refers to the dilatation of the small bowel with a thin outer layer composed of a single bowel wall layer and a thick inner wall due to double wall thickness of opposed bowel loop. The coffee-bean sign is regarded as a specific sign of volvulus in both radiographic and ultrasonic imaging, and 4 cases have reported this finding in the fetus [8, 9].

Interestingly, three of the eight cases reported in this case series tested positive for cystic fibrosis [8]. The association between cystic fibrosis and fetal volvulus has been described by Durand et al. [7], whereby the malfunction of the transmembrane conductance regulator leads to viscous mucous secretions, which then obstructs the bowel and predisposes to volvulus [7].

The recommended management includes referral to a tertiary centre with neonatal surgical services, multidisciplinary team planning for antenatal, intrapartum, and neonatal care. Continued close surveillance of fetal wellbeing is warranted if delivery is not imminent and prompt surgical review and management in the neonatal period [9–13]. The indications for delivery that have been documented in the literature include persistent significant ascites causing cardiac failure, pulmonary hypertension, pleural or pericardial effusions, or hypovolemic shock [13].

Neonatal management includes close observation and supportive therapy [14]. Serial clinical examination, surveillance for sepsis including inflammatory markers, and coagulopathy and assessment for clinical deterioration are indicated by metabolic acidosis and increasing ventilation requirements [14].

Despite improvements in prenatal diagnosis, there are no studies comparing the outcomes of volvulus diagnosed prenatally versus postnatally [15]. Basu and Burge compared antenatal to postnatal diagnosis in relation to small bowel atresia. The authors found in the 31% of cases that were detected prenatally that these cases had a higher rate and longer duration of total parental nutrition (83% versus 44%) [16]. The severity of bowel obstruction may have contributed to the antenatal detection, therefore influencing the outcomes reported in this study. The clear advantage to prenatal diagnosis relates to preparation of the parents and in utero transfer of patients to tertiary centres for delivery, rather than emergent transfers in the neonatal period and potential separation of the mother and her baby [15]. Further studies are required to further delineate between the outcomes of newborns diagnosed in the prenatal versus postnatal period.

The indications for surgical intervention include pneumoperitoneum, intestinal obstruction, progressive peritonitis, sepsis, and fixed intestinal loop on plain abdominal film [14]. Surgical management at the time of laparotomy in the neonatal period for the treatment of volvulus is ideally primary anastomosis over stoma formation to maximise small bowel length [17].

This case highlights the importance of careful assessment of the fetal bowel in the third trimester ultrasound, the complexities surrounding the diagnosis of fetal midgut volvulus along with the multidisciplinary team approach required for prompt recognition and management.

4. Conclusion

With advances in ultrasound technology and its widespread use in the third trimester, the diagnosis of volvulus prenatally may become more common. Timely referral to a tertiary centre with fetal medicine specialists, availability of neonatal intensive care facilities, and paediatric surgical service are paramount to managing this acute bowel complication.

Abbreviations

CTG: Cardiotocography
AFI: Amniotic fluid index
FISH: Fluorescence in situ hybridization
SNP: Single nucleotide polymorphism
CPAP: Continuous positive airway pressure.

Disclosure

This case report was accepted and presented as a Poster at the 21st Annual Congress of the Perinatal Society of Australia and New Zealand (PSANZ) held at the Canberra Convention Centre between April 2 and 5, 2017, Australia.

Acknowledgments

The authors would like to thank the patient and her family for allowing them to put together this case report.

References

[1] S. A. Noreldeen, S. G. Hodgett, and N. Venkat-Raman, "Midgut volvulus with hemorrhagic ascites: a rare cause of fetal anemia," *Ultrasound in Obstetrics & Gynecology*, vol. 31, no. 3, pp. 352–354, 2008.

[2] T. S. Steffensen, E. Gilbert-Barness, K. A. DeStefano, and E. V. Kontopoulos, "Midgut volvulus causing fetal demise in utero," *Fetal and Pediatric Pathology*, vol. 27, no. 4-5, pp. 223–231, 2008.

[3] P. T. Stockmann, "Malrotation," in *Principles and Practice of Pediatric Surgery*, vol. 2, p. 1283, Lippincott Williams & Wilkins, Philadelphia, Penn, USA, 2nd edition, 2005.

[4] K. E. Best, P. W. Tennant, and M. C. Addor, "Epidemiology of small intestinal atresia in Europe: A register-based study," *Archives of Disease in Childhood Fetal and Neonatal Edition*, vol. 97, p. 353, 2012.

[5] H. Komuro, T. Hori, T. Amagai et al., "The etiologic role of intrauterine volvulus and intussusception in jejunoileal atresia," *Journal of Pediatric Surgery*, vol. 39, no. 12, pp. 1812–1814, 2004.

[6] S. Kargl, O. Wagner, and W. Pumberger, "Volvulus without malposition—a single-center experience," *Journal of Surgical Research*, vol. 193, no. 1, pp. 295–299, 2015.

[7] M. Durand, K. Coste, A. Martin et al., "Fetal midgut volvulus as a sign for cystic fibrosis," *Prenatal Diagnosis*, vol. 28, no. 10, pp. 973-974, 2008.

[8] A. Sciarrone, E. Teruzzi, A. Pertusio et al., "Fetal midgut volvulus: Report of eight cases," *The Journal of Maternal-Fetal and Neonatal Medicine*, vol. 29, no. 8, pp. 1322–1327, 2016.

[9] S. G. Jakhere, S. A. Saifi, and A. A. Ranwaka, "Fetal small bowel volvulus without malrotation: The whirlpool & coffee bean signs," *Journal of Neonatal-Perinatal Medicine*, vol. 7, no. 2, pp. 143–146, 2014.

[10] R. M. R. Tan, J. Lee, A. Biswas, and C. Amutha, "Ascites, anemia and (intestinal) atresia," *Journal of Perinatology*, vol. 34, no. 1, pp. 78–80, 2014.

[11] J. Kornacki, M. Czarnecka, M. Błaszczyński et al., "Congenital midgut volvulus associated with fetal anemia," *Fetal Diagnosis and Therapy*, vol. 28, no. 2, pp. 119–122, 2010.

[12] H.-C. Chao, M.-S. Kong, J.-Y. Chen, S.-J. Lin, and J.-N. Lin, "Sonographic features related to volvulus in neonatal intestinal malrotation," *Journal of Ultrasound in Medicine*, vol. 19, no. 6, pp. 371–376, 2000.

[13] R. K. Kitamura, P. Midulla, and T. Mirensky, "Meconium peritonitis following intestinal atresia: A case report," *Journal of Pediatric Surgery Case Reports*, vol. 9, pp. 9-10, 2016.

[14] M. N. de la Hunt, "The acute abdomen in the newborn," *Seminars in Fetal and Neonatal Medicine*, vol. 11, no. 3, pp. 191–197, 2006.

[15] U. Keskin, K. E. Karasahin, M. Ozturk et al., "Prenatal diagnosis of the acute meconium peritonitis secondary to ileum volvulus perforation: A case report," *Fetal and Pediatric Pathology*, vol. 34, no. 1, pp. 9–13, 2015.

[16] R. Basu and D. M. Burge, "The effect of antenatal diagnosis on the management of small bowel atresia," *Pediatric Surgery International*, vol. 20, no. 3, pp. 177–179, 2004.

[17] M. E. Baldassarre, A. Laneve, A. Rizzo et al., "A case of fetal midgut volvulus and jejunal atresia: Nutritional support and maintenance of mucosal function and integrity," *Immunopharmacology and Immunotoxicology*, vol. 30, no. 3, pp. 601–608, 2008.

33

Successful Vaginal Delivery of Naturally Conceived Dicavitary Twin in Didelphys Uterus: A Rare Reported Case

Houda Nasser Al Yaqoubi and Nishat Fatema

Department of Obstetrics and Gynaecology, Ibri Regional Hospital, Ministry of Health, Ibri, Oman

Correspondence should be addressed to Nishat Fatema; nishat.doc.om@gmail.com

Academic Editor: Giampiero Capobianco

Didelphys uterus, or double uterus, is an embryological developmental malformation of the mullerian ducts with the incidence of approximately 8.3% of all müllerian duct abnormalities (MDAs). Didelphys uterus accompanying dicavitary twin gestation is encountered as a very rare entity with overall incidence of about 1 in 1,000,000. We report a rare case of didelphys uterus, diagnosed since her first pregnancy, and during her fourth pregnancy she conceived dicavitary twin naturally without any infertility treatment. Though, the pregnancy course was complicated by preterm labour at 34-week gestation and she delivered simultaneously both fetuses with the cephalic presentation by spontaneous vaginal delivery with good maternal and neonatal outcomes.

1. Introduction

Didelphys uterus is an embryological developmental malformation of the müllerian or Wolffian ducts, characterized by complete failure of the müllerian ducts to fuse, resulting in two separate uterine cavities and cervices. Sometimes a longitudinal or transverse vaginal septum varying from thin and easily displaceable to thick and inelastic may also be associated with didelphys uterus [1, 2].

Among müllerian duct anomalies (MDAs), the septate uterus is the most common (35%) followed by bicornuate uterus (25%), arcuate uterus (20%), then unicornuate (9.6%), and complete agenesis (3%). The occurrence of didelphys uterus is the second least common with the incidence of approximately 8.3% of all MDAs. The prevalence of didelphys uterus is reported to be 1 in 1000–1 in 30,000 women [1].

These uterine anomalies are associated with delayed natural conception and subfertility. In case of infertile women, uterus didelphys has been found around 0.2%. For such cases, successful pregnancies can be achieved by artificial reproductive technique and embryo transfer [2, 3].

Natural twin conception in each cavity of didelphys uterus is a very rare entity and only a handful of cases are reported in the literature to date. Because of its rarity, didelphic uterus accompanying natural dicavitary twin conception

without any fertility treatment has not been researched extensively in the literature, so the exact rate of occurrence is unknown in general population [1, 4].

Dicavitary twin in a double uterus was first described in 1927. The overall incidence of dicavitary twin gestation (ART/Natural conception) in uterus didelphys has been reported approximately 1 in 1,000,000 [1, 3].

Like other MDAs, uterine didelphys is associated with various obstetric complications like spontaneous miscarriages, malpresentation, preterm delivery, preterm rupture of membrane, intrauterine growth restriction, and the need for operative delivery [4, 5].

We are discussing an extremely rare case of a naturally conceived dicavitary twin pregnancy in didelphys uterus, who had a successful vaginal delivery of both fetuses simultaneously without any complications at 34 weeks of gestation.

2. Case Presentation

A 30-year-old G4P1Ab2 woman was diagnosed by MRI to have uterus didelphys with two cervices and longitudinal upper vaginal septum since her first pregnancy. During her fourth pregnancy, she was booked with us at 10 weeks of gestation with a singleton fetus in each cavity (dicavitary twin) of the uterus didelphys.

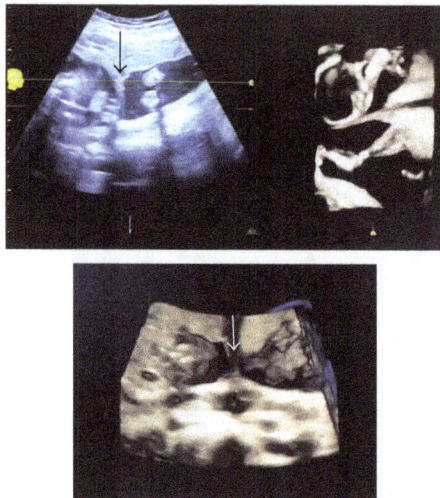

FIGURE 1: Thick septum separating the uterine cavities showing in 2D and 3D ultrasound mode. The arrows showed thick septum separating the uterine cavities showing in 2D and 3d ultrasound mode.

Her past obstetric history revealed that she had two first trimester miscarriages followed by IUI (intrauterine insemination) conception in her third pregnancy. In her third pregnancy, induction of labour (IOL) was done at 36 weeks of gestation in view of intrauterine growth restriction (IUGR). Following IOL, she delivered vaginally an alive preterm baby with the weight of 2 kg. Her medical history is significant for hypothyroidism and she is on Tab. Thyroxin 25 microgram daily.

During her current pregnancy, she conceived naturally without any fertility treatment. After booking, she was referred for routine antenatal care at Maternal-Fetal Medicine (MFM) clinic due to twin gestation and uterine anomaly and for the risks associated with it. On subsequent follow-up in MFM clinic, she was diagnosed as dicavitary twin pregnancy in didelphys uterus by USG (Figure 1). Her blood group was AB +ve and booking hemoglobin was 11.7 gm/dl.

She was started on low dose aspirin (75 mg) in view of the previous history of IUGR baby. She followed up biweekly at the MFM clinic. Detailed anatomical analysis of both fetuses was done by ultrasound during second trimester. The analysis revealed normal amniotic fluid and anteriorly placed placenta for both fetuses. The length of both cervices was within normal limit.

During 33 + 3 weeks of gestation at the time of her routine antenatal follow-up, she complained of intermittent premature contraction, so vaginal examination was performed which revealed left cervix 1.5 cm long os 2 cm dilated membrane intact and station at −3 and the other cervix was closed.

She was admitted for observation; two doses of dexamethasone (12 mg) were given 12 hours apart for fetal lung maturation. Fetal growth for both fetuses by USG: first fetus (right uterus) was with estimated weight 1.7 kg and normal amniotic fluid, and the second fetus (left uterus) estimated weight was 1.9 kg and normal amniotic fluid. Umbilical

artery Doppler for both fetuses was normal (Figure 3). Cardiotocograph tracing for both fetuses was satisfactory. Two days later she was discharged and plan of delivery was discussed with the couple in detail; if both babies remained cephalic and no complications arise, she will be allowed for the trial of vaginal delivery. If there was malpresentation or any element of fetal distress of any one of the fetuses, then the cesarean section would be considered for both fetuses. She and her husband agreed with our plan.

One week after discharge from the hospital, at 34 + 3 weeks of gestation, she was presented with preterm labour. On physical examination, she was vitally stable and was getting the strong uterine contraction and vaginal examination revealed that she was in the second stage of labour. Immediately after admission, the first twin was delivered and after delivery of first twin amniotomy was done for the second twin. Around 11 minutes after the delivery of first twin, the second twin was delivered from the other uterine cavity. Both placentas were removed smoothly from the separate uterine cavities. The neonatal outcomes were good with Apgar scores for both babies of 9 in 1 minute and 10 in 5 minutes. The first baby was a male with weight 1.6 kg, and the second baby was female with weight 2 kg. Neonates were kept in the neonatal intensive care unit for preterm care and observation. Neither the patient nor the neonates have experienced any other complications. Patient's postnatal course was uneventful and on the second postnatal day she was discharged in good condition with her healthy babies.

3. Discussion

We presented a case of known uterus didelphys with naturally conceived dicavitary twin pregnancy which is an extremely rare occurrence.

The failure of fusion of the müllerian ducts results in uterus didelphys. It is a developmental abnormality of müllerian ducts comprised the double uterus with completely developed independent horns including endometrium, myometrium, and serosal layers; two cervices; and longitudinal or transverse vaginal septum (Figure 2(a)). The etiology of uterus didelphys is not known exactly with the frequency from 1 in 1000 to 1 in 30,000 women [4, 5]. Didelphys uterus accompanying naturally conceived twin pregnancy with each fetus in the separate cavity (Figure 2(b)) is a rare entity. Only a few number of cases have been reported, but no large series exist in the literature [1, 6].

To the best of our knowledge, not more than 20 cases of dicavitary twin or multiple gestation in didelphys uterus have been researched to date [6, 7].

The exact incidence of the condition is unknown. The overall incidence of dicavitary twin gestation conceived either spontaneously or by the artificial reproductive technique is estimated approximately 1 in 1,000,000 [1, 6]. It is hypothesized that these twins are biovular in all cases, where the two ova might come from the two follicles of the same ovary or in both ovaries ovulation may occur during the same cycle [8].

Our patient was diagnosed to have didelphys uterus since her first pregnancy and conceived dicavitary twin,

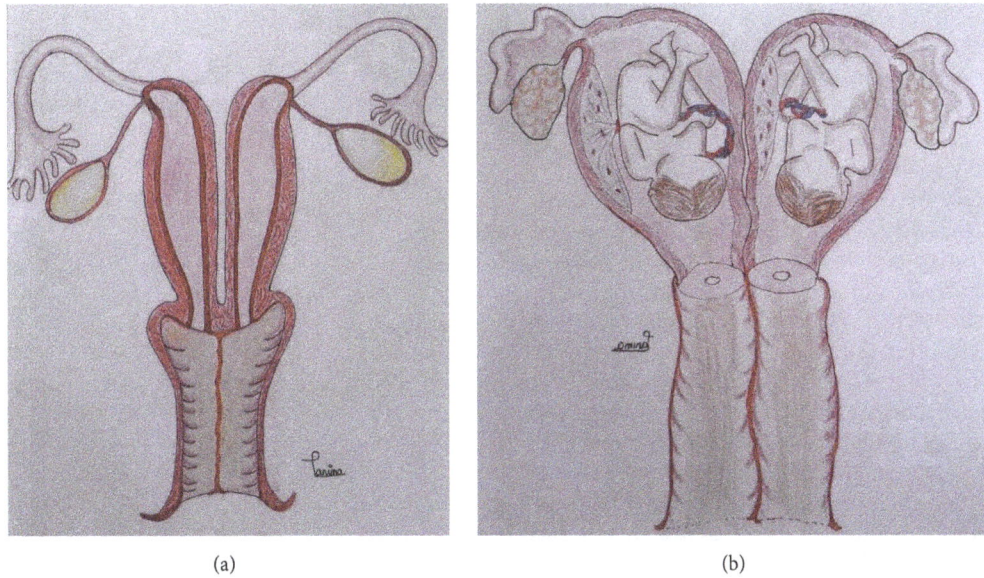

(a)

(b)

FIGURE 2: (a) Schematic diagram of nongravid didelphys uterus and (b) schematic diagram of gravid didelphys uterus with dicavitary twin.

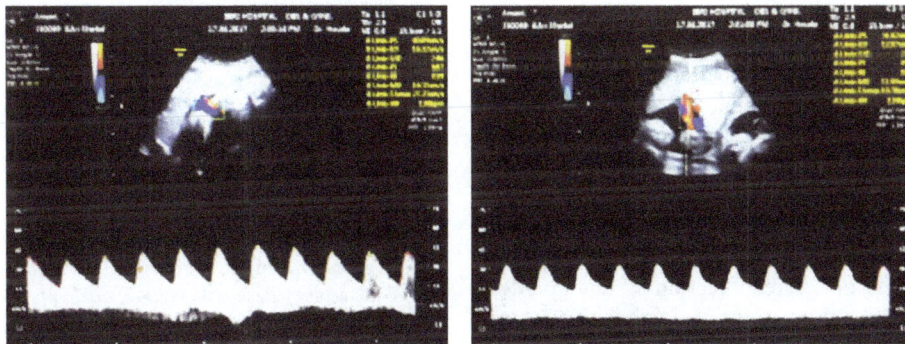

FIGURE 3: Umbilical artery Doppler for both fetuses at 33 weeks of gestation.

naturally without any infertility treatment. Unfortunately, the pregnancy course was complicated by preterm labour at 34 weeks of gestation and she delivered simultaneously both fetuses with the cephalic presentation by spontaneous vaginal delivery. The time interval between deliveries of both fetuses was only 11 minutes.

Similar to our case, Allegrezza reported a case of natural dicavitary twin pregnancy in didelphys uterus, in which the patient had premature rupture of membrane followed by preterm labour at 31 weeks of gestation, both fetuses were cephalic and delivered vaginally without any complications [4].

The contractions of both uteri may not begin simultaneously. There are reported cases where the delivery interval between the twins varies from several hours or even several weeks [8].

One case is reported by Nohara et al. in which one twin was delivered by cesarean section at 25 weeks of gestation due to fetal distress followed by premature rupture of membrane and another one was delivered vaginally with

a 66 days' interval at 35 weeks of gestation. They described that in didelphys uterus as the uterine horns are individually functioning so the initiation of labour could be local rather than systemic control [7].

Maki et al. described another case of dicavitary twins in didelphys uterus that were conceived after fertility treatment, where at 37 weeks of gestation the woman had preterm premature rupture of the membrane of right horn of uterus followed by progression of labour with simultaneous contractions of both horns of the uterus. The fetus in the right horn was delivered by spontaneous vaginal delivery and the second twin was delivered by cesarean section in view of abnormal cardiotocograph (CTG). They analyzed the synchronized contractions of both horns of the didelphys uterus and commented that the primary uterine contractions are caused by the individual rhythms of the bilateral pacemaker sites surrounding the uterotubal junction and subsequently the help of the gap junctions in between both uterine sides resulted in synchronized uterine contractions to expel the uterine contents [6].

In our case, luckily the CTG tracing of both fetuses was reactive, and both were delivered vaginally without any difficulty within an 11-minute time interval.

Only a few cases of twin gestation with didelphys uterus that had spontaneous vaginal delivery are mentioned in the literature [1, 8].

Didelphys uterus is associated with varieties of obstetric complications including early and late miscarriages, malpresentation, intrauterine growth restriction, preterm delivery, and preterm rupture of membrane [4, 5, 9].

Cervical incompetence is not commonly occurred with didelphys uterus so cervical cerclage is not routinely recommended unless there is an evidence of cervical incompetence or dilation either by clinical examination or ultrasonography during early second trimester. A case of didelphys uterus with dicavitary twin was reported with the short cervix at 30 weeks of gestation with uterine contractions. They managed the case by tocolytic therapy with nifedipine until 34 weeks and then at 37 weeks of gestation cesarean section was done for both fetuses due to fetal distress of one twin. They did not observe any adverse effects of tocolytic therapy [1, 2].

The overall obstetric outcome of uterus didelphys is poor but still better than the other MDAs like the septate or bicornuate uterus. The reason behind this occurs is that in didelphys uterus the blood supply through the collateral circulation in between two horns is better in comparison to other MDAs. The successful pregnancy rate with didelphys uterus is 57%, and the fetal survival rate is documented around 64% [2, 4, 10].

In these cases, no specific route of termination of pregnancy is recommended in the literature, though both vaginal and cesarean delivery have been mentioned in the previous studies. The incidence of cesarean section is documented about 82%. If both fetal presentations are cephalic and there are no other associated risk factors, then vaginal delivery can be considered as the mode of delivery [2, 5, 10].

If the cesarean section is indicated then a low midline longitudinal incision is preferable for proper exposure of both uterine cavity to facilitate the delivery of the fetuses [3].

4. Conclusion

Most of the previous studies regarding didelphys uterus with twin gestation had the history of fertility treatment, and the termination of pregnancy was required by cesarean section either due to fetal malpresentation or fetal distress. Our presented case is the dicavitary twin with didelphys uterus, which was conceived naturally, and although the pregnancy was complicated by preterm labour, both fetuses were delivered vaginally with good maternal and neonatal outcomes.

Didelphys uterus is associated with a twin pregnancy is a high-risk pregnancy. The early detection of this anomaly of the uterus and accompanying pregnancy by ultrasonography is of great value. Close monitoring of fetal growth, biophysical profile, and the cervical condition is recommended throughout the pregnancy. The time and mode of delivery should be planned and discussed in detail with the couple during antenatal follow-up [4, 5, 8].

Acknowledgments

The authors would like to thank Dr. Tanima Roy (Bangladesh) for her great effort and support by drawing the schematic diagrams (Figure 2).

References

[1] O. Ozyuncu, M. Turgal, A. Yazicioglu, and A. Ozek, "Spontaneous twin gestation in each horn of uterus didelphys complicated with unilateral preterm labor," *Case Reports in Perinatal Medicine*, vol. 3, no. 1, 2014.

[2] S. Rezai, P. Bisram, I. Lora Alcantara, R. Upadhyay, C. Lara, and M. Elmadjian, "Didelphys uterus: a case report and review of the literature," *Case Reports in Obstetrics and Gynecology*, vol. 2015, Article ID 865821, 5 pages, 2015.

[3] M. Yang, J. Tseng, C. Chen, and H. Li, "Delivery of double singleton pregnancies in a woman with a double uterus, double cervix, and complete septate vagina," *Journal of the Chinese Medical Association*, vol. 78, no. 12, pp. 746–748, 2015.

[4] D. M. Allegrezza, "Uterus didelphys and dicavitary twin pregnancy," *Journal of Diagnostic Medical Sonography*, vol. 23, no. 5, pp. 286–289, 2016.

[5] C. Magudapathi, "Uterus didelphys with longitudinal vaginal septum: normal deliver—case report," *Journal of Clinical Case Reports*, vol. 2, article 13, 2012.

[6] Y. Maki, S. Furukawa, H. Sameshima, and T. Ikenoue, "Independent uterine contractions in simultaneous twin pregnancy in each horn of the uterus didelphys," *Journal of Obstetrics and Gynaecology Research*, vol. 40, no. 3, pp. 836–839, 2014.

[7] M. Nohara, M. Nakayama, H. Masamoto, K. Nakazato, K. Sakumoto, and K. Kanazawa, "Twin pregnancy in each half of a uterus didelphys with a delivery interval of 66 days," *BJOG: An International Journal of Obstetrics & Gynaecology*, vol. 110, no. 3, pp. 331-332, 2003.

[8] R. Kekkonen, M. Nuutila, and T. Laatikainen, "Twin pregnancy with a fetus in each half of a uterus didelphys," *Acta Obstetricia et Gynecologica Scandinavica*, vol. 70, no. 4-5, pp. 373-374, 1991.

[9] J. R. Jackson, B. Williams, and J. Thorp, "Spontaneous triplets carried in a uterus didelphys," *Case Reports in Women's Health*, vol. 3-4, pp. 1-2, 2014.

[10] S. Bhattacharya and P. K. Mistri, *Twin Pregnancy in a Woman with Uterus Didelphys*, 2011, http://cogprints.org/7271/.

34

Oophoropexy for Recurrent Ovarian Torsion

Jennifer Hartley(iD), **Muhammad Akhtar, and Edmond Edi-Osagie**

Saint Mary's Hospital, Central Manchester University Hospitals NHS Foundation Trust, Oxford Road, Manchester M13 9WL, UK

Correspondence should be addressed to Jennifer Hartley; jen1808@doctors.org.uk

Academic Editor: Svein Rasmussen

A 31-year-old nulliparous patient presents with a three-day history of right sided colicky abdominal pain and associated nausea. This patient has previously presented twice with right sided ovarian torsion with the background of polycystic ovaries in the last two consecutive years. Blood tests were normal. Due to previous history, there was a high index of clinical suspicion that this may be a further torsion. Therefore, the patient was taken to theatre for a diagnostic laparoscopy and a further right sided ovarian torsion was noted. At this time, oophoropexy was performed to the uterosacral ligament to prevent further torsion in order to preserve the patients' fertility. In this article, we detail this case and also provide a discussion of ovarian torsion including risk factors, presentation, and current thoughts on management.

1. Introduction

Ovarian torsion is a common gynaecological emergency with the majority of cases occurring in women of reproductive age [1]. Ovarian torsion involves the rotation of the ovary on its ligamentous supports often leading to interruption of its blood supply and in some cases necrosis. Prompt diagnosis is paramount to conserve ovarian and tubal function. Torsion is more likely to occur on the right side–possibly due to the fact that the infundibulopelvic ligament is longer on the right and/or due to the presence of the sigmoid colon preventing torsion on the left [2]. Ovarian torsion is also more likely to occur in adnexa with increased weight or diameter [3]. There have been some case reports linking torsion with polycystic ovarian syndrome due to increased ovarian volume [4]. Some experts advise that oophoropexy should be performed in cases of ovarian torsion in childhood to prevent recurrence particularly when one ovary has been removed [5]. However, there are doubts about the routine use of oophoropexy due to the lack of long-term follow-up studies in regard to its effect on future fertility.

2. Case Presentation

A 31-year-old nulliparous woman known to have polycystic ovaries presents to the emergency department with right sided lower abdominal pain. The patient states that the pain feels "exactly the same as when she previously had an ovarian torsion" with a very high pain score. The patient had suffered from right sided ovarian torsion twice in the last two years and both times had undergone laparoscopic detorsion by different surgeons.

The patient was unable to tolerate ultrasound on the day of admission. Blood tests were unremarkable apart from a mildly raised C-reactive protein (CRP) of 19 mg/L. The differential diagnosis consisted of recurrent ovarian torsion, ectopic pregnancy, tuboovarian abscess, and appendicitis. Ectopic pregnancy was ruled out with a negative serum β-HCG on admission. Tuboovarian abscess was felt unlikely to be the cause as the patient was apyrexial and inflammatory markers were normal. Appendicitis was also unlikely with normal inflammatory markers and no signs of peritonism. However, appendicitis would have been identifiable on the laparoscopy that was planned. Repeat ovarian torsion was the most likely diagnosis given her history and similar symptoms during her previous two admissions.

After informed consent, the patient underwent a diagnostic laparoscopy which revealed that the right ovary and tube had torted twice. The ovary and tube were untwisted (detorsion) and the right ovary was fixed to the right uterosacral ligament using two 1.0 PDS sutures (oophoropexy), as this was the third time she had suffered an ovarian torsion on

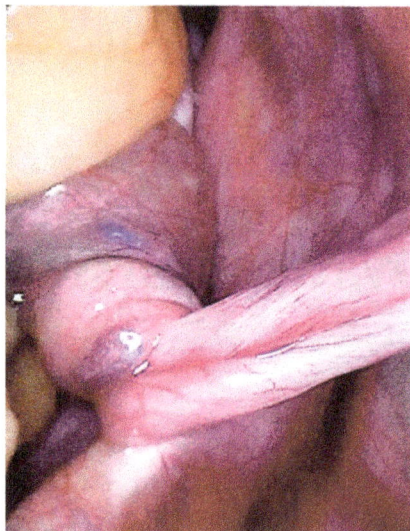

FIGURE 1: 1st admission.

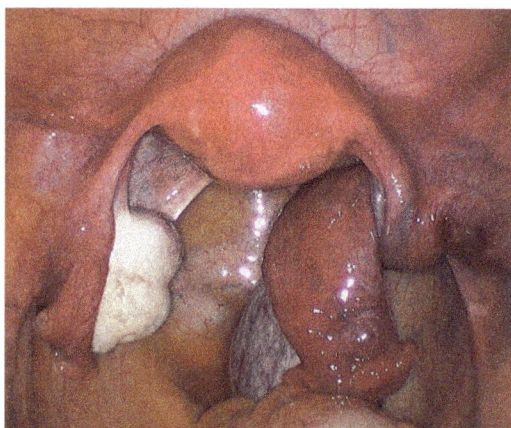

FIGURE 2: 2nd admission.

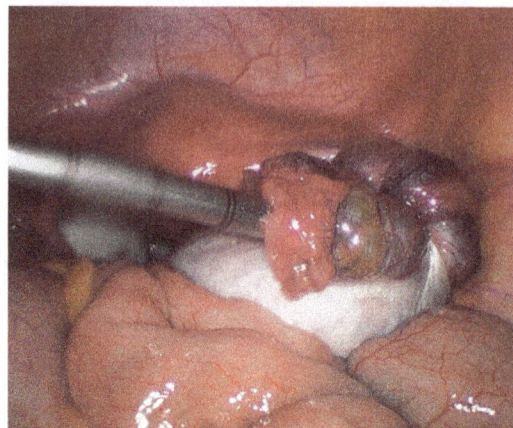

FIGURE 3: 3rd admission.

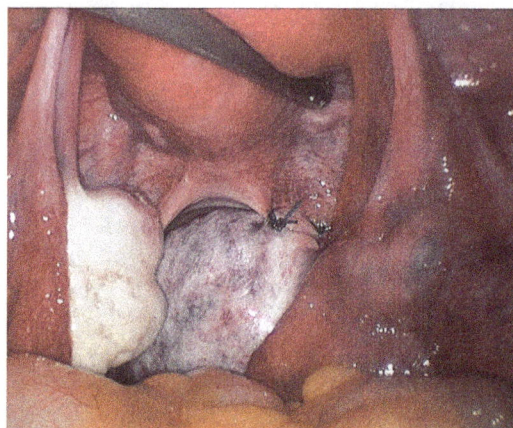

FIGURE 4: Fixation.

the right side. The left tube and ovary were normal and the uterus was normal. The appendix was normal. In this case, this method of oophoropexy was chosen due to the absence of any notable uteroovarian ligament elongation and technical ease. Furthermore, by identifying the ureteric path prior to fixation of the ovary to the uterosacral ligament, we were able to avoid the pelvic side wall and therefore minimise the risk of damage to the ureter and blood vessels (see Figures 1, 2, 3, and 4).

The woman had unremarkable postoperative recovery. She had a pelvic ultrasound five weeks after operation, which showed both ovaries to be normal in size, shape, and echotexture with vascularity demonstrated within both ovaries using colour Doppler. The right ovary measured $34 \times 14 \times 32$ mm.

3. Discussion

Adnexal torsion involves the rotation of the ovary on its ligamentous supports often leading to interruption of its blood supply and in some cases necrosis. Adnexal torsion

accounts for 2.5–5% of all gynaecological emergencies [5]. Adnexal torsion is rare but its frequency is increasing with the increasing use of fertility treatments which can cause ovarian hyperstimulation. A high index of suspicion and subsequent rapid organisation of an emergency laparoscopy would ensure protection of future ovarian function and fertility.

Maintenance of fertility by acting rapidly when adnexal torsion is suspected is of paramount importance when considering that 70–80% of cases are encountered in women of reproductive age. There is an estimated pregnancy coexistence rate of 15–25% [1, 6, 7].

Rarely, delay or misdiagnosis may be responsible for potential fatal thrombophlebitis or peritonitis [3].

Torsion is more likely to occur on the right side, possibly due to the fact that the infundibulopelvic ligament is longer on the right and/or due to the presence of the sigmoid colon preventing torsion on the left [8].

Adnexal torsion is more likely to occur in ovaries with increased ovarian diameter or weight or in those with elongated infundibulopelvic ligaments [9].

Benign ovarian cysts other than endometriomas are more often the cause of torsion than neoplasms. This is thought to

TABLE 1

Surgical techniques for oophoropexy
Fixation of the ovary to posterior abdominal wall [13]
Fixation of the ovary to pelvic side wall [8]
Plication of the uteroovarian ligaments [14]
Uteroovarian ligament shortening by "endoloop application" [4]
Combined approach of fixation of the ovary and shortening of the ligament [5]

be because neoplasms along with endometriomas are often the source of adhesions or invade neighbouring tissues [3].

Benign cystic teratomas are more prone to torsion due to the increased weight and density of these cysts. Similarly polycystic are recognised to have tendencies for adnexal torsion. Tsafrir et al. (2012) reported polycystic ovaries to be present in 7% of 216 cases of torsion.

Torsion in pregnancy can be attributed to the additional weight of the corpus luteum. The corpus luteum produces progesterone required for continuing pregnancy during the first trimester before the placenta takes over production at twelve weeks. Therefore, it is recommended that progesterone is substituted in those women who undergo cystectomy or oophorectomy in the first trimester [8].

The symptoms of adnexal torsion include colicky abdominal pain, nausea, and vomiting. Pain lasting more than ten hours before surgery is associated with an increased rate of adnexal necrosis.

Patients with ovarian torsion can be febrile, particularly in cases of tissue necrosis. Torsion is challenging to diagnose; interestingly some reports have shown that half of all patients with torsion have suffered similar episodes of abdominal pain in the past. This knowledge is useful to consider when attempting differentiating torsion from appendicitis [9].

Doppler sonography remains the most useful investigation as reduced or missing flow in the ovary can provide evidence of torsion. However, Peña et al. (2000) found that 60% of cases of torsion are missed by Doppler, although its positive predictive value is 100% [10]. Doppler sonography is limited in the fact that it can only diagnose interruption of arterial flow. It cannot diagnose interferences in venous flow which can often precede arterial interruptions.

Laparoscopy is the gold standard for diagnosis of adnexal torsion [8].

Laparoscopy in pregnancy has divided opinion. Nezhat et al. (1997) demonstrate the benefits of operative laparoscopy and subsequent successful pregnancy outcomes [11]. Schelling (2000) recommends laparoscopy to be avoided in pregnancy due to complicated access, prolonged operating times, and a theoretical risk of fetal acidosis due to an increased abdominal pressure and consequent decrease in uterine perfusion [12].

Pucci and Seed (1991) report that no adverse fetal effects due to carbon dioxide pneumoperitoneum have been detected [15]. Taking this into consideration, when operating on pregnant women certain steps are recommended. These include monitoring arterial blood gas and carbon dioxide level and avoiding pneumoperitoneum pressure greater than 12 mmHg and left lateral positioning.

Conservative treatment consists of untwisting the adnexa (detorsion). More recently, debate has sparked over the issue of oophoropexy and what the best practice is. Oophoropexy or fixation of the ovary is performed with the aim of reducing the risk of further episodes of torsion, therefore maintaining long-term fertility. However, there is a lack of evidence regarding the long-term outcome of oophoropexy. Theoretical concerns in regard to oophoropexy include concerns over the interference of tubal blood supply or a disruption to the communication between ovary and fallopian tube [16].

There is also debate over the appropriateness of oophoropexy of the contralateral ovary in cases of children who have lost an ovary due to torsion and necrosis. Once a child has lost one ovary they are at risk of asynchronous torsion of the contralateral ovary which can be catastrophic for that child's future reproductive health [9].

Methods of oophoropexy include fixation of the ovary to the pelvic side wall, posterior abdominal wall, or the posterior wall of the uterus. Plication of the uteroovarian ligaments is another method which can be employed to prevent recurrence. On review of the literature, plication of the uteroovarian ligament is the preferred technique of oophoropexy as it supposedly has minimal effect on fertility outcome. A combined approach of fixation of the ovary and shortening of the ligament may be more efficacious in preventing recurrence [5] (see Table 1).

One case report details a patient who suffered six separate episodes of torsion and two failed oophoropexies to the pelvic side wall. This patient subsequently underwent elective uteroovarian ligament shortening with no further episodes. This brings to light the issue of timing when performing oophoropexy due to the potential issue of suture instability in fragile, oedematous, and/or ischaemic tissue when oophoropexy is performed at the time of diagnosis of torsion [5].

4. Conclusion

In conclusion, it is evident that studies comparing long-term results of various methods of oophoropexy are needed. Evidence is also lacking in terms of the preferable timing of oophoropexy and whether the contralateral adnexa should also be fixed. It is also clear that emergency laparoscopy is the only reliable way to detect an adnexal torsion. Proceeding to laparoscopy should be prompt in order to prevent any complications which could have a detrimental effect on the patients' future fertility. In the meantime, a case by case approach should be employed with attention to potential risks of recurrence such as adnexal masses, polycystic ovaries, and the presence of large ovarian cysts.

Oophoropexy is an effective surgical method to prevent recurrence after two or more episodes of ovarian torsion; plication of uteroovarian ligaments remains the most anatomically feasible method.

The efficacy and safety of oophoropexy are not well established.

Evidence is based upon small case series and anecdotal case reports of different approaches of oophoropexy.

The impact of oophoropexy on subsequent fertility and its efficacy to prevent future recurrences merit further study.

Additional Points

This case occurred at Saint Mary's Hospital, Manchester. The patient was under the care of Mr. Edi-Osagie, Consultant Gynaecologist. Both Dr. Hartley and Dr. Akhtar were trainees involved in the management. This case is relevant as it is unusual to see a case of recurrent torsion three times in the same patient. Our review demonstrates that we lack evidence on the best approach to take in regard to recurrent ovarian torsion.

Consent

Written consent has been obtained from the patient for publication.

References

[1] G. Oelsner, S. B. Cohen, D. Soriano, D. Admon, S. Mashiach, and H. Carp, "Minimal surgery for the twisted ischaemic adnexa can preserve ovarian function," *Human Reproduction*, vol. 18, no. 12, pp. 2599–2602, 2003.

[2] V. N. Weitzman, A. J. DiLuigi, D. B. Maier, and J. C. Nulsen, "Prevention of recurrent adnexal torsion," *Fertility and Sterility*, vol. 90, no. 5, 2008.

[3] C. Huchon and A. Fauconnier, "Adnexal torsion: a literature review," *European Journal of Obstetrics & Gynecology and Reproductive Biology*, vol. 150, no. 1, pp. 8–12, 2010.

[4] Z. Tsafrir, J. Hasson, I. Levin, E. Solomon, J. B. Lessing, and F. Azem, "Adnexal torsion: cystectomy and ovarian fixation are equally important in preventing recurrence," *European Journal of Obstetrics & Gynecology and Reproductive Biology*, vol. 162, no. 2, pp. 203–205, 2012.

[5] E. Simsek, E. Kilicdag, H. Kalayci, S. Yuksel Simsek, and A. Parlakgumus, "Repeated ovariopexy failure in recurrent adnexal torsion: Combined approach and review of the literature," *European Journal of Obstetrics & Gynecology and Reproductive Biology*, vol. 170, no. 2, pp. 305–308, 2013.

[6] B. W. Rackow and P. Patrizio, "Successful pregnancy complicated by early and late adnexal torsion after in vitro fertilization," *Fertility and Sterility*, vol. 87, no. 3, pp. e9–e12, 2007.

[7] S. S. Thakore, M. J. Chun, and K. Fitzpatrick, "Recurrent Ovarian Torsion due to Paratubal Cysts in an Adolescent Female," *Journal of Pediatric & Adolescent Gynecology*, vol. 25, no. 4, pp. e85–e87, 2012.

[8] D. Djavadian, W. Braendle, and F. Jaenicke, "Laparoscopic oophoropexy for the treatment of recurrent torsion of the adnexa in pregnancy: case report and review," *Fertility and Sterility*, vol. 82, no. 4, pp. 933–936, 2004.

[9] E. Kurtoglu, A. Kokcu, and M. Danaci, "Asynchronous bilateral ovarian torsion. A case report and mini review," *Journal of Pediatric & Adolescent Gynecology*, vol. 27, no. 3, pp. 122–124, 2014.

[10] J. E. Peña, D. Ufberg, N. Cooney, and A. L. Denis, "Usefulness of Doppler sonography in the diagnosis of ovarian torsion," *Fertility and Sterility*, vol. 73, no. 5, pp. 1047–1050, 2000.

[11] F. R. Nezhat, S. Tazuke, C. H. Nezhat, D. S. Seidman, D. R. Phillips, and C. R. Nezhat, "Lapa- roscopy during pregnancy: a literature review," *J soclaparoendoscsurg*, vol. 1, no. 1, pp. 17–27, 1997.

[12] M. Schelling, Adnextumoren in der Schwangerschaft. 2000. In: Schneider H, Husslein P, Schneider KTM, eds. Geburtshilfe. Heidelburg: Springer-Verlag.

[13] M. Abeş and H. Sarihan, "Oophoropexy in children with ovarian torsion," *European Journal of Pediatric Surgery*, vol. 14, no. 3, pp. 168–171, 2004.

[14] M. M. Germain, T. Rarick, and E. Robins, "Management of intermittent ovarian torsion by laparoscopic oophoropexy," *Obstetrics & Gynecology*, vol. 88, no. 4, pp. 715–717, 1996.

[15] R. O. Pucci and R. W. Seed, "Case report of laparoscopic cholecystectomy in the third trimester of pregnancy," *American Journal of Obstetrics & Gynecology*, vol. 165, no. 2, pp. 401–402, 1991.

[16] N. Fuchs, N. Smorgick, Y. Tovbin et al., "Oophoropexy to Prevent Adnexal Torsion: How, When, and for Whom?" *Journal of Minimally Invasive Gynecology*, vol. 17, no. 2, pp. 205–208, 2010.

35

Atrial Fibrillation as a Rare Complication of the Use of Nifedipine as a Tocolytic Agent: A Case Report and Review of the Literature

Nikolina P. Docheva ⓘ, Emily D. Slutsky ⓘ, Roger Sandelin ⓘ, and James W. Van Hook

Department of Obstetrics and Gynecology, University of Toledo, Toledo, OH, USA

Correspondence should be addressed to Nikolina P. Docheva; nikolina.docheva@utoledo.edu

Academic Editor: Giampiero Capobianco

Calcium channel blockers are commonly used tocolytic agents on Labor and Delivery units worldwide as part of the management of preterm labor. Despite their overall reassuring safety profile, rare cardiovascular complications have been reported. In this report, we describe the case of threatened preterm labor managed with nifedipine with subsequent development of atrial fibrillation. This type of cardiac arrhythmia may have considerable consequences for both the mother and the fetus. The aim of this case report and comprehensive review of the literature is to raise awareness.

1. Introduction

Normal maternal physiologic adaptations that occur during pregnancy can predispose to cardiac arrhythmias. Some of these adaptations are increased circulating blood volume and cardiac output with subsequent myocardial stretching, reduced systemic vascular resistance, modest decline in blood pressure, high plasma catecholamine concentrations, and adrenergic receptor sensitivity [1–5]. Studies have shown that the most common arrhythmias in pregnancy are ectopic premature contractions and nonsustained arrhythmias [6, 7]. Atrial fibrillation is rare in pregnancy with prevalence of 2 per 100,000 pregnancies and accounts for 1% of all hospital admissions for arrhythmia in the pregnant patient [7]. Most of the cases described in the literature occur in women with preexisting heart conditions such as congenital heart disease, hyperthyroidism, electrolyte disturbances, or the use of either recreational or prescribed drugs [8–10]. Atrial fibrillation, in the absence of structural heart disease or known cause, also known as "lone atrial fibrillation," is even more rare [10–16]. We present a case report of a patient without any structural cardiac defects who developed atrial fibrillation following the administration of nifedipine as a tocolytic agent.

2. Case Presentation

A 25-year-old African American woman, Gravida 7, Para 1, Aborta 5, presented at 29 weeks and 2 days with threatened preterm labor. The patient initially sought care at an outside facility where she received 0.25 mg of terbutaline SC for tocolysis and 12 mg IM of betamethasone for lung maturation. The patient was transferred to our tertiary facility with strong, regular uterine contractions. She underwent a transvaginal ultrasonogram which showed a normal cervical length of 3.4 cm. The patient was placed on continuous cardiotocographic monitoring and started on nifedipine (Procardia) 20 mg every 4 hours, with subsequent administration of the second dose of 12 mg IM betamethasone. Her pregnancy was complicated by opioid abuse, normocytic anemia (hemoglobin on admission 9.9 g/dL), and history of low transverse cesarean section for breech presentation. During the course of her hospitalization, she complained of heart palpitations and chest pain that radiated to her neck. On examination, her pulse palpated as irregularly irregular and vitals revealed a tachycardia into the 140 s. A twelve-lead ECG confirmed atrial fibrillation with rapid ventricular response. Cardiology was consulted. The patient was transferred to the intensive care unit and began on diltiazem drip and

TABLE 1: Laboratory results.

Laboratory test	Result	Normal range
Hemoglobin (g/dL)	10.4	11.7–15.5
Hematocrit (%)	30.8%	35–47%
CK-MB (ng/mL)	1.0	0.0–4.9
Total CK (U/L)	15	24–170
Ck relative index (Units)	6.7	0.0–2.4
Troponin I (ng/mL)	<0.01	0.00–0.04
Sodium (mmol/L)	134–146	142
Potassium (mmol/L)	4.2	3.5–5.0
D-dimer (ng/mL)	<255	340
AST (U/L)	17	0–41
ALT (U/L)	8	0–31
Magnesium (mg/dL)	1.7	1.8–2.6
TSH (uIU/mL)	1.95	0.49–4.67
T4 (ng/dL)	0.76	0.61–1.60

intravenous metoprolol for rate control. She received a total of six doses of nifedipine during her admission before discontinuation of the medication. Her symptoms occurred within 20 hours from the first dose of nifedipine. Workup included an echocardiogram, lower extremities venous Doppler, troponin levels, thyroid function test, electrolytes, liver function tests, and a repeat urine drug test. All results were normal apart from borderline magnesium of 1.7 mg/dL (see Table 1 for further results). The patient converted to normal sinus rhythm in less than 24 hours with a CHA_2DS_2-VASc score of 1 and anticoagulation with 81 mg aspirin was started. After transfer out of the intensive care unit the patient remained in sinus rhythm for the remainder of the hospitalization. Discharge medications included metoprolol 25 mg twice daily for rate control with close outpatient follow-up with MFM and cardiology.

The pregnancy culminated with a repeat low-transverse cesarean section at 39-week gestation resulting in a live-born male infant with Apgar scores of 9 and 9 at 1 and 5 minutes, respectively, and birthweight of 3400 grams. Continuous cardiac monitoring for 24 hours following delivery showed sinus rhythm. Per cardiology recommendations she was continued on metoprolol for prophylactic rate control and 81 mg aspirin in the postpartum period until she was seen as an outpatient. During that visit, metoprolol was discontinued.

3. Discussion

It is well known that atrial fibrillation predisposes to hemodynamic abnormalities and thromboembolic events leading to significant morbidity and mortality [17]. Pregnancy is a hypercoagulable state [18, 19] with an increased cardiac workload and therefore an increased susceptibility to arrhythmias [1–5]. Women with a history of any type of arrhythmia prior to pregnancy are at an increased risk of cardiac related morbidity, such as stroke and heart failure, during pregnancy [20]. However, because atrial fibrillation is rare in pregnancy, as are the sequela, it is difficult to adequately study the

related adverse events. Lee et al. studied atrial fibrillation in pregnancy; of 264,730 pregnancies, atrial fibrillation was noted in only 157 [21]. The results suggest that older women (≥30 years of age) had higher odds of developing atrial fibrillation, and the odds significantly increased with increasing age [e.g., age 30–34 OR 4.1 95% CI (2.0–9.4), $p < 0.001$, and age ≥40 OR 5.2 95% CI (2.0–14.10), $p < 0.001$]. They also reported an increased prevalence among White and Black women as compared to Asian and Hispanic patients (111.6, 101.7, 45.0, and 34.3 per 100,000, resp.). Moreover, the odds for atrial fibrillation were higher during the third trimester compared to the first trimester of pregnancy [3.2 95% CI (1.5–7.7), $p = 0.002$]. In addition, there was no difference in birthweight among fetuses born to mothers with or without atrial fibrillation. However, the rate of admission to the neonatal intensive care unit was higher in the atrial fibrillation group (10.8% versus 5.1% $p = 0.003$) [21].

The case described *here-in* of threatened preterm labor depicts a common scenario seen in Labor and Delivery units worldwide. Preterm birth affects 5 to 18% of pregnancies and is a leading cause of infant morbidity and mortality [22]. Inhibition of uterine contractility with tocolytic agents is central to the treatment for preterm labor. Many different agents are available to inhibit uterine contractions including calcium channel blockers, magnesium sulfate, nonsteroidal anti-inflammatory drugs, beta-adrenergic receptor agonists, and oxytocin antagonists. The choice of a tocolytic agent is largely based on its contraindications. A recent systematic review and meta-analysis of randomized controlled trials ($N = 2,179$ women) showed that nifedipine was associated with a significant reduction in the risk of preterm delivery within 7 days of starting treatment, when initiated before 34-week gestation, compared with beta-adrenergic receptor agonists. The analysis also showed that there was no difference between the tocolytic efficacy of nifedipine and magnesium sulfate. However, nifedipine had significantly less maternal adverse events than magnesium sulfate and beta-adrenergic receptor agonists [23].

Nifedipine is a dihydropyridine calcium channel blocker that causes smooth muscle relaxation with vasodilatory action in the peripheral vasculature. There is a potential to provoke a compensatory adrenergic drive in order to maintain cardiac output, resulting in reflex tachycardia [24]. As previously mentioned the maternal physiologic adaptations of pregnancy predispose to arrhythmias and the additional effects of nifedipine on the maternal cardiovascular system can increase the risk of developing an arrhythmia. Despite the relatively safe profile of nifedipine, case reports have been published in the literature which described patients developing myocardial infarction [25, 26], severe hypotension leading to fetal demise [27], maternal hypoxia [28], and pulmonary edema associated with nifedipine [29, 30]. Moreover, a study showed cases of nifedipine-associated maternal dyspnea in patients with twin pregnancies underscoring a concern for administering nifedipine in women with compromised cardiovascular conditions which could be due to multiple gestation, maternal hypertension, cardiac disease, or intrauterine infection [24]. Our patient received a total of 6 doses of nifedipine 20 mg and we believe that this predisposed her to develop paroxysmal atrial fibrillation. In addition, she was anemic, further increasing the strain on the myocardium and potentiating the effects of the nifedipine. Parasuraman et al. [31] published the first case report in which a patient with threatened preterm labor was treated with nifedipine and developed atrial fibrillation that responded to DC cardioversion, whereas Cheung et al. [32] described a case of maternal atrial fibrillation after sequential use of nifedipine and atosiban for the treatment of preterm labor. de Heus et al. reported, in a multicenter prospective cohort study, that, among the 542 women treated with nifedipine, 5 (0.9%) had a serious adverse side effect and 6 (1.1%) had a mild adverse side effect [33]. In addition, Khan et al., in a systematic review and meta-regression analysis, evaluated the safety of nifedipine as a tocolytic agent in preterm labor and as an antihypertensive agent in the treatment of hypertension in pregnancy. The results showed that adverse events were the highest among women given more than 60 mg total dose of nifedipine [OR 3.78, 95% CI (1.27–11.2), $p = 0.017$] and in reports from case series compared to controlled studies [OR 2.45, 95 CI (1.17–5.15), $p = 0.018$] [34]. Outside pregnancy, short acting nifedipine has been associated with increased risk of myocardial infarction and mortality when used to treat hypertension. This is believed to be due to the hypotension and reflex tachycardia that can predispose to an arrhythmia [35]. The FDA states that atrial or ventricular dysrhythmias can occur in less than 1% of patients on short acting nifedipine [36].

This case report provides a lesson for physicians in the field of high risk obstetrics. Caution must be taken when administering tocolytic agents such as nifedipine. Even though the medication is overall safe and the aforementioned side effects are rare, there is a small subset of patients that develop severe side effects such as atrial fibrillation, which may lead to significant maternal and fetal morbidity.

References

[1] W. M. Barron, S. K. Mujais, M. Zinaman, E. L. Bravo, and M. D. Lindheimer, "Plasma Catecholamine Responses to Physiologic Stimuli in Normal Human Pregnancy," *Obstetric Anesthesia Digest*, vol. 154, no. 1, pp. 80–84, 1986.

[2] J. H. McAnulty, M. J. Morton, and K. Ueland, "The heart and pregnancy," *Current Problems in Cardiology*, vol. 13, no. 9, pp. 594–665, 1988.

[3] S. Hunter and S. C. Robson, "Adaptation of the maternal heart in pregnancy," *British Heart Journal*, vol. 68, no. 6, pp. 540–543, 1992.

[4] G. J. Gilson, S. Samaan, M. H. Crawford, C. R. Qualls, and L. B. Curet, "Changes in hemodynamics, ventricular remodeling, and ventricular contractility during normal pregnancy: a longitudinal study," *Obstetrics & Gynecology*, vol. 89, no. 6, pp. 957–962, 1997.

[5] J. G. Ouzounian and U. Elkayam, "Physiologic changes during normal pregnancy and delivery," *Cardiology Clinics*, vol. 30, no. 3, pp. 317–329, 2012.

[6] A. Shotan, E. Ostrzega, A. Mehra, J. V. Johnson, and U. Elkayam, "Incidence of arrhythmias in normal pregnancy and relation to palpitations, dizziness, and syncope," *American Journal of Cardiology*, vol. 79, no. 8, pp. 1061–1064, 1997.

[7] J.-M. Li, C. Nguyen, J. A. Joglar, M. H. Hamdan, and R. Page, "Frequency and outcome of arrhythmias complicating admission during pregnancy: Experience from a high-volume and ethnically-diverse obstetric service," *Clinical Cardiology*, vol. 31, no. 11, pp. 538–541, 2008.

[8] P. Szekely and L. Snaith, "Atrial fibrillation and pregnancy," *British Medical Journal*, vol. 1, no. 5237, pp. 1407–1410, 1961.

[9] L. T. A. Dicarlo-Meacham and L. J. Dahlke, "Atrial fibrillation in pregnancy," *Obstetrics & Gynecology*, vol. 117, no. 2, pp. 489–492, 2011.

[10] N. Sauvé, É. Rey, and A. Cumyn, "Atrial Fibrillation in a Structurally Normal Heart during Pregnancy: A Review of Cases From a Registry and From the Literature," *Journal of Obstetrics and Gynaecology Canada*, vol. 39, no. 1, pp. 18–24, 2017.

[11] R. M. Gowda, G. Punukollu, I. A. Khan et al., "Lone atrial fibrillation during pregnancy [9]," *International Journal of Cardiology*, vol. 88, no. 1, pp. 123-124, 2003.

[12] K. M. Kuczkowski, "New onset transient lone atrial fibrillation in a healthy parturient: Déjà vu [9]," *International Journal of Cardiology*, vol. 97, no. 2, p. 339, 2004.

[13] C.-H. Lin and C.-N. Lee, "Atrial fibrillation with rapid ventricular response in pregnancy," *Taiwanese Journal of Obstetrics and Gynecology*, vol. 47, no. 3, pp. 327–329, 2008.

[14] C. A. Walsh, T. Manias, and C. Patient, "Atrial fibrillation in pregnancy," *European Journal of Obstetrics & Gynecology and Reproductive Biology*, vol. 138, no. 1, pp. 119-120, 2008.

[15] L. Cacciotti, G. S. Camastra, and G. Ansalone, "Atrial fibrillation in a pregnant woman with a normal heart," *Internal and Emergency Medicine*, vol. 5, no. 1, pp. 87-88, 2010.

[16] C. J. Sengheiser and K. C. Channer, "Recurrent atrial flutter and fibrillation in pregnancy," *BMJ Case Reports*, vol. 2011, 2011.

[17] C. T. January et al., "Correction to 2017 ACC/AHA/HRS Guideline for the Evaluation and Management of Patients With Syncope: Executive Summary: A Report of the American College of Cardiology/American Heart Association Task Force on Clinical Practice Guidelines and the Heart Rhythm Society," *Circulation*, vol. 136, no. 16, pp. e269–e270, 2017.

[18] K. A. Bremme, "Haemostatic changes in pregnancy," *Best Practice & Research Clinical Haematology*, vol. 16, no. 2, pp. 153–168, 2003.

[19] M. Franchini, "Haemostasis and pregnancy," *Thrombosis and Haemostasis*, vol. 95, no. 3, pp. 401–413, 2006.

[20] S. C. Siu, M. Sermer, J. M. Colman et al., "Prospective multicenter study of pregnancy outcomes in women with heart disease," *Circulation*, vol. 104, no. 5, pp. 515–521, 2001.

[21] M. Lee, W. Chen, Z. Zhang et al., "Atrial Fibrillation and Atrial Flutter in Pregnant Women—A Population-Based Study," *Journal of the American Heart Association*, vol. 5, no. 4, p. e003182, 2016.

[22] R. Romero, S. K. Dey, and S. J. Fisher, "Preterm labor: one syndrome, many causes," *Science*, vol. 345, no. 6198, pp. 760–765, 2014.

[23] A. Conde-Agudelo, R. Romero, and J. P. Kusanovic, "Nifedipine in the management of preterm labor: a systematic review and metaanalysis," *American Journal of Obstetrics & Gynecology*, vol. 204, no. 2, pp. 134.e1–134.e20, 2011.

[24] H. P. Van Geijn, J. E. Lenglet, and A. C. Bolte, "Nifedipine trials: Effectiveness and safety aspects," *BJOG: An International Journal of Obstetrics & Gynaecology*, vol. 112, no. 1, pp. 79–83, 2005.

[25] S. G. Oei, S. K. Oei, and H. A. Brölmann, "Myocardial infarction during nifedipine therapy for preterm labor," *The New England Journal of Medicine*, vol. 340, no. 2, p. 154, 1999.

[26] D. Verhaert and R. van Acker, "Acute myocardial infarction during pregnancy," *Acta Cardiologica*, vol. 59, no. 3, pp. 331–339, 2004.

[27] A. J. Van Veen, M. J. Pelinck, M. G. Van Pampus, and J. J. H. M. Erwich, "Severe hypotension and fetal death due to tocolysis with nifedipine," *BJOG: An International Journal of Obstetrics & Gynaecology*, vol. 112, no. 4, pp. 509-510, 2005.

[28] R. Hodges, A. Barkehall-Thomas, and C. Tippett, "Maternal hypoxia associated with nifedipine for threatened preterm labour," *BJOG: An International Journal of Obstetrics & Gynaecology*, vol. 111, no. 4, pp. 380-381, 2004.

[29] O. M. Abbas, A. H. Nassar, N. A. Kanj, and I. M. Usta, "Acute pulmonary edema during tocolytic therapy with nifedipine," *American Journal of Obstetrics & Gynecology*, vol. 195, no. 4, pp. e3–e4, 2006.

[30] M. S. Kutuk, M. T. Ozgun, S. Uludag, M. Dolanbay, and A. Yildirim, "Acute pulmonary failure due to pulmonary edema during tocolytic therapy with nifedipine," *Archives of Gynecology and Obstetrics*, vol. 288, no. 4, pp. 953-954, 2013.

[31] R. Parasuraman, M. M. Gandhi, and N. H. Liversedge, "Nifedipine tocolysis associated atrial fibrillation responds to DC cardioversion," *BJOG: An International Journal of Obstetrics & Gynaecology*, vol. 113, no. 7, pp. 844-845, 2006.

[32] C. S.-Y. Cheung, T. K.-T. Li, and C.-P. Lee, "Maternal atrial fibrillation after sequential use of nifedipine and atosiban for treatment of preterm labor: Case report," *European Journal of Obstetrics & Gynecology and Reproductive Biology*, vol. 166, no. 2, p. 229, 2013.

[33] R. de Heus, B. W. Mol, J. H. Erwich et al., "Adverse drug reactions to tocolytic treatment for preterm labour: prospective cohort study," *BMJ*, vol. 338, no. mar05 2, pp. b744–b744, 2009.

[34] K. Khan, J. Zamora, R. F. Lamont et al., "Safety concerns for the use of calcium channel blockers in pregnancy for the treatment of spontaneous preterm labour and hypertension: A systematic review and meta-regression analysis," *The Journal of Maternal-Fetal and Neonatal Medicine*, vol. 23, no. 9, pp. 1030–1038, 2010.

[35] C. D. Furberg, B. M. Psaty, and J. V. Meyer, "Nifedipine: Dose-related increase in mortality in patients with coronary heart disease," *Circulation*, vol. 92, no. 5, pp. 1326–1331, 1995.

[36] "PROCARDIA® (nifedipine) CAPSULES For Oral Use".

Unusual Case of a Torted Mesenteric Fibroid

Rawan Bajis⊙[1] and Gregg Eloundou[2]

[1]*King Edward Memorial Hospital, Australia*
[2]*Joondalup Health Campus, Australia*

Correspondence should be addressed to Rawan Bajis; rawan.bajis@health.wa.gov.au

Academic Editor: Giampiero Capobianco

Extrauterine leiomyomas are very rare and present a clinical and diagnostic challenge due to their unusual growth patterns and behaviours. A 47-year-old woman was transferred to our tertiary specialist obstetrics and gynaecology hospital with acute abdominal pain and a palpable abdominal mass. She was taken immediately to theatre with the presumptive diagnosis of an ovarian torsion. Intraoperatively, a large necrotic mass originating from the mesentery and attachments to the bowel at the ileocaecal junction was noted. When converted to laparotomy due to limited access and poor visualisation, the uterus, ovaries, and tubes were found to be normal. A right partial hemicolectomy was performed with the assistance of the colorectal surgeon due to suspicion of bowel malignancy. Histology revealed a benign infarcted leiomyoma with adhesions to the adjacent ileum. The diagnosis of a primary torted mesenteric fibroid was made.

1. Introduction

Leiomyomas (fibroids) are histologically distorted smooth muscle tumours, which are thought to arise from the genitourinary tract and are almost always benign [1]. They are very common, occurring in up to 65% of women and are incidentally found in approximately 80% of all uterine specimens at hysterectomy [2, 3]. They are estrogen and progesterone dependent which might explain their prevalence in the female reproductive years as well as their regression following menopause [2]. They represent the most common gynaecological tumour and cause severe clinical symptoms in up to 30% of women [4]. Women with uterine fibroids often present with a variety of symptoms depending on their anatomical location and size. These could range from abnormal vaginal bleeding, pelvic pain, and pressure symptoms against neighbouring organs, to subfertility [5–7]. Rarely, fibroids can occur and grow in unusual locations outside the uterus and in doing so present a clinical and diagnostic challenge [8]. Due to their unusual growth patterns and behaviours, patients present with a wide variety of symptoms and on occasions can be acutely unwell, mimicking other gynaecological or nongynaecological conditions and in some cases mimicking other malignancies. As a result, the diagnosis of most extrauterine fibroids is often only made intraoperatively, either during diagnostic laparoscopy for acute presentations of pain or during surgery for management of other previously diagnosed abdominal-pelvic masses. They can also be diagnosed incidentally on various imaging modalities such as ultrasound, CT, or MRI performed for unrelated conditions [8].

Little is known about these rare extrauterine growths. In fact, it is often only after histological assessment of the resected specimen that a diagnosis of a leiomyoma is made. It has been postulated that these atypical leiomyomas develop secondary to cell spillage and seeding during morcellation at hysterectomy or myomectomy [9, 10]. Rarely, as in this case, have extrauterine fibroids been reported in the absence of previous fibroid surgery and hence why the physiopathology of primary solitary mesenteric leiomyoma development in a "virgin" abdomen is not clearly recognised or understood.

We present a case of a 46-year-old woman with a torted mesenteric fibroid; her puzzling presentation, intraoperative findings, and suggested theories behind the possible development are also discussed.

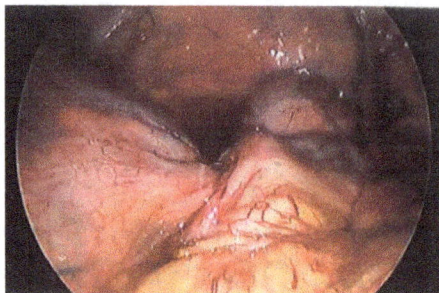

FIGURE 1: Laparoscopic view of fibroid (right) and its attachment to the bowel (left). Area of torsion noted in between.

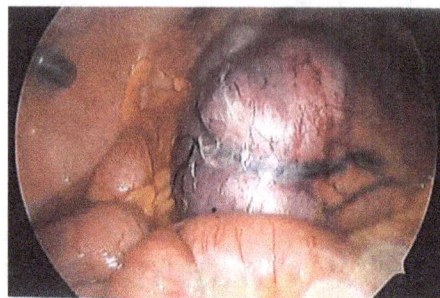

FIGURE 2: Laparoscopic view of infarcted fibroid.

2. Case Presentation

A 47-year-old para 2 presented to the general hospital emergency department with a 3-day history of severe abdominal pain, nausea, and vomiting. This was her first hospital presentation with abdominal pain. Her past medical history included two previous caesarean sections but no other abdominal surgeries. A month prior to this presentation, she had visited her primary healthcare provider complaining of a distended abdomen. An ultrasound performed at the time had reported a large pedunculated uterine fibroid measuring 126x104x108mm. The left ovary was normal but the right ovary was not visualised. Unfortunately, this information was not readily available to the treating team at the time of her acute presentation.

A FAST scan (focused assessment with sonography for trauma) done in the general hospital had reported a moderate amount of free fluid in the right iliac fossa and a large pelvic mass. The presumed diagnosis was an ovarian cyst torsion and formed the premise for transfer to our tertiary specialist obstetrics and gynaecology hospital.

On arrival to our specialist hospital, the patient was haemodynamically stable and afebrile. On palpation of her abdomen, a large, firm, mobile, and tender mass was noted, extending to her umbilicus. She had a negative pregnancy test. Besides a raised CRP of 77ml/L, the rest of her blood profile was normal.

Given the acute nature of her presentation and the ultrasound findings, she was transferred to theatre for laparoscopic management of a torted ovarian cyst. At laparoscopy, performed through Palmers point entry due to the large mass extending to the umbilicus, a large 25cm multilobulated necrotic mass occupying the entire lower abdomen and pelvis was found. The mass was mobile with attachments to the bowel at the right iliac fossa. Due to limited laparoscopic accessibility, it was impossible to fully explore the rest of the pelvic organs safely. Laparoscopy was converted to a laparotomy and a transverse lower abdominal incision was made for a safer inspection. A large necrotic mass originating from the mesentery of the ileocaecal junction was noted (Figure 1). Its borders were confluent with the walls of the terminal ileum at the ileocaecal junction, which in itself had become necrotic having axially rotated under the weight of the growth (Figure 2). This raised the suspicion of a bowel malignancy. The appendix could not be clearly visualised. The

uterus, ovaries, and tubes appeared normal. Specifically, the uterus showed no areas of detachment. The on-call colorectal surgeon was contacted to assist with the remainder of the surgery due to extensive bowel involvement. The right colon and terminal ileum were mobilized and the mesentery was dissected to the level of the origin of the ileocolic vessels. A right partial hemicolectomy was performed with a primary ileocolic anastomosis and the mesenteric defect closed. A frozen section was considered, however, due to the large nature of the necrotic mass and extensive bowel involvement with adjacent necrosis, the entire specimen was resected en bloc. Postoperatively, she had a five-day hospital stay complicated by an ileus requiring nasogastric tube placement. She made a full recovery and was discharged home with outpatient clinic follow-up.

On macroscopic histopathology, a large mass attached to the serosal surface of the ileocaecal junction with a 10mm vascular stalk was reported. Microscopically, a circumscribed mass composed of interlacing bundles of smooth muscle with large areas of necrosis and infarction was noted. Adhesions made up of fibrofatty tissue, between the mass and the caecum, were present. The smooth muscle cells stained positive for desmin and actin and showed a low Ki-67 staining pattern. Features of a benign leiomyoma with extensive infarction were confirmed. Adhesions between the leiomyoma and the adjacent ileum and caecum were extensively present, supporting the diagnosis of a torted extrauterine mesenteric fibroid.

3. Discussion

Extrauterine fibroids are extremely rare and poorly understood. They develop outside the uterus and arise as proliferation of smooth muscle cells with behaviours and histological characteristics identical to their uterine leiomyoma counterparts [8]. Their diagnosis is complicated by their nonspecific clinical presentation. A history of a hysterectomy or fibroid surgery with morcellation is often an associated finding and may be suggestive of the diagnosis and aetiology [11]. Extrauterine fibroids usually present with acute pain and complications secondary to compression affects as a consequence of their location [8]. Common presentations include bowel obstruction, haemorrhage, and, as in this case, infarction resulting in an acute abdomen and severe pain. Their appearance may mimic that of malignancy dictating the need for a wide resection.

Unusual extrauterine fibroid growth patterns described in the literature to date include peritoneal leiomyomatosis, intravenous leiomyomas, benign metastasizing leiomyomas, retroperitoneal leiomyomas, and parasitic leiomyomas. Although various theories and hypothesis exist regarding the mechanism behind these manifestations, no established conclusive pathophysiology has been made. It is important however to consider the heterogeneous theories that do exist regarding the bizarre manifestations of these extrauterine leiomyomas, before considering the diagnosis of our case.

Disseminated peritoneal leiomyomatosis, first described by Taubert et al. in 1965, is a rare condition characterized by innumerable diffuse vascular peritoneal nodules that grow along submesothelial tissues in the abdominopelvic peritoneum. It is thought that these multiple growths arise from smooth muscle metaplasia of submesothelial mesenchymal cells, the embryological origins of the peritoneum that line the female reproductive tract [12]. These are almost always benign but sarcomatous transformations have been described [13]. Hormonal factors have also been implicated in their pathogenesis as case reports of these extrauterine masses have been documented in association with pregnancy, hormone secreting ovarian tumours, and the combined contraceptive pill [14, 15].

Another rare extrauterine pathology exists in the form of Intravenous leiomyomas. These manifest as intramural proliferation of leiomyomas that occur within intrauterine and systemic veins [16]. They are believed to grow within vessels of the myometrium and parametrium with reported cases of extensions to the inferior vena cava and the heart [17]. These are almost always associated with previous uterine fibroid surgery.

Benign metastasizing leiomyomas, as first described in 1939, manifest as nodules of well-differentiated benign leiomyomatous tissue located at distal sites to the uterus, mimicking metastatic disease [18]. Most commonly, these benign metastatic lesions are located in the lung and have been noted up to 20 years after surgery for known uterine fibroids [1, 19]. These are hormone receptor positive tumours and have been reported to self-resolve in postmenopausal patients. It is on this premise that hormone modulators may provide the rationale behind treatment of symptomatic individuals [20, 21]. Lymphovascular embolization of uterine leiomyomatous tissue at distant sites is the most commonly recognised theory [21].

As first described in the literature by Kelly et al. in 1909, parasitic leiomyomas are a rare type of migratory leiomyoma. It was first hypothesised that pedunculated subserosal leiomyomas could adhere to surrounding structures, detach from the uterus, and develop axillary blood supplies, thus explaining the diagnoses of leiomyomas at sites distal to a myomatous uterus [22]. Although rare, they have been reported to occur more frequently in the broad ligament, pelvic peritoneum, and omentum [1]. A second hypothesis exists whereby cell spillage and seeding take place during morcellation at time of surgical resection of the uterine fibroid or at hysterectomy. Kho et al. reported a case series of 12 parasitic myomas in 2009, noting several leiomyomas adherent to nearby bowel mesentery, appendix, anterior abdominal wall, and rectovaginal septum [10]. In all but two cases, women had previously undergone abdominal surgery for known fibroid or endometriosis. This case series supported the previously hypothesised theory that prior surgery, specifically hysterectomy or myomectomy with morcellation, is a potential risk factor for the development of extrauterine fibroids, specifically iatrogenic parasitic myomas. As such, the Food and Drug Administration of USA has recently advised against the continued use of power morcellators in treatment of uterine fibroids [23]. Although a review regarding the use of morcellation therapy was initially sparked due to the increased reports of iatrogenic abdominal and peritoneal seeding of uterine sarcoma, the increased prevalence of extrauterine fibroids has also played a part in discouraging its use [24]. Parasitic myomas remain rare but may become more frequently reported with increased use of laparoscopic surgery in gynaecology. Therefore, it should be considered as a differential in any female presenting with acute abdominal pain or with an abdominal-pelvic mass with known history of fibroid surgery [11].

Our case presented a diagnostic dilemma and left us puzzled as to the possible pathophysiological explanation. The most probable mechanism for her diagnosis would be that of a parasitic myoma. This is reinforced by the fact that she had had two previous caesarean sections and an ultrasound scan a month prior to her presentation reporting the presence of a subserosal pedunculated fibroid. However, caesarean sections have not yet been postulated as a potential source for seeding. Also, at the time of surgery, the uterus appeared normal with no area of detachment noted. Given the degree of dense adhesion to bowel and mesentery, and the short length of time that had elapsed between her scan and presentation, it is possible that the migration theory could not be the sole explanation. This case could therefore represent a solitary primary mesenteric fibroid.

In the literature to date, there is little evidence of primary mesenteric fibroids in an unmorcellated abdomen. In a case series published by Dan et al. in 2012 of two patients who required right hemicolectomies for extrauterine fibroids, one patient had no prior history of abdominal surgery, whereas the other had a history of a laparoscopic myomectomy just eleven days prior [25]. Whether there is predilection for the right abdomen is unclear; however, in this case series and the one we report here, all three patients had right hemicolectomies for leiomyoma's morbidly adherent to the mesentery of the right-sided colon.

What is even rarer is the presence of a torted extrauterine leiomyoma. In our case, the fibroid had rotated along a stalk morbidly adherent to underlying mesentery and bowel. There are few reported cases in the literature describing torted parasitic fibroids in the absence of having had previous abdominal surgeries [26–28]. Similar to our case, however, Yeh et al. in 1999 published a case report of a woman who presented with a torted fibroid of the broad ligament with no uterine wall attachment and no prior history of abdominal surgery [28]. That too could be considered a primary extrauterine fibroid similar to the one we are presenting. Whatever the definition, the mechanism remains a mystery.

It is important to consider the possibility of an extrauterine fibroid as a differential diagnosis in any female presenting with an intra-abdominal and pelvic mass, especially with a history of previous surgery for fibroids. It is also important to recognise the need for prompt exploratory surgery in any premenopausal patient presenting with acute abdominal pain and the clinical suspicion of torsion.

Our case highlights the complexity of the diagnosis of extrauterine fibroids and adds to the body of literature describing and reporting extrauterine fibroids. As they remain rare and grossly misunderstood, it is prudent to continue reporting cases in order to create a database which could be used to formulate a better understanding of the clinical presentation, diagnosis, and management.

Consent

Patient has given written informed consent for this case to be published in a medical journal.

References

[1] M. S. Mahmoud, K. Desai, and F. R. Nezhat, "Leiomyomas beyond the uterus; benign metastasizing leiomyomatosis with paraaortic metastasizing endometriosis and intravenous leiomyomatosis: a case series and review of the literature," *Archives of Gynecology and Obstetrics*, vol. 291, no. 1, pp. 223–230, 2015.

[2] S. E. Bulun, "Uterine fibroids," *The New England Journal of Medicine*, vol. 369, no. 14, pp. 1344–1355, 2013.

[3] S. F. Cramer and A. Patel, "The frequency of uterine leiomyomas," *American Journal of Clinical Pathology*, vol. 94, no. 4, pp. 435–438, 1990.

[4] W. H. Catherino, E. Parrott, and J. Segars, "Proceedings from the National Institute of Child Health and Human Development Conference on the Uterine Fibroid Research Update Workshop," *Fertility and Sterility*, vol. 95, no. 1, pp. 9–12, 2011.

[5] A. Zimmermann, D. Bernuit, C. Gerlinger, M. Schaefers, and K. Geppert, "Prevalence, symptoms and management of uterine fibroids: an international internet-based survey of 21,746 women," *BMC Women's Health*, vol. 12, no. 1, article 6, 11 pages, 2012.

[6] K. Puri, A. O. Famuyide, P. J. Erwin, E. A. Stewart, and S. K. Laughlin-Tommaso, "Submucosal fibroids and the relation to heavy menstrual bleeding and anemia," *American Journal of Obstetrics & Gynecology*, vol. 210, no. 1, pp. 38-e1–38-e7, 2014.

[7] B. Kroon, N. Johnson, M. Chapman, A. Yazdani, R. Hart, and Australasian CREI Consensus Expert Panel on Trial Evidence (ACCEPT) Group, "Fibroids in infertility—consensus statement from ACCEPT (Australasian CREI Consensus Expert Panel on Trial evidence)," *Australian and New Zealand Journal of Obstetrics and Gynaecology*, vol. 51, no. 4, pp. 289–295, 2011.

[8] N. Fasih, A. K. P. Shanbhogue, D. B. Macdonald et al., "Leiomyomas beyond the uterus: unusual locations, rare manifestations," *RadioGraphics*, vol. 28, no. 7, pp. 1931–1948, 2008.

[9] R. Sinha, M. Sundaram, S. Lakhotia, P. Kadam, G. Rao, and C. Mahajan, "Parasitic myoma after morcellation," *Journal of Gynecological Endoscopy and Surgery*, vol. 1, no. 2, pp. 113–115, 2009.

[10] K. A. Kho and C. Nezhat, "Parasitic myomas," *Obstetrics & Gynecology*, vol. 114, no. 3, pp. 611–615, 2009.

[11] D. Larraín, B. Rabischong, C. K. Khoo, R. Botchorishvili, M. Canis, and G. Mage, "'Iatrogenic' parasitic myomas: unusual late complication of laparoscopic morcellation procedures," *Journal of Minimally Invasive Gynecology*, vol. 17, no. 6, pp. 719–724, 2010.

[12] H.-D. Taubert, S. E. Wissner, and A. L. Haskins, "Leiomyomatosis peritonealis disseminata: An unusual complication of genital leiomyomata," *Obstetrics & Gynecology*, vol. 25, no. 4, pp. 561–574, 1965.

[13] W. H. Parker, Y. S. Fu, and J. S. Berek, "Uterine sarcoma in patients operated on for presumed leiomyoma and rapidly growing leiomyoma," *Obstetrics & Gynecology*, vol. 83, no. 3, pp. 414–418, 1994.

[14] F. A. Tavassoli and H. J. Norris, "Peritoneal leiomyomatosis (leiomyomatosis peritonealis disseminata): A clinicopathologic study of 20 cases with ultrastructural observations," *International Journal of Gynecological Pathology*, vol. 1, no. 1, pp. 59–74, 1982.

[15] J. R. Willson and A. R. Peale, "Multiple peritoneal leiomyomas associated with a granulosa-cell tumor of the ovary," *American Journal of Obstetrics & Gynecology*, vol. 64, no. 1, pp. 204–208, 1952.

[16] E. N. Consamus, M. J. Reardon, A. G. Ayala, M. R. Schwartz, and J. Y. Ro, "Metastasizing leiomyoma to heart," *Methodist DeBakey Cardiovascular Journal*, vol. 10, no. 4, pp. 251–254, 2014.

[17] M. J. Kocica, M. R. Vranes, D. Kostic et al., "Intravenous leiomyomatosis with extension to the heart: Rare or underestimated?" *The Journal of Thoracic and Cardiovascular Surgery*, vol. 130, no. 6, pp. 1724–1726, 2005.

[18] P. E. Steiner, "Metastasizing fibroleiomyoma of the uterus: report of a case and review of the literature," *The American Journal of Pathology*, vol. 15, no. 1, article 89, 1939.

[19] Y.-I. Kwon, T.-H. Kim, J. W. Sohn, H. J. Yoon, D. H. Shin, and S. S. Park, "Benign pulmonary metastasizing leiomyomatosis: Case report and a review of the literature," *Korean Journal of Internal Medicine*, vol. 21, no. 3, pp. 173–177, 2006.

[20] A. O. Awonuga, M. Rotas, A. N. Imudia, C. Choi, and N. Khulpateea, "Recurrent benign metastasizing leiomyoma after hysterectomy and bilateral salpingo-oophorectomy," *Archives of Gynecology and Obstetrics*, vol. 278, no. 4, pp. 373–376, 2008.

[21] M. M. Beck, B. Biswas, A. D'Souza, and R. Kumar, "Benign metastasising leiomyoma after hysterectomy and bilateral salpingo-oophorectomy," *Hong Kong Medical Journal*, vol. 18, no. 2, pp. 153–155, 2012.

[22] H. A. Kelly and T. S. Cullen, *Myomata of the Uterus*, Saunders, 1909.

[23] FDA Safety Communication, *UPDATED Laparoscopic Uterine Power Morcellation in Hysterectomy and Myomectomy*, 2014.

[24] M. W. Beckmann, I. Juhasz-Böss, D. Denschlag et al., "Surgical methods for the treatment of uterine fibroids - risk of uterine sarcoma and problems of morcellation: position paper of the DGGG," *Geburtshilfe und Frauenheilkunde*, vol. 75, no. 2, pp. 148–164, 2015.

[25] D. Dan, D. Harnanan, S. Hariharan, R. Maharaj, I. Hosein, and V. Naraynsingh, "Extrauterine leiomyomata presenting with sepsis requiring hemicolectomy," *Revista Brasileira de Ginecologia e Obstetrícia*, vol. 34, no. 6, pp. 285–289, 2012.

[26] D. M. Narasimhulu, E. Eugene, and S. Sumit, "Torsion of an iatrogenic parasitic fibroid related to power morcellation for specimen retrieval," *Journal of the Turkish German Gynecology Association*, vol. 16, no. 4, pp. 259–262, 2015.

[27] D. S. Park, J. Y. Shim, S. J. Seong, and Y. W. Jung, "Torsion of parasitic myoma in the mesentery after myomectomy," *European Journal of Obstetrics & Gynecology and Reproductive Biology*, vol. 169, no. 2, pp. 414-415, 2013.

[28] H.-C. Yeh, M. Kaplan, and L. Deligdisch, "Parasitic and pedunculated leiomyomas: Ultrasonographic features," *Journal of Ultrasound in Medicine*, vol. 18, no. 11, pp. 789–794, 1999.

37

Pregnancy Complications in a-Thalassemia (Hemoglobinopathy H): A Case Study

Marianna Politou [iD],[1] **Giorgos Dryllis,**[1] **Maria Efstathopoulou,**[1]
Serena Valsami,[1] **Faidra-Evangelia Triantafyllou,**[1] **Athanasia Tsaroucha,**[2]
Antonios Kattamis,[3] **and Nikos F. Vlahos** [iD][4]

[1]*Department of Hematology and Blood Transfusion Unit, Aretaieion Hospital, School of Medicine,*
 National and Kapodistrian University of Athens, Greece
[2]*Anesthesiology Clinic, Aretaieion General Hospital, School of Medicine, University of Athens,*
 National and Kapodistrian University of Athens, Greece
[3]*Second Department of Obstetrics and Gynecology, Aretaieion General Hospital, School of Medicine,*
 National and Kapodistrian University of Athens, Greece
[4]*First Department of Pediatrics, University General Hospital "Attikon", School of Medicine,*
 National and Kapodistrian University of Athens, Greece

Correspondence should be addressed to Marianna Politou; mpolitou@med.uoa.gr

Academic Editor: Giovanni Monni

Thalassemia intermedia (TI) is a clinical definition which represents a wide spectrum of thalassemia genotypes but mainly includes patients who do not require or only occasionally require transfusion. An uncommon case of a 32-year-old Greek woman, para 1, at the 22nd week + day 3 of gestation with thalassemia intermedia (she was splenectomized), where her pregnancy was complicated with portal vein thrombosis, splenic thrombosis, and partial HELLP, is described. This is a generally uncommon event in thalassemia intermedia. She had no transfusion as her hematologist consulted and she took anticoagulation therapy. Thus, we present for the first time in the literature a case of HbH a-thalassemia pregnant woman whose pregnancy was complicated with portal vein thrombosis, splenic vein thrombosis, and partial HELLP; she was treated with anticoagulation therapy and she had a successful outcome.

1. Introduction

Thalassemias are hereditary disorders that result from the quantitative changes of alpha or beta chains of hemoglobin. Thalassemia intermedia (TI) or NTDT (Nontransfusion Dependent Thalassemia) is a clinical definition which includes patients with a wide spectrum of both alpha and beta thalassemia genotypes, who do not require lifelong regular transfusions for survival, although they may require occasional transfusions in certain clinical settings and for defined periods of time. HbH disease is the result of absence of the three α-globin genes (--/-α) due to deletional or nondeletional mutations. The phenotypic expression of the disease is wide and the clinical symptoms are a result of both hemolytic anemia and ineffective erythropoiesis [1, 2].

Progress in the management of TI patients enabled increasing rates of pregnancies among TI women [3]. Patients with TI have an increased risk of thrombosis [4] and pregnancy, as a hypercoagulable state increases that risk further. We here present a woman with TI a-thalassemia (hemoglobinopathy H), whose pregnancy was complicated with portal vein thrombosis and partial HELLP.

2. Case Study

A 32-year-old Greek woman, para 1, at the 22nd week + day 3 of gestation, was referred to the A&Es with a 1-week history of abdominal discomfort and persistent vomiting. The woman had HbH disease (thalassemia intermedia) with a - a 3.7/Hb Icaria a genotype. She was splenectomized at the age of 6.5 years and she maintained a Hb around 8 g/dl without blood transfusions. Her medical history included incidents of superficial-vein thrombosis in 2005, 2008, and 2009 (with negative family history of thrombosis) for which she was receiving acenocoumarol. Since the confirmation of pregnancy she was receiving Salospir 100 mg p.o. and Enoxaparin 40 mg sc.

Laboratory exams revealed moderate hypochromic microcytic anemia (Ht 28.1%, Hb 8.46 g/dL, MCV: 67.2, and MCH: 20.2), mild thrombocytosis (PLTs: 519 × 109/L), and leukocytosis: WBC 27 × 109/L (neu: 87%, lymph: 9%, and mono: 4%). The C-reactive protein was 11.4 mg/L. INR and aPTT were within normal limits but fibrinogen was high, 519.9 mg/L, and D-dimers were >5000 μg/L. The rest of the biochemistry showed the following: TBil: 1.50 mg/dl; dBil: 0.8 mg/dl; SGOT 110 IU/L; SGPT 176 IU/L; ALP 165 IU/L; γ-GT 46 IU/L; and ferritin: 63 ng/ml, indicative of hepatic impairment. An abdominal ultrasound revealed portal vein and spleen-vein thrombosis. The patient underwent a thrombophilia testing which was negative for hereditary thrombophilia (FV Leiden, FIIG20210A) as well as for anticardiolipins antibodies. Because of the site of the thrombosis (visceral), latent myeloproliferative neoplasms (MPN) were also excluded (she was negative for the JAK2V617F mutation).

The patient was treated with enoxaparin 60 mg bd, sc, and Salospir 100 mg p.o. o.d. Transaminases were normalized two weeks later and a new abdominal ultrasound, performed two months later, showed chronic portal vein and chronic spleen-vein thrombosis.

At the 35th week + day 3, the liver enzymes and the rest of the biochemistry were as follows: SGOT 466 IU/L, SGPT 931 IU/L, ALP 220 IU/L, γ-GT 41 IU/L, TBil: 1.80 mg/dl, Ht 38%, Hb 10.2 g/dL, WBC 12.3 × 109/L, and PLTs: 487 × 109/L. The abdominal ultrasound showed no new findings. With the clinical suspicion of partial HELLP syndrome (the patient had only elevated liver enzymes) an urgent caesarian section (C-section) was performed. Anticoagulation bridging with heparin was used perioperatively. During the C-section, the patient developed hypertension episode [blood pressure: 190 (systolic)/ 110 (diastolic) mmHg] and she was treated with hydralazine. The premature newborn was 1810 gr but healthy and stayed in the neonatal ICU for 7 days.

Mother's liver enzymes were normalized within five days after the delivery and the patient was discharged. The patient is now on long-term anticoagulant therapy with acenocoumarol. The imaging of splenic veins is unchanged.

3. Discussion

The clinical manifestations of thalassemia intermedia result from ineffective erythropoiesis, chronic anemia, and iron overload. HbH which is a form of NTDT has a diverse phenotypic presentation depending on the degree of alpha globin chain deficiency which in turn relates to the underlying a-thalassemia mutations with hemolysis being the dominant clinical symptom [1]. Our patient had HbH disease and

she was compound heterozygote for deletional and nondeletional mutations ($--\alpha$ 3.7/αIcaria α). She had an intermediate phenotype that is characterized by a diagnosis at age between 2 and 4 years, maintenance of a Hb above 8.0 g/dl without transfusions, and moderate splenomegaly. She had a component of both hemolysis and ineffective erythropoiesis since ineffective erythropoiesis is more severe in nondeletional genotypes [5].

Most data in the literature concerning thrombosis in thalassemia come from b-thalassemia. Thromboembolic events occur in both b-thalassemia major and NTDT patients [6]. Thromboembolic events happen in TM and TI thalassemia patients with a frequency of 4.3% $\kappa\alpha\iota$ 5.2%, respectively [7, 8]. The prevalence of thromboembolic events is even higher in transfusion-independent, splenectomized patients (29%), as in our case, compared to regularly transfused TM patients (2%) [9].

The underlying mechanisms that cause a hypercoagulable state in thalassemia include the oxidative damage of the red blood cell membrane proteins (due to hemolysis), endothelial impairment, platelet activation, and strong inflammatory reaction involving cytokines, adhesion molecules, and neutrophil activation. Splenectomy increases platelet counts and induces membranes abnormalities that further increase hypercoagulability [10].

In general, pregnancy in thalassemia intermedia patients can be complicated with automatic miscarriages, fetal loss, preterm delivery, IUGR, and thrombosis [11]. Oxidative stress due to iron overload and placental hypoxia caused by maternal anemia seem to provoke such complications. Pregnancy in HbH disease may be complicated mainly with anemia [12]. A study by Tongsong et al. has shown that common obstetric complications such as antepartum hemorrhage, preeclampsia, and postpartum hemorrhage are not significantly associated with HbH disease [13] but Tantiweerawong et al. have found that HbH may adversely affect maternal health [14].

However, our patient delivered at term and her fetus was not small for gestational age.

It is of interest that despite the established association of pregnancy with a hypercoagulable state, existing studies in TI pregnant women have not reported an increased risk of thromboembolic complications compared to nonpregnant TI women [3].

In our study, pregnancy was complicated with portal vein thrombosis, a generally uncommon event in NTDT. The patient underwent an extended investigation for the putative underlying cause of thrombosis that included hereditary and acquired thrombophilia tests along with tests for the exclusion of a latent myeloproliferative disorder and paroxysmal nocturnal hemoglobinemia because of the site of thrombosis (visceral). The absence of any other possible known prothrombotic factor supports the notion that thrombosis could be associated with splenectomy and the component of ineffective erythropoiesis in our patient (carrier of a-icaria mutation).

Furthermore, in this study the patient presented a partial HELLP syndrome (elevated liver enzymes). The well-known pathophysiological mechanism of HELLP syndrome is based on the release of various placental factors such as soluble vascular endothelial growth factor receptor-1 (sVEGFR-1), which then binds vascular endothelial growth factor (VEGF) and placental growth factor (PGF), causing endothelial cell and placental dysfunction by preventing them from binding to endothelial cell receptors. The result is hypertension, proteinuria, and increased platelet activation and aggregation which cause thrombotic events during pregnancy. The multi-organ microvascular injury and hepatic necrosis causing liver dysfunction further contribute to the development of HELLP.

Anemia requiring transfusion often complicates pregnancy in TI patients. However, no study has evaluated obstetric outcomes based on Hb levels in TI, and therefore the decision to transfuse should be individualized depending on maternal and fetal indications. While a significant proportion of pregnancies in TI women was complicated by IUGR in a Lebanese study, blood transfusions during pregnancy do not seem to decrease the risk of IUGR as well as other complications [15]. On the contrary, Tongsong et al. demonstrated that there are several benefits of frequent transfusions during pregnancy in HbH disease, like the prevention of growth restriction, suggesting that a strict control of hemoglobin levels could result in better outcome [13]. Data from nonthalassemic cohorts suggests that hemoglobin levels above 10 g/dL during gestation are recommended for optimal fetal growth and preclusion of preterm delivery [16]. However, targeting the 10 g/dL cutoff proved being of clinical benefit to only 78% of the pregnant NTDT patients and their fetuses in an Italian case series, while the fetuses of the other 22% suffered from IUGR [17]. There is no solid Hb cutoff for blood transfusion in pregnant TI women and the only determining factors are the cardiac function and general condition of the mother and the growth status of the fetus. Blood transfusions can increase the risk of developing alloimmune antibodies that would exacerbate any preexisting hemolytic anemia, such as thalassemia [18]. As such, our patient had no transfusion as per her obstetrician's judgment, which was primed by fetal growth and maternal cardiac status and overall well-being, and after consulting with the patient's treating hematologist.

There are no specific guidelines regarding thromboprophylaxis in pregnant TI patients. Thrombophylaxis might be essential during pregnancy and the postpartum period in cases of NTDT with splenectomy or a history of recurrent abortions. According to recent data, low-dose aspirin seems to be effective in preventing thromboembolic events during pregnancy without posing a major safety risk to mother or fetus [11]. Therefore, splenectomized women, as in our case, or those with a serum platelet count above 600×10^9/L should begin or continue taking aspirin at a dose of 75 mg/day. For splenectomized women with a platelet count above 600×10^9/L it is highly recommended to administrate low-molecular-weight heparin. We could suggest that for pregnant women receiving long-term vitamin-K antagonists before their pregnancy, like in this case, it is better to receive adjusted-dose of LMWH or a therapeutic dose of LMWH, rather than prophylactic-dose, throughout pregnancy followed by resumption of long-term anticoagulants postpartum.

4. Conclusion

In conclusion we present for the first time in the literature a pregnant woman with HbH disease whose pregnancy was complicated with both visceral thrombosis and partial HELLP, who was treated with anticoagulation and had a successful outcome.

References

[1] E. P. Vichinsky, "Clinical manifestations of α-thalassemia.," *Cold Spring Harbor Perspectives in Medicine*, vol. 3, no. 5, p. a011742, 2013.

[2] E. Kanavakis, I. Papassotiriou, M. Karagiorga et al., "Phenotypic and molecular diversity of haemoglobin H disease: a Greek experience," *British Journal of Haematology*, vol. 111, no. 3, pp. 915–923, 2000.

[3] E. Voskaridou, A. Balassopoulou, E. Boutou et al., "Pregnancy in beta-thalassemia intermedia: 20-year experience of a Greek thalassemia center," *European Journal of Haematology*, vol. 93, no. 6, pp. 492–499, 2014.

[4] M. D. Cappelini, K. M. Musallam, E. Pogiiiali, and A. T. Taher, "Hypercoagulability in non –tranfusion –dependent thalassemia," *Blood Reviews*, vol. 6 Suppl 1, pp. S20–S23, 2012.

[5] E. P. Vichinsky, "Alpha thalassemia major–new mutations, intrauterine management, and outcomes.," *Hematology / the Education Program of the American Society of Hematology. American Society of Hematology. Education Program*, pp. 35–41, 2009.

[6] A. T. Taher, K. M. Musallam, M. Karimi et al., "Overview on practices in thalassemia intermedia management aiming for lowering complication rates across a region of endemicity: the optimal care study," *Blood*, vol. 115, no. 10, pp. 1886–1892, 2010.

[7] C. Borgna Pignatti, V. Carnelli, V. Caruso et al., "Thromboembolic events in beta thalassemia major: an Italian multicenter study," *Acta Haematologica*, vol. 99, no. 2, pp. 76–79, 1998.

[8] S. Moratelli, V. De Sanctis, D. Gemmati et al., "Thrombotic risk in thalassemic patients," *Journal of Pediatric Endocrinology and Metabolism*, vol. 11, supp 3, pp. 915–921, 1998.

[9] M. D. Cappellini, L. Robbiolo, B. M. Bottasso, R. Coppola, G. Fiorelli, and P. M. Mannucci, "Venous thromboembolism and hypercoagulability in splenectomized patients with thalassaemia intermedia," *British Journal of Haematology*, vol. 111, no. 2, pp. 467–473, 2000.

[10] S. E. Crary and G. R. Buchanan, "Vascular complications after splenectomy for hematologic disorders," *Blood*, vol. 114, no. 14, pp. 2861–2868, 2009.

[11] G. Petrakos, P. Andriopoulos, and M. Tsironi, "Pregnancy in women with thalassemia: Challenges and solutions," *International Journal of Women's Health*, vol. 8, pp. 441–451, 2016.

[12] M. Rabiee, J.-A. Shams, and N. Zafargandie, "The adverse effects of pregnancies complicated by hemoglobin H (HBH) disease," *Iranian Journal of Pathology*, vol. 10, no. 4, pp. 318–321, 2015.

[13] T. Tongsong, K. Srisupudit, and S. Luewan, "Outcomes pregnancies affected by hemoglobin H disease," *International Journal of Gynecology & Obstetrics*, vol. 104, no. 3, pp. 206–209, 2009.

[14] N. Tantiweerawong, A. Jaovisidha, and N. Israngura Na Ayud-hya, "Pregnancy outcome of hemoglobin H disease," *International Journal of Gynecology and Obstetrics*, vol. 90, no. 3, pp. 236-237, 2005.

[15] A. H. Nassar, I. M. Usta, J. B. Rechdan, S. Koussa, A. Inati, and A. T. Taher, "Pregnancy in patients with beta-thalassemia intermedia: outcome of mothers and newborns," *American Journal of Hematology*, vol. 81, no. 7, pp. 499–502, 2006.

[16] A. Levy, D. Fraser, M. Katz, M. Mazor, and E. Sheiner, "Maternal anemia during pregnancy is an independent risk factor for low birthweight and preterm delivery," *European Journal of Obstetrics & Gynecology and Reproductive Biology*, vol. 122, no. 2, pp. 182–186, 2005.

[17] R. Origa, A. Piga, G. Quarta et al., "Pregnancy and β-thalassemia: an Italian multicenter experience," *Haematologica*, vol. 95, no. 3, pp. 376–381, 2010.

[18] D. M. Townsley, "Hematologic complications of pregnancy," *Seminars in Hematology*, vol. 50, no. 3, pp. 222–231, 2013.

38

Fetal Sirenomelia Associated with an Abdominal Cyst Originating from a Saccular Cloaca

Yui Kinjo,[1] Hitoshi Masamoto (iD),[1] Hayase Nitta,[1] Tadatsugu Kinjo,[1] Tomoko Tamaki,[2] Naoki Yoshimi (iD),[2] and Yoichi Aoki (iD)[1]

[1]Department of Obstetrics and Gynecology, Graduate School of Medicine, University of the Ryukyus, Okinawa, Japan
[2]Department of Pathology and Oncology, Graduate School of Medicine, University of the Ryukyus, Okinawa, Japan

Correspondence should be addressed to Hitoshi Masamoto; masamoto@eve.u-ryukyu.ac.jp

Academic Editor: Giovanni Monni

A 40-year-old pregnant woman presented with a fetal abdominal cyst and oligohydramnios. Color Doppler scan revealed a single blood vessel from the fetal aorta into a single umbilical artery. Severe oligohydramnios limited ultrasonographic evaluation of the fetal lower limbs, kidneys, or bladder. The pregnancy was terminated; the fetus showed fused lower limbs, bulging abdomen, and absent external genitalia and was diagnosed with type III sirenomelia. On autopsy, no normal bladder was observed, but duodenal atresia, anorectal atresia, and right renal agenesis were found. An intra-abdominal cyst, diagnosed histologically as a saccular cloaca, occupied the abdominal cavity. Ultrasonographic diagnosis of fetal sirenomelia is difficult due to poor depiction of the lower limbs. A vitelline artery leading to a single umbilical artery and a fetal abdominal cyst occupying most of the abdominal cavity are considered fetal sirenomelia associated with large defects of the gastrointestinal and genitourinary tracts.

1. Introduction

Sirenomelia is a rare and lethal congenital anomaly characterized by fusion of the lower limbs and additional malformations, including renal agenesis, anorectal atresia, oligohydramnios, and a single umbilical artery. Most infants die within one or two days after birth. Two main pathogenic hypotheses have been proposed for sirenomelia. One is defective blastogenesis hypothesis: the result of a defect in the development of caudal mesoderm during the gastrulation stage occurring in the third week of gestation, and the other is the vascular steal theory: a persistent vitelline artery and abnormalities of the abdominal vasculature lead to a deficient blood flow and nutrient supply to the caudal part of the embryo [1–3].

We experienced a rare case of fetal sirenomelia associated with an abdominal cyst and a single umbilical artery.

2. Case Presentation

A 40-year-old pregnant woman, gravida 1 para 0, presented with a fetal abdominal cystic lesion with a diameter of 17 mm by ultrasonography at 13 weeks of gestation and was referred to our hospital at 14 weeks of gestation. This was an in vitro fertilization pregnancy. She had a history of aortic dissection at the age of 31 and underwent aortic valve replacement. Thereafter, spironolactone and carvedilol were continuously administered. She underwent ultrasonography on admission, and a fetal abdominal cyst with a size of 34 × 24 mm and oligohydramnios were found (Figure 1). The fetal bladder and bilateral kidneys were not visualized. Also, a single blood vessel running from the aorta anteriorly along the abdominal mass and coursing into the single umbilical artery was seen on color Doppler ultrasonography. Bilateral iliac arteries were not identified. At 17 weeks of gestation, the abdominal mass was enlarged to 46 × 16 mm in size and an amniotic cavity could barely be seen. Precise ultrasonographic evaluation of the fetal lower limbs was limited due to the severe oligohydramnios; the bilateral kidneys and normal bladder were not depicted. We suspected fetal gastrointestinal or urinary tract malformation.

Fetal therapy was difficult in this case and the infant's prognosis was considered as extremely poor due to the early severe oligohydramnios. The patient and her husband chose

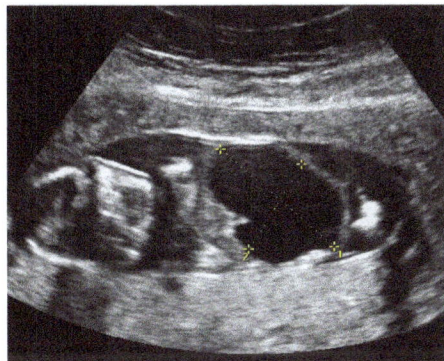

FIGURE 1: Ultrasonographic findings of the fetus at 14 weeks of gestation. A fetal intra-abdominal cyst (34 × 24 mm in size) and oligohydramnios are observed.

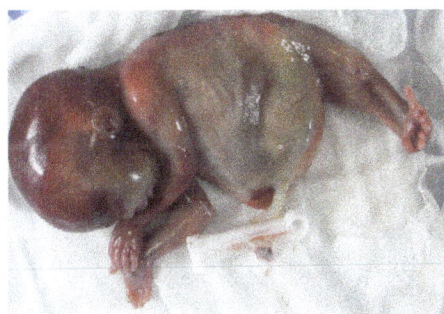

FIGURE 2: Sirenomelia with fused lower limbs and a bulging abdomen.

a termination of pregnancy. A fetus weighing 226 g was delivered vaginally at 19 weeks of gestation. The fetus showed fused lower limbs, a bulging abdomen, and absent external genitalia (Figure 2). Two femurs, two tibias, and absent fibulae were found on inspection and palpation of the fused lower limbs, so we arrived at a diagnosis of type III sirenomelia on the Stocker and Heifetz classification [4].

The parents agreed to an autopsy, which revealed a normal stomach, liver, pancreas, and left kidney. Malformations were duodenal atresia, anorectal atresia, and agenesis of the right kidney. The abdominal cavity was occupied by the intra-abdominal cyst, which included clear serous fluid. Histopathological examination revealed that the cyst comprised small intestine epithelium in the anterior region and bladder epithelium and urothelium in the posterior, which turned out to be a saccular cloaca (Figure 3). Fetal karyotyping by chorionic villus sampling resulted in a 46,XY/46,XY del(10)(q11.1) mosaicism fetus.

3. Discussion

Infants with sirenomelia are born at an approximate rate of 1 in 100,000 births. Twinning, maternal diabetes, and maternal age less than 20 years are reported as risk factors [5–7]. Maternal exposure to some drugs during pregnancy is a risk factor for fetal sirenomelia. Associations of vitamin A and

cocaine with fetal sirenomelia have been reported [8, 9]. Our patient took spironolactone and carvedilol during early pregnancy due to her history of aortic dissection. In rats treated with a high dose of spironolactone, feminization of male rat fetuses was observed [10]. One case report described ambiguous genitalia in a human newborn of a mother treated with spironolactone during pregnancy [11]. However, no association with sirenomelia is known for the two drugs given to our case.

The etiology of the sirenomelia is still unknown. Stevenson et al. [1] advocate "vascular steal theory" as one option. In a persistent vitelline artery, the blood supply for caudal development of the fetus is directed to the placenta, causing caudal blastodermal hypoperfusion. As a result, renal agenesis, bladder and ureteral hypoplasia, deficiency of the genitalia, intestinal dysplasia, anorectal atresia, synsacrum hypoplasia, and malformations of lower limbs are thought to occur.

One of the most consistent vascular features of sirenomelia is the presence of an aberrant umbilical artery derived from a persistent vitelline artery. In our case, an aberrant vitelline artery that developed from the aorta ran alongside the intra-abdominal mass, coursing into the single umbilical artery. It is sufficient for a diagnosis of sirenomelia to depict a persistent vitelline artery and its continuation by using color and power Doppler imaging [2, 12].

There are a few reports of sirenomelia associated with an intra-abdominal cyst. Schiesser et al. [13] reported a case of sirenomelia detected in the first trimester and associated with a fetal intra-abdominal cystic structure. They supposed the cystic lesion to be an expression of the complex malformation of the lower abdomen or the sonographic appearance of necrosis but did not examine the histology of the cyst. Van Keirsbilck et al. [14] reported a case of fetal sirenomelia with a cystic pelvic structure shown by MRI at 14 weeks of gestation, which originated from a dilated sigmoid colon associated with rectal atresia.

In the pathologic findings of our case, the fetal intra-abdominal cyst was found to be comprised of small intestinal epithelium in the anterior region and bladder epithelium in the posterior region and turned out to be a saccular cloaca. In viviparity, at 5 weeks, the midgut and allantoic membrane, as primordia of the small intestine and bladder, form a continued alveus with the hindgut and cloaca. In this case, the fetal intra-abdominal cyst was thought to be originating from this immature structure. There are few reports of histological examination of intra-abdominal cysts in sirenomelia.

It has been reported that ultrasonographic diagnosis of fetal sirenomelia is feasible during the first trimester because of the usually normal amniotic fluid volume, but in the second trimester it becomes difficult due to severe oligohydramnios associated with renal agenesis, resulting in poor depiction of the lower limbs [14, 15]. Oligohydramnios, an aberrant vitelline artery leading to a single umbilical artery, and a fetal abdominal cyst that occupies most of the abdominal cavity in the second trimester are considered as fetal sirenomelia associated with large defects of the gastrointestinal and genitourinary tracts, and the fetus is more likely to be incompatible with life.

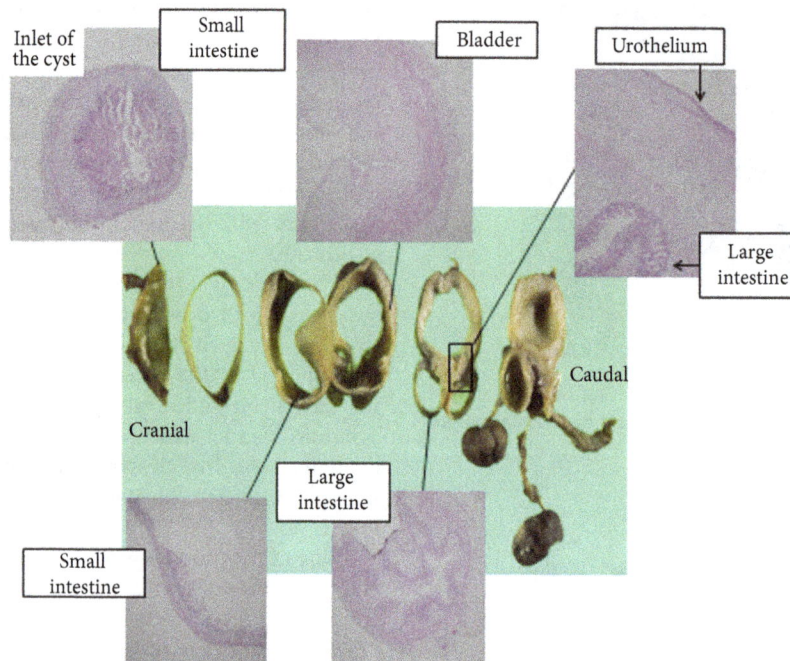

FIGURE 3: Sections of the specimen of the fetal abdominal cyst and histologic findings (hematoxylin and eosin staining, ×40).

Consent

Written informed consent was obtained from the patient for publication of this case report and any accompanying images.

Acknowledgments

The authors would like to acknowledge Enago (https://www.enago.jp) for the English language review.

References

[1] R. E. Stevenson, K. L. Jones, M. C. Phelan et al., "Vascular steal: The pathogenetic mechanism producing sirenomelia and associated defects of the viscera and soft tissues," *Pediatrics*, vol. 78, no. 3, pp. 451–457, 1986.

[2] W. Sepulveda, R. Romero, P. G. Pryde, H. M. Wolfe, J. R. Addis, and D. B. Cotton, "Prenatal diagnosis of sirenomelus with color Doppler ultrasonography," *American Journal of Obstetrics & Gynecology*, vol. 170, no. 5 I, pp. 1377–1379, 1994.

[3] C. Garrido-Allepuz, E. Haro, D. González-Lamuño, M. L. Martínez-Frías, F. Bertocchini, and M. A. Ros, "A clinical and experimental overview of sirenomelia: Insight into the mechanisms of congenital limb malformations," *Disease Models & Mechanisms*, vol. 4, no. 3, pp. 289–299, 2011.

[4] J. T. Stocker and S. A. Heifetz, "Sirenomelia. A morphological study of 33 cases and review of the literature.," *Perspectives in Pediatric Pathology*, vol. 10, pp. 7–50, 1987.

[5] I. M. Orioli, E. Amar, J. Arteaga-Vazquez et al., "Sirenomelia: An epidemiologic study in a large dataset from the International Clearinghouse of Birth Defects Surveillance and Research, and literature review," *American Journal of Medical Genetics Part C: Seminars in Medical Genetics*, vol. 157, no. 4, pp. 358–373, 2011.

[6] M. L. Martínez-Frías, E. Bermejo, E. Rodríguez-Pinilla, L. Prieto, and J. L. Frías, "Epidemiological analysis of outcomes of pregnancy in gestational diabetic mothers," *American Journal of Medical Genetics*, vol. 78, no. 2, pp. 140–145, 1998.

[7] M. Al-Haggar, S. Yahia, D. Abdel-Hadi, F. Grill, and A. Al Kaissi, "Sirenomelia (symelia apus) with Potteri's syndrome in connection with gestational diabetes mellitus: A case report and literature review," *African Health Sciences*, vol. 10, no. 4, pp. 395–399, 2010.

[8] E. Von Lennep, N. El Khazen, G. De Pierreux, J. J. Amy, F. Rodesch, and N. Van Regemorter, "A case of partial sirenomelia and possible vitamin A teratogenesis," *Prenatal Diagnosis*, vol. 5, no. 1, pp. 35–40, 1985.

[9] S. Sarpong and V. Headings, "Sirenomelia accompanying exposure of the embryo to cocaine," *Southern Medical Journal*, vol. 85, no. 5, pp. 545–547, 1992.

[10] A. Hecker, S. H. Hasan, and F. Neumann, "Disturbances in sexual differentiation of rat foetuses following spironolactone treatment," *Acta Endocrinologica*, vol. 95, no. 4, pp. 540–545, 1980.

[11] A. Shah, Ambiguous genitalia in a newborn with spironolactone exposure. 93rd Annual Meeting of the Endocrine Society Boston 2011-06.

[12] S. Patel and I. Suchet, "The role of color and power Doppler ultrasound in the prenatal diagnosis of sirenomelia," *Ultrasound in Obstetrics & Gynecology*, vol. 24, no. 6, pp. 684–691, 2004.

[13] M. Schiesser, W. Holzgreve, O. Lapaire et al., "Sirenomelia, the mermaid syndrome - Detection in the first trimester," *Prenatal Diagnosis*, vol. 23, no. 6, pp. 493–495, 2003.

[14] J. Van Keirsbilck, M. Cannie, C. Robrechts et al., "First trimester diagnosis of sirenomelia," *Prenatal Diagnosis*, vol. 26, no. 8, pp. 684–688, 2006.

[15] O. Akbayir, K. Gungorduk, S. Sudolmus, A. Gulkilik, and C. Ark, "First trimester diagnosis of sirenomelia: A case report and review of the literature," *Archives of Gynecology and Obstetrics*, vol. 278, no. 6, pp. 589–592, 2008.

39

The Rising Triad of Cesarean Scar Pregnancy, Placenta Percreta, and Uterine Rupture: A Case Report and Comprehensive Review of the Literature

Nikolina Docheva (ID),[1] **Emily D. Slutsky** (ID),[1] **Nicolette Borella,**[2] **Renee Mason,**[3] **James W. Van Hook,**[1] **and Sonyoung Seo-Patel**[1]

[1]*Department of Obstetrics and Gynecology, University of Toledo, Toledo, Ohio, USA*
[2]*Mercyhurst University, Department of Biology, Eerie, Pennsylvania, USA*
[3]*Promedica Physicians Obstetrics-Gynecology, Maumee, Ohio, USA*

Correspondence should be addressed to Emily D. Slutsky; emily.slutsky@utoledo.edu

Academic Editor: Giampiero Capobianco

As the rate of cesarean sections continues to rapidly rise, knowledge of diagnosis and management of cesarean scar pregnancies (CSPs) is becoming increasingly more relevant. CSPs rest on the continuum of placental abnormalities which include morbidly adherent placenta (accreta, increta, and percreta). A CSP poses a clinical challenge which may have significant fetal and maternal morbidity. At this point, no clear management guidelines and recommendations exist. *Herein* we describe the case of a second trimester CSP with rapid diagnosis and management in a tertiary care center. The case underscores the need for well-coordinated mobilization of resources and a multidisciplinary approach. A review of the literature is performed and deficits in universal management principles are underscored.

1. Introduction

Over the last two decades there has been a rapid growth of the number of cesarean sections performed and, in 2014, 1 in 3 women who gave birth in the USA did so by cesarean section [1]. This trend has been largely attributed to the rise of the "primary cesarean section," with a corresponding decrease in operative vaginal deliveries [1, 2]. Yet, no significant decrease in maternal and neonatal morbidity and mortality has been observed [3]. Even though vaginal delivery after a cesarean section is endorsed by ACOG for appropriate candidates, the rate of repeat cesarean deliveries is now close to 91% [2].

A cesarean section is not a benign procedure and is associated with an increased risk of maternal and fetal morbidity and mortality [4]. A rare complication of cesarean section is a "cesarean scar pregnancy" (CSP), which is also known as "cesarean ectopic pregnancy," and "cesarean delivery scar pregnancy."

2. Case Presentation

A 34-year-old Gravida 11 Para 3073 at 16 weeks and 1 day gestation presented to the emergency room of an outside hospital with a 2-day history of progressively worsening nausea, vomiting, and diarrhea, exacerbated by eating. The pregnancy had been unremarkable. Her past medical history included endometriosis and infertility. Her past surgical history was significant for two cesarean sections and left salpingo-oophorectomy secondary to an ectopic pregnancy. Physical exam elicited severe, diffuse abdominal tenderness. Fetal heart tones were taken to be in the 140s and positive fetal movement was reported. Laboratory investigations, including complete blood count, comprehensive metabolic panel, amylase, and lipase, were within normal limits. The ER physician's leading differential diagnosis was of gastrointestinal etiology. An MRI and MRCP were performed to rule out appendicitis and gallbladder disease. The MRI was notable for a large amount of intraperitoneal fluid of unknown etiology; an intrauterine fetus was visualized.

The patient continued to experience intractable pain, worse with movement and breathing, despite IV pain medication. At that point she has been at the outside facility for approximately 12 hours. The patient was transferred to our facility under the joint care of the Obstetrics/Gynecology and General Surgery teams. Upon arrival, the patient's hemodynamic status had deteriorated. She presented with tachycardia, dyspnea, chest pain, and worsening abdominal pain. Her hemoglobin had fallen from 11.7 g/dL to 7.9 g/dL. Transabdominal ultrasound imaging revealed a single intrauterine pregnancy that was positioned low in the uterus, with marked thinning of the anterior myometrium at the site of the pregnancy, and significant hemoperitoneum. Fetal heart tones were steady in the 140s. The MRI images were reevaluated prior to surgery (see Figure 1).

At this point, the patient was taken for emergency laparotomy and the staff Gynecologic Oncologist was consulted. The patient underwent a modified radical hysterectomy with right ureteral lysis and cystotomy with bladder repair. The intraoperative findings were consistent for a placenta percreta and uterine rupture with a 2 x 1 cm defect in the right lower uterine segment. There were significant intraabdominal blood and evidence of invasion of the placenta into the posterior aspect of the bladder. Total estimated blood loss for the surgery was 3,150 mL. The patient received 900 mL of cell saver and 1 unit packed red blood cells (PRBC) intraoperatively.

The patient was admitted to the ICU following surgery. She was transferred out of the unit on postoperative day 1. Two more units of PRBC were transfused over the course of the postoperative period. She was discharged on postoperative day 4 after having met her postoperative milestones. Due to the cystotomy, she was discharged with Foley urinary catheter in place for a minimum of 7 days with cystogram scheduled prior to removal. Patient was referred for grief counseling.

Pathologic examination of the uterus included placenta percreta with uterine rupture (see Figure 2 for gross specimen). There was absence of decidua identified in the lower uterine segment in the area of the uterine rupture.

3. Discussion

A CSP is not an "ectopic" pregnancy and instead involves the implantation (part or whole) of the gestation and the placenta into the niche (dehiscence at the hysterotomy site) or scar of the prior cesarean section [5, 6]. The estimated incidence of CSP is reported to range from 1 in 1,800 to 1 in 2,500 of all cesarean deliveries performed [6, 7].

It has been proposed that, in CSPs, invasion of the conceptus occurs through a defect or microscopic dehiscence in the scar or niche. This is believed to be secondary to the poor vascularization with fibrosis of the lower uterine segment [7].

Another complication of cesarean section and CSP is the morbidly adherent placenta (accreta, increta, and percreta).

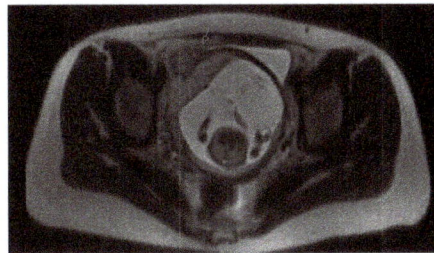

FIGURE 1: Cross-sectional MRI showing intrauterine pregnancy and CSP with suggestion of placental invasion to the bladder.

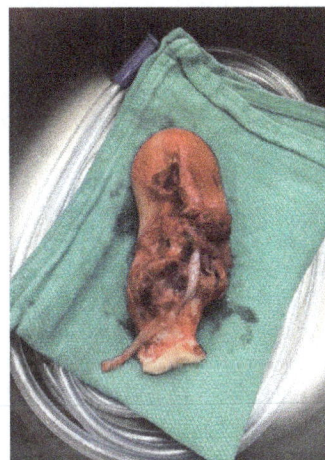

FIGURE 2: Gross specimen showing uterine rupture.

As more cases are now reported in the literature, it is believed that CSP and a morbidly adherent placenta are on a continuum spectrum of implantation abnormalities starting with CSP and progressing to deeper placental invasion as the gestation advances. This is supported by evidence which shows that these entities are indistinguishable histopathologically [8].

CSP is a clinical challenge as it can manifest broadly in two ways: (1) during the time of an ultrasound examination in a patient with a prior cesarean section and (2) as an acute emergency as described in this case report [4, 6, 7]. Due to its rarity, however, the natural history of CSP has proven difficult to study and most of what we know has been based on case reports and case series. Wellknown complications from CSP include morbidly adherent placenta, uterine rupture, hemorrhage, preterm labor, fetal demise, arteriovenous malformation, need for uterine artery embolization, hysterectomy, and even maternal death [6, 7, 9].

Rotas et al. in their review of cases of CSPs, showed that 36.8% (21/57) of patients were asymptomatic, 38.6% (22/57) had painless vaginal bleeding, 15.8% (9/57) had abdominal pain with bleeding, and 8.8% (5/57) had only abdominal pain [7]. This heterogenous presentation of patients with CSPs can be attributed to the continuum of the condition, the gestational age, the type of CSP, and implantation in the scar versus implantation in the niche. Patients with CSP implanted in the fully healed scar have a better outcome than those with CSP implanted in the niche [5].

Diagnosis of CSP is based on combination of patient's history, clinical manifestations, and imaging. Accurate and prompt diagnosis of the condition is crucial as it can be life-threatening [6, 7]. Transvaginal ultrasound is the main imaging modality for the diagnosis of CSP with a sensitivity of 84.6% (95% CI 0.763-0.905) [7]. Color Doppler imaging, 3-dimensional power Doppler ultrasonography, and 3-dimensional vocal imaging systems have also been used to evaluate the flow, resistance, and pulsatility indices of the vasculature at or in the area of the hysterotomy [6, 7]. Other diagnostic imaging modalities such as MRI can be used as an adjuvant to ultrasound as well as aid in preparation for surgery and intraoperative orientation. In addition, endoscopic modalities such as cystoscopy can be used to rule out bladder invasion and hysteroscopy can be used for improved visualization. In our case, the patient had two ultrasounds early in the pregnancy, one to confirm viability and the second for nuchal translucency. However, in both of those the lower uterine segment was not evaluated. When she presented to the outside hospital, her initial symptoms were worrisome for a gastrointestinal etiology of pain. Recommendation from Radiology included performing MRCP and MRI, thereby avoiding CT scan. The MRI revealed free intraperitoneal fluid. The patient was then transferred to our hospital, a tertiary care center, where ultrasound was used to reevaluate the pain of the patient and monitor the fetal status. The transabdominal imaging confirmed hemoperitoneum and suspected uterine rupture. The patient was promptly taken to the operating room for an exploratory laparotomy. The MRI was beneficial to the surgical team because it allowed them to perform placental mapping and evaluate the invasion of the bladder. Ultrasound remains the first-line imaging modality, as it provides results in timely fashion, has high sensitivity, is accessible, and is highly cost-effective.

Currently, there is no consensus on the treatment and management of CSP. It is clear that early diagnosis and treatment are ideal for minimizing complications and preserving fertility. There is currently no recommendation or literature which supports expectant management and thus treatment must be pursued. Currently, treatment is individualized and inconsistent as CSPs are rare and physicians are often underexperienced in the area [10].

The role for systemic methotrexate (MTX) is limited to gestational age <8 weeks, absence of fetal cardiac activity, and beta-human chorionic gonadotropin (beta-hCG) levels < 12,000 mIU/mL [11]. When criteria are met, this is considered first-line treatment. Multidose MTX treatment regimens have not been formally studied. Additionally, local MTX is associated with a success rate of 61.1% and can be applied to pregnancies with beta-HCG < 20,000 mIU/mL and a mass less than 3 cm in diameter [12].

Timor-Tritsch et al. advocated for the adjuvant use of an inflatable Foley catheter following MTX injection as prevention of hemorrhage however noted the risk of balloon expulsion within 3 days of placement [13]. The subsequent introduction of the double-balloon catheter, however, addressed

balloon expulsion with better ability to tamponade bleeding. The double-balloon catheter was also used to successfully terminate the pregnancy [14].

Local embryocides, such as potassium chloride, crystalline trichosanthin with mifepristone, and hyperosmolar glucose, have been similarly used, although with a high failure rate and need for rescue hysterectomies to control hemorrhage [15–19].

Uterine artery embolization (UAE) has been studied as a conservative therapy for various gynecologic and obstetric indications such as postpartum hemorrhage and uterine fibroids. It has been used for the treatment of CSP, in combination with local MTX therapy [20, 21] or curettage [22]. Because one of the goals of CSP management is the preservation of fertility, the use of UAE has been met with hesitancy. UAE can contribute to hypomenorrhea secondary to uterine and endometrial necrosis. No large-scale studies on long-term fertility following UAE have been completed to this point.

Hysteroscopy alone can rarely successfully be used – and not many cases have been published with standalone hysteroscopic treatment [23] The criteria for successful hysteroscopic management include (1) gestational sac with or without fetal pole; (2) presence or absence of fetal heartbeat; (3) location of sac in the anterior part of the uterine isthmus; (4) an empty uterine cavity without contact with the sac; (5) a clearly visible cervical canal; and (6) absence of a defect in the myometrial tissue between the bladder and the sac [24, 25]. Bleeding can be successfully controlled with coagulation or Foley catheter tamponade [26]. Follow-up should be diligently performed with serial beta-HCG levels. Hysteroscopy has also proven useful as an adjunct when systemic methotrexate had been insufficiently effective in controlling vaginal bleeding [27].

Dilation and curettage is not only rarely successful as the sole management technique—21 cases were identified by Rotas et al. with only five as not requiring any further treatment or intervention. 23.8% or 3/21 required hysterectomy after severe hemorrhage [7]. Dilation and curettage as a treatment option results in significant complications requiring additional and more invasive measures such as hysterectomy, laparoscopy, or systemic methotrexate.

Laparoscopic removal of a CSP has been reported in a few case reports as well with precautions to minimize bleeding. Wang et al. describe a case in which successful laparoscopic evacuation of a CSP hinged on the use of bilateral uterine artery ligation before excision [28]. Additional successful laparoscopic case reports advocated the use of hysteroscopy as diagnostic confirmation [29]. Also, vasopressin may be used to minimize bleeding at the time of the procedure [30]. There have been strides in the field to begin using robotic assisted laparoscopy for the surgical excision of CSPs [31].

As we strive to improve identification and diagnosis of CSP by early trimester ultrasound and Doppler imaging, a standardized, evidence-based approach to CSP management should be clarified. The techniques described above have been successfully and unsuccessfully used in combination. The individualization of approaches is not yet clear but hinges on gestational age, hemodynamic stability, anatomical complications, and surgeon's comfort level and access to resources.

The aim of minimally invasive techniques is the avoidance of the peripartum hysterectomy, which is associated with substantial risk—damage to the bladder, bowel, and ureters with potential for short-term and long-term complications [32, 33]. The psychological weight of simultaneously losing a pregnancy and a loss of future fertility can provide a huge burden to patients.

If laparotomy is indicated, the Triple-P procedure has been offered as a reasonable alternative, particularly with a morbidly adherent placenta. Chandraharan describes the surgery as follows: perioperative placental localization and delivery of the fetus via transverse uterine incision above the upper border of the placenta, pelvic devascularization, and placental nonseparation with myometrial excision and reconstruction of the uterine wall [34]. Multiple successful cases were described [35].

There are several case reports which described presentation of second trimester CSPs as uterine rupture. Common initial findings including acute abdomen, hemodynamic instability, and acute blood loss require resuscitative measures. In all cases, emergency laparotomy was performed with significant extravasation of blood within the peritoneal cavity [36–38].

A case series included the use of suction dilation and curettage in the management of early second trimester CSPs. Two of the three cases culminated in hysterectomies due to pathologically adherent placentas [39].

Patients who undergo treatment must ideally adhere to close long-term surveillance. On average, resolution of beta-hCG levels occurred over the course of 88.6 days (range: 26-177) when treatment took place with any method outside of hysterectomy and UAE [6]. Beta-hCG will initially increase, as observed when following ectopic pregnancies. One suggested mechanism for this is the resulting necrosis of trophoblastic cells and the release of stored beta-hCG within the cells [6]. Timor-Tritsch et al. also recommend the use of 3-dimensional ultrasound with power Doppler to compare the vascular density over time [6]. This has not been thoroughly studied yet.

There is a crucial need for counseling patients accurately about the risks of subsequent pregnancy in this population. Regardless of minimally invasive treatment technique, patients with previous CSP are at high risk of future uterine rupture, hemorrhage secondary to placenta implantation abnormalities, and recurrence of CSP. Out of 27 patients cited in recent literature, 19 subsequent pregnancies went to term [40]. A review of the literature by Gao et al. found that uneventful term intrauterine pregnancies occurred following all the above described modalities of treatment of CSPs, despite the risks involved [41]. The successful pregnancy rate was 87.5% with the rate of recurrence of CSP at 11.1%. Live birth rate was 62.5%. Of note, uterine defect repair did not significantly improve outcomes [41]. Timing of delivery was inconsistent; Gao et al. suggest that repeat cesarean section should occur when fetal lung maturity was confirmed, while other publications reported positive outcomes with performing term repeat cesarean sections [41, 42].

Although there have been case reports and series of CSPs carried to term [43], with even live births in patients with several recurrent CSPs [44], the overarching theme remains that perinatal and maternal risks are significant. The CSPs that do continue to term have overwhelmingly resulted in placenta percreta and hysterectomy.

Acknowledgments

The authors would like to thank the Radiology Department of Promedica Toledo Hospital for input on MRI frame selection.

References

[1] B. E. Hamilton, J. A. Martin, M. J. Osterman, S. C. Curtin, and T. J. Matthews, "Births: Final Data for 2014," *National Vital Statistics Reports*, vol. 64, no. 12, pp. 1–64, 2015.

[2] F. Menacker and B. E. Hamilton, "Recent trends in cesarean delivery in the United States," *NCHS Data Brief*, no. 35, pp. 1–8, 2010.

[3] A. B. Caughey, A. G. Cahill, J. Guise, and D. J. Rouse, "American College of O, Gynecologists, Society for Maternal-Fetal M," *American Journal of Obstetrics & Gynecology*, vol. 210, no. 3, pp. 179–193, 2014.

[4] I. E. Timor-Tritsch, N. Khatib, A. Monteagudo, J. Ramos, R. Berg, and S. Kovács, "Cesarean scar pregnancies: Experience of 60 cases," *Journal of Ultrasound in Medicine*, vol. 34, no. 4, pp. 601–610, 2015.

[5] A. Kaelin Agten, G. Cali, A. Monteagudo, J. Oviedo, J. Ramos, and I. Timor-Tritsch, "The clinical outcome of cesarean scar pregnancies implanted "on the scar" versus "in the niche"," *American Journal of Obstetrics & Gynecology*, vol. 216, no. 5, pp. e1–e6, 2017.

[6] I. E. Timor-Tritsch, A. Monteagudo, R. Santos, T. Tsymbal, G. Pineda, and A. A. Arslan, "The diagnosis, treatment, and follow-up of cesarean scar pregnancy," *American Journal of Obstetrics & Gynecology*, vol. 207, no. 1, pp. 44.e1–44.e13, 2012.

[7] M. A. Rotas, S. Haberman, and M. Levgur, "Cesarean scar ectopic pregnancies: etiology, diagnosis, and management," *Obstetrics & Gynecology*, vol. 107, no. 6, pp. 1373–1381, 2006.

[8] I. E. Timor-Tritsch, A. Monteagudo, G. Cali et al., "Cesarean scar pregnancy and early placenta accreta share common histology," *Ultrasound in Obstetrics & Gynecology*, vol. 43, no. 4, pp. 383–395, 2014.

[9] G. Calì, I. E. Timor-Tritsch, J. Palacios-Jaraquemada et al., "Outcome of Cesarean scar pregnancy managed expectantly: systematic review and meta-analysis," *Ultrasound in Obstetrics & Gynecology*, vol. 51, no. 2, pp. 169–175, 2018.

[10] N. Gonzalez and T. Tulandi, "Cesarean Scar Pregnancy: A Systematic Review," *Journal of Minimally Invasive Gynecology*, vol. 24, no. 5, pp. 731–738, 2017.

[11] S. Bodur, O. Özdamar, S. Kiliç, and I. Gün, "The efficacy of the systemic methotrexate treatment in caesarean scar ectopic pregnancy: A quantitative review of English literature," *Journal of Obstetrics & Gynaecology*, vol. 35, no. 3, pp. 290–296, 2015.

[12] T. Cok, H. Kalayci, H. Ozdemir, B. Haydardedeoglu, A. H. Parlakgumus, and E. Tarim, "Transvaginal ultrasound-guided local methotrexate administration as the first-line treatment for cesarean scar pregnancy: follow-up of 18 cases," *Journal of Obstetrics and Gynaecology Research*, vol. 41, no. 5, pp. 803–808, 2015.

[13] I. E. Timor-Tritsch, G. Cali, A. Monteagudo et al., "Foley balloon catheter to prevent or manage bleeding during treatment for cervical and Cesarean scar pregnancy," *Ultrasound in Obstetrics & Gynecology*, vol. 46, no. 1, pp. 118–123, 2015.

[14] I. E. Timor-Tritsch, A. Monteagudo, T.-A. Bennett, C. Foley, J. Ramos, and A. Kaelin Agten, "A new minimally invasive treatment for cesarean scar pregnancy and cervical pregnancy," *American Journal of Obstetrics & Gynecology*, vol. 215, no. 3, pp. 351.e1–351.e8, 2016.

[15] H. Roberts, C. Kohlenber, V. Lanzarone, and H. Murray, "Ectopic pregnancy in lower segment uterine scar," *Australian and New Zealand Journal of Obstetrics and Gynaecology*, vol. 38, no. 1, pp. 114–116, 1998.

[16] W. Weimin and L. Wenqing, "Effect of early pregnancy on a previous lower segment cesarean section scar," *International Journal of Gynecology and Obstetrics*, vol. 77, no. 3, pp. 201–207, 2002.

[17] J. Hartung and J. Meckies, "Management of a case of uterine scar pregnancy by transabdominal potassium chloride injection [1]," *Ultrasound in Obstetrics & Gynecology*, vol. 21, no. 1, pp. 94-95, 2003.

[18] L. J. Salomon, H. Hernandez, A. Chauveaud, S. Doumerc, and R. Frydman, "Successful management of a heterotopic Caesarean scar pregnancy: Potassium chloride injection with preservation of the intrauterine gestation: Case report," *Human Reproduction*, vol. 18, no. 1, pp. 189–191, 2003.

[19] H. F. Yazicioglu, S. Turgut, R. Madazli, M. Aygün, Z. Cebi, and S. Sönmez, "An unusual case of heterotopic twin pregnancy managed successfully with selective feticide [1]," *Ultrasound in Obstetrics & Gynecology*, vol. 23, no. 6, pp. 626-627, 2004.

[20] E. L. Hois, J. F. Hibbeln, M. J. Alonzo, M. E. Chen, and M. G. Freimanis, "Ectopic pregnancy in a cesarean section scar treated with intramuscular methotrexate and bilateral uterine artery embolization," *Journal of Clinical Ultrasound*, vol. 36, no. 2, pp. 123–127, 2008.

[21] X.-Y. Yang, H. Yu, K.-M. Li, Y.-X. Chu, and A. Zheng, "Uterine artery embolisation combined with local methotrexate for treatment of caesarean scar pregnancy," *BJOG: An International Journal of Obstetrics & Gynaecology*, vol. 117, no. 8, pp. 990–996, 2010.

[22] B. Zhang, Z.-B. Jiang, M.-S. Huang et al., "Uterine artery embolization combined with methotrexate in the treatment of cesarean scar pregnancy: Results of a case series and review of the literature," *Journal of Vascular and Interventional Radiology*, vol. 23, no. 12, pp. 1582–1588, 2012.

[23] A. Ash, A. Smith, and D. Maxwell, "Caesarean scar pregnancy," *BJOG: An International Journal of Obstetrics & Gynaecology*, vol. 114, no. 3, pp. 253–263, 2007.

[24] D. L. Fylstra, "Ectopic pregnancy within a cesarean scar: a review," *Obstetrical & Gynecological Survey* , vol. 57, no. 8, pp. 537–543, 2002.

[25] K.-M. Seow, L.-W. Huang, Y.-H. Lin, M. Y.-S. Lin, Y.-L. Tsai, and J.-L. Hwang, "Cesarean scar pregnancy: Issues in management," *Ultrasound in Obstetrics & Gynecology*, vol. 23, no. 3, pp. 247–253, 2004.

[26] R. Deans and J. Abbott, "Hysteroscopic management of cesarean scar ectopic pregnancy," *Fertility and Sterility*, vol. 93, no. 6, pp. 1735–1740, 2010.

[27] A. Chao, T.-H. Wang, C.-J. Wang, C.-L. Lee, and A.-S. Chao, "Hysteroscopic management of cesarean scar pregnancy after unsuccessful methotrexate treatment," *Journal of Minimally Invasive Gynecology*, vol. 12, no. 4, pp. 374–376, 2005.

[28] C. Wang, L. Yuen, C. Yen, C. Lee, and Y. Soong, "Three-Dimensional Power Doppler Ultrasound Diagnosis and Laparoscopic Management of a Pregancy in a Previous Cesarean Scar," *Journal of Laparoendoscopic & Advanced Surgical Techniques*, vol. 14, no. 6, pp. 399–402, 2004.

[29] M. Noe, G. Kunz, M. Herbertz, G. Mall, and G. Leyendecker, "The cyclic pattern of the immunocytochemical expression of oestrogen and progesterone receptors in human myometrial and endometrial layers: characterisation of the endometrial-subendometrial unit," *Human Reproduction*, vol. 14, no. 1, pp. 190–197, 1999.

[30] A. Ades and S. Parghi, "Laparoscopic Resection of Cesarean Scar Ectopic Pregnancy," *Journal of Minimally Invasive Gynecology*, vol. 24, no. 4, pp. 533–535, 2017.

[31] M. T. Siedhoff, L. D. Schiff, J. K. Moulder, T. Toubia, and T. Ivester, "Robotic-assisted laparoscopic removal of cesarean scar ectopic and hysterotomy revision," *American Journal of Obstetrics & Gynecology*, vol. 212, no. 5, pp. 681–681.e4, 2015.

[32] E. Shin, M. Fadel, E. Sewart, and W. Yoong, ""Re: Campbell S, Corcoran P, Manning E, Greene R, for the Irish Maternal Morbidity Advisory Group. Peripartum hysterectomy incidence, risk factors and clinical characteristics in Ireland" [Eur. J. Obstet. Gynecol. Reprod. Biol. 207 (2016) 56–61]," *European Journal of Obstetrics & Gynecology and Reproductive Biology*, vol. 212, pp. 193-194, 2017.

[33] T. Van Den Akker, C. Brobbel, O. M. Dekkers, and K. W. M. Bloemenkamp, "Prevalence, Indications, Risk Indicators, and Outcomes of Emergency Peripartum Hysterectomy Worldwide: A Systematic Review and Meta-analysis," *Obstetrics & Gynecology*, vol. 128, no. 6, pp. 1281–1294, 2016.

[34] E. Chandraharan, S. Rao, A.-M. Belli, and S. Arulkumaran, "The Triple-P procedure as a conservative surgical alternative to peripartum hysterectomy for placenta percreta," *International Journal of Gynecology and Obstetrics*, vol. 117, no. 2, pp. 191–194, 2012.

[35] M. Teixidor Vinas, A. M. Belli, S. Arulkumaran, and E. Chandraharan, "Prevention of postpartum hemorrhage and hysterectomy in patients with morbidly adherent placenta: a cohort study comparing outcomes before and after introduction of the Triple-P procedure," *Ultrasound in Obstetrics & Gynecology*, vol. 46, no. 3, pp. 350–355, 2015.

[36] A. Honig, L. Rieger, F. Thanner, M. Eck, M. Sutterlin, and J. Dietl, "Placenta percreta with subsequent uterine rupture at 15 weeks of gestation after two previous cesarean sections," *Journal of Obstetrics and Gynaecology Research*, vol. 31, no. 5, pp. 439–443, 2005.

[37] M. C. Fleisch, J. Lux, M. Schoppe, K. Grieshaber, and M. Hampl, "Placenta percreta leading to spontaneous complete uterine rupture in the second trimester: Example of a fatal complication of abnormal placentation following uterine scarring," *Gynecologic and Obstetric Investigation*, vol. 65, no. 2, pp. 81–83, 2008.

[38] R. T. Overcash and Z. H. Khackician, "Late-first-trimester cesarean section scar ectopic pregnancy with placenta increta: A case report," *Obstetrics, Gynaecology and Reproductive Medicine*, vol. 57, no. 1, pp. 61–64, 2012.

[39] L. A. M. Dickerhoff, A. S. Mahal, C. K. Stockdale, and A. J. Hardy-Fairbanks, "Management of cesarean scar pregnancy in the second trimester: a report of three cases," *The Journal of Reproductive Medicine*, vol. 60, no. 3-4, pp. 165–168, 2015.

[40] K.-M. Seow, J.-L. Hwang, Y.-L. Tsai, L.-W. Huang, Y.-H. Lin, and B.-C. Hsieh, "Subsequent pregnancy outcome after conservative treatment of a previous cesarean scar pregnancy," *Acta Obstetricia et Gynecologica Scandinavica*, vol. 83, no. 12, pp. 1167–1172, 2004.

[41] L. Gao, Z. Huang, X. Zhang, N. Zhou, X. Huang, and X. Wang, "Reproductive outcomes following cesarean scar pregnancy - A case series and review of the literature," *European Journal of Obstetrics & Gynecology and Reproductive Biology*, vol. 200, pp. 102–107, 2016.

[42] J. Ben Nagi, S. Helmy, D. Ofili-Yebovi, J. Yazbek, E. Sawyer, and D. Jurkovic, "Reproductive outcomes of women with a previous history of Caesarean scar ectopic pregnancies," *Human Reproduction*, vol. 22, no. 7, pp. 2012–2015, 2007.

[43] I. Timor-Tritsch, A. Monteagudo, G. Cali et al., "OP34.02: Sonographically-proven Caesarean scar pregnancies (CSP) can result in a live offspring and morbidly adherent placenta (MAP)," *Ultrasound in Obstetrics & Gynecology*, vol. 44, no. S1, pp. 178-178, 2014.

[44] T.-A. Bennett, J. Morgan, I. E. Timor-Tritsch, C. Dolin, M. Dziadosz, and M. Tsai, "Fifth recurrent Cesarean scar pregnancy: observations of a case and historical perspective," *Ultrasound in Obstetrics & Gynecology*, vol. 50, no. 5, pp. 658–660, 2017.

40

Sonographic Demonstration of Intracranial Hemorrhage in a Fetus with Hydrops Fetalis due to Rh Alloimmunization after Intrauterine Intravascular Transfusion: A Case Report and Review of the Literature

Rauf Melekoglu ⑩,[1] **Ebru Celik,**[2] **and Hasim Kural**[1]

[1]*Department of Obstetrics and Gynecology, Faculty of Medicine, The University of Inonu, 44280 Malatya, Turkey*
[2]*Department of Obstetrics and Gynecology, Faculty of Medicine, The University of Koc, 34010 İstanbul, Turkey*

Correspondence should be addressed to Rauf Melekoglu; rmelekoglu@gmail.com

Academic Editor: Maria Grazia Porpora

Intrauterine transfusion is the most common and successful intrauterine procedure for the treatment of fetal anemia due to red cell alloimmunization. Fetal intracranial hemorrhage is a very rare complication of intrauterine transfusion in patients with Rh(D) alloimmunization and it has been demonstrated only in a few case reports in the literature. Herein, we described a case of grade IV intraventricular hemorrhage that was diagnosed following the first intrauterine transfusion and reviewed the literature about the fetal intracranial hemorrhage that occurred after intrauterine intravascular transfusion procedure.

1. Introduction

Intrauterine transfusion (IUT) is the most common and successful intrauterine procedure for the treatment of fetal anemia due to red cell alloimmunization [1]. The beneficial effect of in utero therapy on perinatal survival has been demonstrated clearly in several observational studies [2, 3]. Despite the dramatic decrease in the IUT requirement due to the widespread use of prophylactic Rh(D) immune globulin, the procedure continues to be a gold standard for treatment of severe fetal anemia [4]. While intrauterine intravascular transfusion has remarkable effect on the treatment of fetal red blood cell alloimmunization, the total procedure-related complication rate has been reported approximately 3.1 percent and commonly indicated as fetal death, neonatal death, emergency cesarean delivery, infection, and premature rupture of membranes [5]. Fetal brain injury is a very rare complication of IUT that has been demonstrated only in a few case reports in the literature [6]. To the best of our knowledge, the literature does not include any cases of a grade IV intraventricular hemorrhage due to IUT.

Herein, we described a case of grade IV intraventricular hemorrhage that was diagnosed following the first IUT and reviewed the literature about the fetal intracranial hemorrhage that occurred after intrauterine intravascular transfusion procedure in patients with Rh(D) alloimmunization. We searched PubMed, Scopus, Embase, and Google Scholar databases using the keywords Rh isoimmunization "OR" intrauterine transfusion "AND" intracranial hemorrhage "OR" brain injury "OR" brain damage. We found only two papers that define three cases of intracranial hemorrhage associated with intrauterine transfusion due to Rh alloimmunization. The initial platelet value was not noted in the third case. Author, case number, patient's age, gestational age, pretransfusion hemoglobin value, pretransfusion platelet value, neurosonogram after the first intrauterine transfusion, and the outcome were summarized in Table 1. In this paper, we have compared our case with the other three cases we have found in the literature.

2. Case Presentation

A 34-year-old woman, gravida 3, para 2, with a history of an intrauterine death at 32 weeks of gestation due to hydrops fetalis as a result of Rh alloimmunization in the previous

TABLE 1: Summary of the reported fetal intracranial hemorrhage cases related to intrauterine transfusion due to Rh alloimmunization.

Authors	Case number	Maternal age	Gestational age	Pretransfusion hemoglobin value (g/dl)	Pretransfusion platelet value (/μl)	Neurosonogram after the first intrauterine transfusion	Outcome
Ghi et al. 2004	Case 1	30	20	1.2	168000	Intraventricular and cerebellar hemorrhage	Termination of pregnancy. Pathological confirmation of cerebellar hemorrhage
	Case 2	25	23	1.6	177000	Cerebellar hemorrhage	Progressive hypoplasia of one cerebellar hemisphere. Delivery at 34 weeks after six IUTs. Normal neurological development at 2 years
Simonazzi et al. 2016	Case 3	32	22	4	-	Suspicious cerebellar infarction	Hemosiderin staining in the cerebellum bilaterally, reflecting prior hemorrhage in postnatal brain MRI. Normal neurological development at 14 months
Current study	Case 4	34	28	2.9	154000	Echogenic collection in the right lateral ventricle and extending to the surrounding cerebral parenchyma compatible with grade IV intraventricular hemorrhage	Diffuse echogenicity extending from the inferior left caudate nucleus to the left ventricle that leads left ventricular dilatation (intraventricular grade IV hemorrhage). Normal neurological development at 6 months

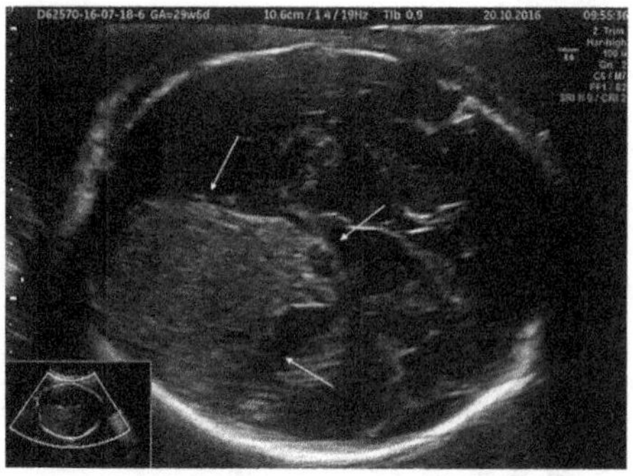

FIGURE 1: Axial view of the fetal head after intrauterine transfusion procedure. A large echogenic collection involving right lateral ventricle and extending to the surrounding parenchyma that suggests grade IV intraventricular hemorrhage.

pregnancy was referred to our center at 13 weeks of gestations. There were no pathologic findings in her physical examination, laboratory findings, and obstetric ultrasonography. Gray-scale and color Doppler ultrasonography evaluation was performed to detect the findings of anemia and hydrops with a two-week interval starting from the 18th gestational week in the Prenatal Diagnosis and Treatment Unit by a protocol defined by Society for Maternal-Fetal Medicine for the pregnant women complicated with Rh alloimmunization [7]. Her obstetric follow-up was unremarkable until 29 weeks of gestation. At 29 weeks of gestation, mid-cerebral artery peak systolic velocity (MCA-PSV) was detected as 80.6 cm/sn [>1.5 multiple of the median (MoM)] in her obstetric Doppler ultrasonography that suggests fetal anemia with ascites, cardiomegaly, and pericardial effusion. An intrauterine intravascular transfusion was performed, and the hemoglobin concentration before the procedure was detected as 2.9 g/dL. 40 ml O Rh(D)-negative red blood cell that was freshly prepared and underwent irradiation and leukodepletion was transfused to the fetus via the umbilical vein in the portion of the umbilical cord near its insertion into the placenta by a 22-gauge needle with no complication. Posttransfusion hemoglobin was detected as 8.1 g/dl. The initial and posttransfusion platelet count was detected in normal range (154000/μl and 163000/μl, resp.). A few days later, ultrasound examination revealed the presence of an echogenic collection involving right lateral ventricle and extending to the surrounding cerebral parenchyma compatible with grade IV intraventricular hemorrhage (Figure 1). The couple was counseled, and they opted for the continuation of in utero therapy. The second IUT was scheduled after ten days. At 30 + 4 weeks of pregnancy, the second IUT was performed. The initial hemoglobin value was detected as 4.9 g/dl. Persistent fetal bradycardia was noted during the procedure, and an emergency cesarean section was performed. APGAR score 4/7, 1315 g, 43 cm male infant was delivered by cesarean section. Neonate was transferred to the neonatal intensive care unit. Exchange transfusion, phototherapy, and intravenous immunoglobulin treatment were applied. Postnatal cranial ultrasonography showed diffuse echogenicity extending from the inferior left caudate nucleus to the left ventricle that

leads to left ventricular dilatation compatible with intraventricular grade IV hemorrhage. The intracranial hemorrhage was gradually regressed in the subsequent ultrasonographic examinations and completely disappeared at the end of the first month, and the neonate was discharged from the hospital after healing two months after birth. At the time of writing this paper, the baby was showing normal neurological development at 6 months.

3. Discussion

Intrauterine transfusion has been reported as the most successful fetal therapy procedure with 95% perinatal survival rate [8]. The overall survival rate after this antenatal treatment procedure varies with experience of center, development of fetal anemia before 20 weeks of gestation, and occurrence of fetal hydrops [9]. The presence of fetal hydrops during the first IUT reduces the success of the treatment. Lindenburg et al. reported the perinatal outcome of 491 fetuses who underwent 1422 intrauterine intravascular transfusion procedure during the antenatal period. They demonstrated that perinatal survival rate was 83% and 95% in hydropic and nonhydropic fetuses, respectively [10]. Although IUT contributes to the reduction of perinatal mortality, concerns about the neurological morbidities associated with this procedure have been considered only in a few studies [11]. Fetal intracranial hemorrhage as a short-term neurological morbidity was reported by Ghi et al. for the first time in 2003 [12]. They described four cases with intracranial hemorrhage related to the fetal anemia (two immune hydrops due to Rh D alloimmunization, two monochorionic twins complicated with the death of the cotwin). Consistently with the case currently reported, each of the cases related to Rh alloimmunization had very low initial hemoglobin values in the first IUT (1.2 g/dl and 1.6 g/dl, resp.). They suggested that disruption of intracranial vessels may be responsible in the pathophysiology of brain injury in severe anemic fetuses and noticed the importance of fetal neurosonography in pregnancies with severe anemia due to Rh alloimmunization undergoing IUT. In 2004, the same group reported multiplanar neurosonography results of seven consecutive hydropic fetuses undergoing intrauterine transfusion procedure due to Rh alloimmunization [13]. In addition to the previously reported two cases, they described a case of periventricular leukomalacia and a case of unilateral ventriculomegaly that was noticed after the first IUT. They speculated that hypoxia/ischemia and the hyperdynamic circulation in fetal anemia cause the brain vessel disruption that leads to intracranial hemorrhage. They also considered that altered coagulation due to IUT might be responsible for intracranial hemorrhage. In our case, the initial and posttransfusion platelet values were detected in the normal range (154000/μl and 163000/μl, resp.), and there was no sign of increasing bleeding time such as excessive bleeding from the umbilical cord after withdrawal of the needle. Furthermore, we hypothesized that preservative-anticoagulant system such as additive solution-1 (AS-1), AS-3, AS-5, citrate-phosphate-dextrose-adenine-1 (CPDA-1), citrate-phosphate-dextrose (CPD), and citrate-phosphate-dextrose-dextrose (CP2D) that were used in red blood cell preparation might predispose to intracranial hemorrhage by altering the coagulation system of the fetus. Thus, we proposed that removing these anticoagulants from the transfusion aliquots before intrauterine transfusion by centrifugation and volume reduction could have a beneficial effect on preventing the hemorrhagic complication of this treatment.

Simonazzi et al. demonstrated the risk of cerebellar damage in fetuses with severe anemia due to RhD alloimmunization after intrauterine intravascular transfusion procedure [14]. They reported three cases of intracranial hemorrhage involving cerebellum that two of them were previously reported by Ghi et al. In the third case, they performed first IUT at 22 weeks of gestation and after two weeks they noted suspicious cerebellar infarction in prenatal ultrasonography. In postnatal magnetic resonance imaging, bilateral cerebellar hemosiderin staining suggested prior hemorrhage. They emphasized that intracranial hemorrhage occurred at the infratentorial part of the brain particularly in intracerebellar hemispheres in all of the tree cases. Furthermore, in addition to hypoxia/ischemia, they also noticed the possible serious effect of sudden fluctuations in cerebral blood flow and arterial blood pressure (hyperdynamic circulation) on the intracranial hemorrhage. In our case, fetal anemia and hydrops were detected at the 28th week of gestation that was developed later compared with the other cases previously reported. Moreover, intracranial hemorrhage was identified in the right lateral ventricle and extending to the surrounding cerebral parenchyma compatible with grade IV intraventricular hemorrhage. Therefore, we considered that intracranial hemorrhage risk is not related to gestational week of the first IUT in the presence of Rh(D) alloimmunization and posttransfusion intracranial hemorrhage is not specific only the infratentorial region of the brain. Also it has been suggested that, in pregnancies complicated with the severe fetal hemolytic disease, an initial extremely low value of hematocrit (≤15%) should be increased gradually for the risk of fetal cardiovascular decompensation due to the acute changes in blood volume and viscosity. In such cases, the planning of the second procedure is recommended after 48 hours of the first transfusion to normalize the fetal hematocrit value [15, 16]. Consistently with the other cases reported previously, intracranial hemorrhage occurred after the first intrauterine intravascular transfusion. Consequently, we concluded that reduction of first transfusion volume might be beneficial to avoid sudden fluctuations in cerebral blood flow and arterial blood pressure.

In conclusion, in this study, a case of intracranial hemorrhage in a fetus with hydrops fetalis due to Rh alloimmunization after intrauterine intravascular transfusion has been presented and a comprehensive, up-to-date review has been performed. Although intracranial hemorrhage is a rare complication of IUT, clinicians should be aware of increased risk of brain damage in fetuses with Rh(D) alloimmunization undergoing this procedure. Detailed sonographic examination of the fetal central nervous system before and after the treatment should be performed in patients that are planning IUT. Also, communicating with blood bank to decrease the additive anticoagulant agents as minimal as possible in the preparation process of red blood cells and reduction of first transfusion volume to avoid sudden fluctuations in cerebral blood flow may be helpful to prevent this complication.

Consent

Written informed consent was obtained from the patient to publish this case report.

Disclosure

No author received any specific grant from any funding agency in the public, commercial, or nonprofit sectors. The abstract of this study was presented as poster presentation during the 16th World Congress in Fetal Medicine 25–29 June 2017.

References

[1] K. J. Moise Jr, "Management of rhesus alloimmunization in pregnancy," *Obstetrics & Gynecology*, vol. 112, no. 1, pp. 164–176, 2008.

[2] D. Deka, V. Dadhwal, A. K. Sharma et al., "Perinatal survival and procedure-related complications after intrauterine transfusion for red cell alloimmunization," *Archives of Gynecology and Obstetrics*, vol. 293, no. 5, pp. 967–973, 2016.

[3] I. L. Van Kamp, F. J. C. M. Klumper, R. H. Meerman, D. Oepkes, S. A. Scherjon, and H. H. H. Kanhai, "Treatment of fetal anemia due to red-cell alloimmunization with intrauterine transfusions in the Netherlands, 1988-1999," *Acta Obstetricia et Gynecologica Scandinavica*, vol. 83, no. 8, pp. 731–737, 2004.

[4] J. Bowman, "Thirty-five years of Rh prophylaxis," *Transfusion*, vol. 43, no. 12, pp. 1661–1666, 2003.

[5] I. L. Van Kamp, F. J. C. M. Klumper, D. Oepkes et al., "Complications of intrauterine intravascular transfusion for fetal anemia due to maternal red-cell alloimmunization," *American Journal of Obstetrics & Gynecology*, vol. 192, no. 1, pp. 171–177, 2005.

[6] L. M. Leijser, N. Vos, F. J. Walther, and G. van Wezel-Meijler, "Brain ultrasound findings in neonates treated with intrauterine transfusion for fetal anaemia," *Early Human Development*, vol. 88, no. 9, pp. 717–724, 2012.

[7] G. Mari, M. E. Norton, J. Stone et al., "Society for Maternal-Fetal Medicine (SMFM) Clinical Guideline #8: The fetus at risk for anemia-diagnosis and management," *American Journal of Obstetrics & Gynecology*, vol. 212, no. 6, pp. 697–710, 2015.

[8] V. E. H. J. Smits-Wintjens, F. J. Walther, and E. Lopriore, "Rhesus haemolytic disease of the newborn: Postnatal management, associated morbidity and long-term outcome," *Seminars in Fetal and Neonatal Medicine*, vol. 13, no. 4, pp. 265–271, 2008.

[9] C. Zwiers, I. T. M. Lindenburg, F. J. Klumper, M. de Haas, D. Oepkes, and I. L. Van Kamp, "Complications of intrauterine intravascular blood transfusion: lessons learned after 1678 procedures," *Ultrasound in Obstetrics & Gynecology*, vol. 50, no. 2, pp. 180–186, 2017.

[10] I. T. M. Lindenburg, I. L. Van Kamp, and D. Oepkes, "Intrauterine blood transfusion: Current indications and associated risks," *Fetal Diagnosis and Therapy*, vol. 36, no. 4, pp. 263–271, 2014.

[11] I. T. Lindenburg, V. E. Smits-Wintjens, J. M. Van Klink et al., "Long-term neurodevelopmental outcome after intrauterine transfusion for hemolytic disease of the fetus/newborn: The LOTUS study," *American Journal of Obstetrics & Gynecology*, vol. 206, no. 2, pp. 141–e8, 2012.

[12] T. Ghi, G. Simonazzi, A. Perolo et al., "Outcome of antenatally diagnosed intracranial hemorrhage: case series and review of the literature," *Ultrasound in Obstetrics & Gynecology*, vol. 22, no. 2, pp. 121–130, 2003.

[13] T. Ghi, L. Brondelli, G. Simonazzi et al., "Sonographic demonstration of brain injury in fetuses with severe red blood cell alloimmunization undergoing intrauterine transfusions," *Ultrasound in Obstetrics & Gynecology*, vol. 23, no. 5, pp. 428–431, 2004.

[14] G. Simonazzi, D. Bernabini, A. Curti et al., "Fetal cerebellar damage in fetuses with severe anemia undergoing intrauterine transfusions," *The Journal of Maternal-Fetal and Neonatal Medicine*, vol. 29, no. 3, pp. 389–392, 2016.

[15] N. Papantoniou, S. Sifakis, and A. Antsaklis, "Therapeutic management of fetal anemia: Review of standard practice and alternative treatment options," *Journal of Perinatal Medicine*, vol. 41, no. 1, pp. 71–82, 2013.

[16] G. Mari, K. J. Moise, R. L. Deter, and R. J. Carpenter, "Flow velocity waveforms of the umbilical and cerebral arteries before and after intravascular transfusion," *Obstetrics & Gynecology*, vol. 75, no. 4, pp. 584–589, 1990.

41

Atypical Distant Metastasis of Breast Malignant Phyllodes Tumors: A Case Report and Literature Review

Tiphaine de Foucher,[1] Hélène Roussel,[2] Mikael Hivelin,[3,4] Léa Rossi,[1,4] Caroline Cornou,[1,4] Anne-Sophie Bats,[1,4] Myriam Deloménie,[1] Fabrice Lécuru,[1,4] and Charlotte Ngô[1,4]

[1]Department of Breast and Gynecological Surgical Oncology, Hôpital Européen Georges Pompidou, AP-HP, Paris, France
[2]Department of Pathology, Hôpital Européen Georges Pompidou, AP-HP, Paris, France
[3]Department of Plastic and Reconstructive Surgery, Hôpital Européen Georges Pompidou, AP-HP, Paris, France
[4]Paris Descartes University, Sorbonne Paris Cité, Paris, France

Correspondence should be addressed to Charlotte Ngô; charlotte.ngo@aphp.fr

Academic Editor: Erich Cosmi

Malignant phyllodes tumors (MPT) are rare breast neoplasms. Preoperative diagnosis is often challenging due to the unspecific clinical, radiological, and histological characteristics of the tumor. Dissemination pathways are local with chest wall invasion, regional with lymph nodes metastasis, and distant, hematogenous, mostly to the lungs, bones, and brain. Distant metastasis (DM) can be synchronous or appear months to years after the diagnosis and initial management. The current report describes the case of a 57-year-old woman presenting with a giant/neglected MPT of the breast, with no DM at initial staging, treated by radical modified mastectomy. Motor disorders due to medullar compression by a paravertebral mass appeared at short follow-up, also treated surgically. The patient died from several DM of rapid evolution. To our knowledge, this is the only case described of MPT with metastases to soft tissue causing medullar compression. We present a literature review on unusual metastatic localizations of MPT.

1. Introduction

Phyllodes tumors (PT) are fibroepithelial tumors characterized by a double-layered epithelial component arranged in clefts surrounded by an overgrowing mesenchymal component organized in leaf-like structures. Grading between benign, borderline, or malignant depends on histological criteria: stromal cellularity, cellular pleomorphism, mitotic activity, margin appearance, and stromal distribution [1]. The average annual incidence rate of malignant phyllodes tumors (MPT) is 2.1 per 1 million women [2].

Surgery allowing tumor-free margins ≥ 1 cm is the first line of treatment [3]. Axillary lymph node dissection is recommended in case of palpable nodes [4]. Radiotherapy and chemotherapy can be options in case of high metastatic risk or recurrence.

Considering all PT, local recurrence (LR) and distant metastases (DM) rates are estimated around 20% and 3.5%, respectively [5]. Considering MPT, LR occurs in 40% and DM in 27% of the cases, mostly to lungs, bones, brain, and liver [6–9]. The estimated 5-, 10-, and 15-year rates of cause-specific survival for women operated for primary nonmetastatic MPT are 91%, 89%, and 89%, respectively [3].

We report the case of a woman with an atypical metastasis from a MPT with a rapidly fatal outcome. We present a literature review about unusual localizations of MPT metastasis.

2. Case Presentation

A 57-year-old menopausal woman presented herself to our institution with a giant necrotic breast tumor and ipsilateral axillary lymphadenopathy (Figure 1). Radical mastectomy with axillary node dissection and partial pectoral muscle resection was performed. Bulk size was 10,6 × 5,9 × 6,3 inches and it weighted 4.2 kg. The majority of the lesion was composed of a benign PT but a focal area presented a bulging

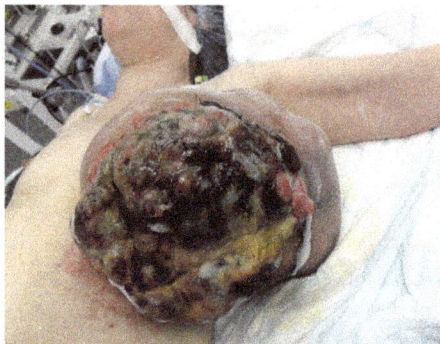

FIGURE 1: Picture of the left breast mass at diagnosis.

high grade malignant PT with severity criteria: infiltrative borders, high mitotic count, marked stromal overgrowth, and marked stromal cellularity (Figure 2). Axillary lymph nodes were disease-free. Postoperative PET-CT showed no distant metastasis.

Few weeks later, the patient came back with cervical and back pain. She also showed a delirious melancholic episode, successfully treated with neuroleptics.

The spinal MRI revealed several paravertebral lesions: a right paravertebral soft tissue tumor extending from C3 to C5 causing spine displacement and a mass in T11-T12 causing mass effect on the conus medullaris (Figure 3). The occurrence of a cauda equina syndrome indicated an emergency surgery. Histopathological analysis showed a high malignancy tumor proliferation with clusters of spindle shaped cells. The phenotype was unspecific but comparable to the breast tumor (Figure 2).

She then presented multiple and rapidly growing metastasis in soft tissues. Chemotherapy with Adriamycin was initiated but she died rapidly, 4 months after primary diagnosis.

3. Discussion and Literature Review

We presented an unusual case of rapidly fatal metastatic evolution of a breast MPT with atypical distant metastasis to paravertebral tissues.

In their retrospective analysis of 295 patients, Mitus et al. found that five-year DFS was 96.9% in patients with benign PT, 83.3% in patients with borderline PT, and 71.7% in patients with malignant PT [7]. 95% of deaths were related to distant metastasis of malignant PT. The mean survival in case of metastasis was 7 months [range 2–17]. These results are consistent with other articles, which show that metastatic PT carries a poor prognosis, with an average survival time of less than 2 years [3, 6, 10].

Several grading systems have been proposed, but the three-tiered system including benign, borderline, and malignant PT is preferred [11]. The grading is based on semi-quantitative assessment of infiltrative borders, stromal overgrowth, stromal cellularity, stromal pleomorphism, mitotic count (≥ 5 mitoses per 10 HPF), and the presence of a malignant heterologous component [9, 12, 13]. In our case,

in the primary tumor, the histologic criteria of MPT were a high mitotic count with marked stromal overgrowth, high stromal cellularity, and atypia. No malignant heterologous component was found.

The patient waited for more than 18 months before consulting. She demonstrated a strong denial of the disease and of the treatments that were planned. In addition, this patient was in a situation of socioeconomic deprivation. Observing low-income women, Nonzee et al. studied the reasons of delayed breast cancer screening, follow-up, and treatment [14]. They showed that despite equal access to cancer care-related services, common explanations for nonadherence included limited knowledge about preventive or cancer care resources and denial or fear. Furthermore, it appears that women with locally advanced breast cancer are more likely to suffer from psychiatric comorbidity and more often live alone [15]. In our case, the melancholic episode may have delayed the diagnosis of soft tissue metastases, due to the denial of imaging and medical treatment of the patient. A more effective comanagement of the patient involving both surgeons and psychiatrists might have improved care.

Selection of review of literature for unusual metastasis is summarized in Figure 4. We finally retrieved 17 articles reporting 17 cases. Three patients suffered of cardiac localizations [16–18]. Four patients had gastrointestinal localizations [19–22]. One patient presented with a borderline PT of the right breast and simultaneous pancreatic tail metastasis [23]. Five patients presented with ENT metastasis [24–28]. One patient presented with a thyroid mass two years after a simple mastectomy for a MPT [29]. One case of left kidney metastasis has been reported [30] and one case of adrenal metastasis [31]. The last patient presented with thoracic vertebra and rib metastasis, as well as a pelvic mass [32]. Cases are summarized in Table 1. Mean DFS was 25 months; mean OS was 49 months. 15 patients were dead at the time of publication because of the disease. This highlights the very poor prognosis of patient with unusual DM of MPT.

In case of initially nonmetastatic MPT with high risk of recurrence, adjuvant therapy including radiotherapy and/or different chemotherapeutic agents (ifosfamide, etoposide, doxorubicin, or cisplatin) can be used, although their role is uncertain [4]. Here the rapid apparition of multiple metastases, despite a negative postoperative PET-CT and free surgical margins, raises the question of systematic postoperative radiotherapy and chemotherapy in case of large MPT. In case of distant metastasis, chemotherapy can be used, as well as postoperative radiation therapy as palliation for pain relief, but with limited efficacy [33]. In our case, chemotherapy was quickly started after metastases diagnosis, but the progression of the disease was so fast that the patient died after only one cycle.

Recently, the potential key role of genomic markers in the characterization of PT has been highlighted. MED12 somatic mutations have been identified as a highly recurrent event in fibroadenomas (FAs) and phyllodes tumors (PTs), with an inverse correlation between the frequency of this mutation and histologic grade [34–36]. Laé et al. identified a limited number of altered signaling pathways associated

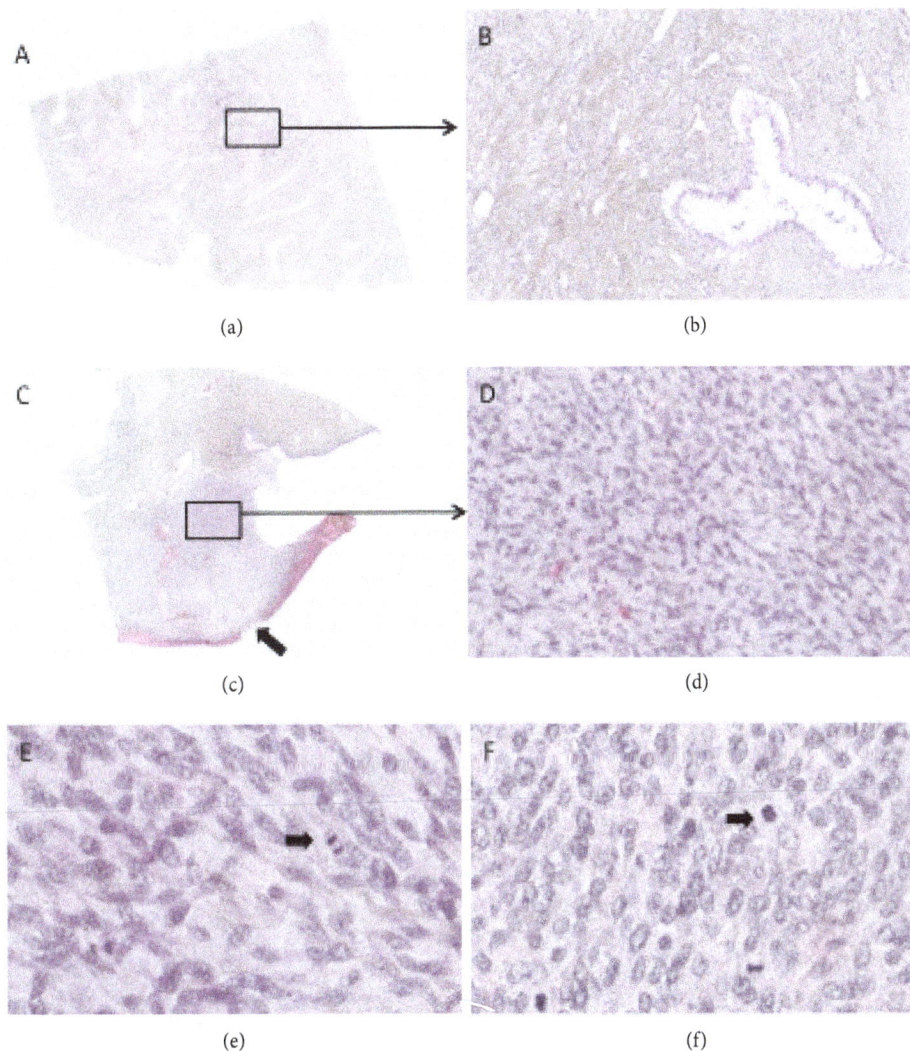

FIGURE 2: Microscopic aspect of the primary tumor (a, b, c, d, e) and medullar metastasis (f). (a, b) Predominant benign PT component. The stroma is more cellular than a fibroadenoma. Stromal cellularity may be higher in the zone adjacent to epithelium without atypia and mitosis ((a) magnification ×2, (b) magnification ×200), (c, d) malignant PT component observed near the cutaneous ulceration (arrow). We observed a high stromal cellularity with atypia and mitosis without epithelial structure. There was no involvement of the tissue beneath the nipples nor lymphovascular or neural invasion. ((c) magnification ×2, (d) magnification ×200), (e, f) malignant primary (e), and medullar metastasis (f) PT at magnification ×400. We observed a similar histologic pattern: a cellular stromal proliferation with atypia and mitosis (arrows). No epithelial components. All immunostainings were negative (estrogen receptor, progesterone receptor, pankeratin AE1, AE3, and PS100, desmin, CD34, caldesmon, and CD99) except for a focal staining with Smooth Muscle Actin antibody.

with this mutation, suggesting the use of these findings as diagnostic and prognostic tools [37]. Focusing on MPT, other authors used molecular profiling to identify overexpressed biomarkers of angiogenesis, EGFR, and immune checkpoints, which points the way toward the use of new targeted therapies [38].

MPT are uncommon breast neoplasm, whose prognosis can be very poor in case of DM. Medullar compression due to soft tissue metastasis is extremely rare. This strengthens the value of an accurate initial diagnosis, so as to enable the identification of high-risk patients. Their management,

including monitoring and treatment, is yet to be determined, as the efficiency of treatments used for DM is still low.

Consent

Consent for publication was obtained from the husband of the deceased patient.

TABLE 1: Summary of the review of literature.

Year of publication	Author	Site of distant metastasis	Delay between primary and metastasis (months)	Treatment	OS and DFS (months)
Present case	T. de Foucher	Paravertebral tissue	1	CT	OS = 4
2016	Yoshiba [24]	Left mandible	36	RT	DFS = 18, OS = 42
2016	Shan [32]	Pelvis	53	Surgery and CT	DFS = 16, OS = 72
2016	Choi [19]	Stomach	64	Endoscopy and PPI	DFS = 35, OS = 68
2015	Karczmarek-Borowska [30]	Left kidney	10	Surgery, palliative RT CT	DFS = 10, OS = 17
2015	Yoshidaya [16]	Heart	4	Surgery	DFS = 4, OS = 6
2014	Wei [23]	Pancreas		Surgery and CT	DFS = 39, OS = 41
2014	Sano [25]	Left tonsil	71	Surgery	DFS = 3
2013	Collin [31]	Adrenal gland	96	Surgery	DFS = 12, OS = 108
2012	Bilen [20]	Jejunum	12	Surgery	DFS = 13
2011	Garg [17]	Heart	36	Surgery	DFS = 5, OS = 36
2010	Nakatsu [18]	Heart	108	Surgery	DFS = 108, OS = 111
2010	Morcos [21]	Jejunum	13	Surgery	DFS = 13, OS = 31
2006	Masmoudi [26]	Gingiva	24	Unknown	DFS = 24, OS = 25
2006	Asoglu [22]	Duodenum	72	Surgery	DFS = 24
2003	Deeming [27]	Mandible	108	Palliative RT	DFS = 72, OS = 114
2003	Staton [28]	Mandible	12	Palliative RT	DFS = 12, OS = 13
2002	Giorgadze [29]	Thyroid	24	Surgery	DFS = 24, OS = 48

OS, overall survival; DFS, disease-free survival; CT, chemotherapy; RT, radiotherapy; PPI, proton pump inhibitors.

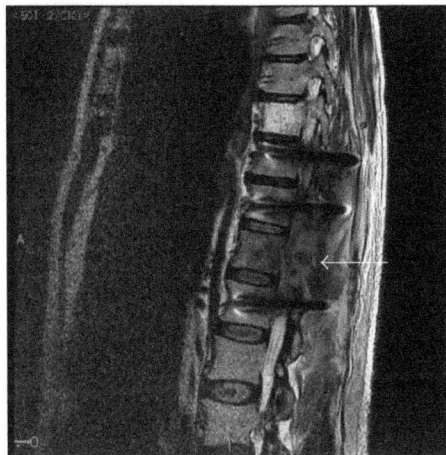

FIGURE 3: Spinal MRI revealing paravertebral lesions between T11-T12 causing significant mass effect on the conus medullaris.

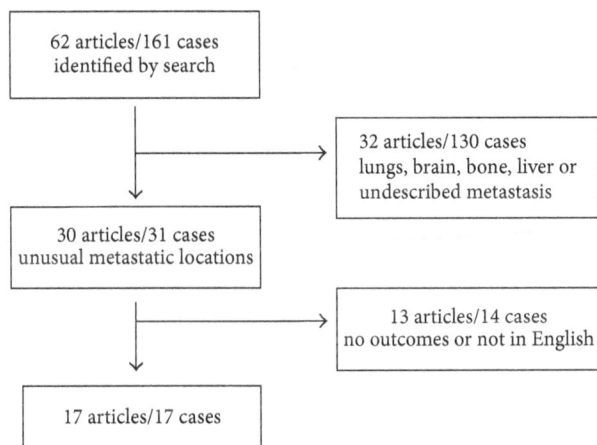

FIGURE 4: Selection for review of literature: references were obtained from the PubMed database, using the keywords "phyllodes tumor metastasis".

Acknowledgments

The authors thank Mr. Matthew Selwyn for his English grammar corrections.

References

[1] F. A. Tavassoli, *Pathology and genetics of tumours of the breast and female genital organs*, World Health Organization Classification of Tumors, 2003, http://www.iarc.fr/en/publications/pdfd-online/pat-gen/bb4/bb4-chap1.pdf.

[2] L. Bernstein, D. Deapen, and R. K. Ross, "The descriptive epidemiology of malignant cystosarcoma phyllodes tumors of the breast," *Cancer*, vol. 71, no. 10, pp. 3020–3024, 1993.

[3] O. K. Macdonald, C. M. Lee, J. D. Tward, C. D. Chappel, and D. K. Gaffney, "Malignant phyllodes tumor of the female breast: association of primary therapy with cause-specific survival from the surveillance, epidemiology, and end results (SEER) program," *Cancer*, vol. 107, no. 9, pp. 2127–2133, 2006.

[4] P. Khosravi-Shahi, "Management of non metastatic phyllodes tumors of the breast: Review of the literature," *Surgical Oncology*, vol. 20, no. 4, pp. e143–e148, 2011.

[5] Y. Belkacémi, G. Bousquet, and H. Marsiglia, "Phyllodes tumor of the breast," *International Journal of Radiation Oncology, Biology and Physics*, vol. 70, no. 2, pp. 492–500, 2008.

[6] I. Kapiris, N. Nasiri, R. A'Hern, V. Healy, and G. P. H. Gui, "Outcome and predictive factors of local recurrence and distant metastases following primary surgical treatment of high-grade malignant phyllodes tumours of the breast," *European Journal of Surgical Oncology*, vol. 27, no. 8, pp. 723–730, 2001.

[7] J. W. Mitus, P. Blecharz, T. Walasek, M. Reinfuss, J. Jakubowicz, and J. Kulpa, "Treatment of patients with distant metastases from phyllodes tumor of the breast," *World Journal of Surgery*, vol. 40, no. 2, pp. 323–328, 2016.

[8] S. Kim, J.-Y. Kim, D. H. Kim, W. H. Jung, and J. S. Koo, "Analysis of phyllodes tumor recurrence according to the histologic grade," *Breast Cancer Research and Treatment*, vol. 141, no. 3, pp. 353–363, 2013.

[9] M. Reinfuss, J. Mituś, K. Duda, A. Stelmach, J. Ryś, and K. Smolak, "The treatment and prognosis of patients with phyllodes tumor of the breast: An analysis of 170 cases," *Cancer*, vol. 77, no. 5, pp. 910–916, 1996.

[10] J. Mitus, M. Reinfuss, and J. W. Mitus, "Malignant phyllodes tumor of the breast: treatment and prognosis," *The Breast Journal*, vol. 20, no. 6, pp. 639–644, 2014.

[11] S. Lakhani, I. Ellis, and S. Schnitt, *WHO classification of tumours of the breast*, IARC Press, Lyon, 4th edition, 2012.

[12] A. V. Barrio, B. D. Clark, J. I. Goldberg et al., "Clinicopathologic features and long-term outcomes of 293 phyllodes tumors of the breast," *Annals of Surgical Oncology*, vol. 14, no. 10, pp. 2961–2970, 2007.

[13] G. Cohn-Cedermark, L. E. Rutqvist, I. Rosendahl, and C. Silfverswärd, "Prognostic factors in cystosarcoma phyllodes. A clinicopathologic study of 77 patients," *Cancer*, vol. 68, no. 9, pp. 2017–2022, 1991.

[14] N. J. Nonzee, D. M. Ragas, T. Ha Luu et al., "Delays in cancer care among low-income minorities despite access," *Journal of Women's Health*, vol. 24, no. 6, pp. 506–514, 2015.

[15] W. A. G. El-Charnoubi, J. B. Svendsen, U. B. Tange, and N. Kroman, "Women with inoperable or locally advanced breast cancer what characterizes them? A retrospective review of 157 cases," *Acta Oncologica*, vol. 51, no. 8, pp. 1081–1085, 2012.

[16] F. Yoshidaya, N. Hayashi, K. Takahashi et al., "Malignant phyllodes tumor metastasized to the right ventricle: a case report," *Surgical Case Reports*, vol. 1, no. 1, 2015.

[17] N. Garg, N. Moorthy, S. K. Agrawal, S. Pandey, and N. Kumari, "Delayed cardiac metastasis from phyllodes breast tumor resenting as cardiogenic shock," *Texas Heart Institute Journal*, vol. 38, no. 4, pp. 441–444, 2011.

[18] T. Nakatsu, T. Koshiji, Y. Sakakibara et al., "Pulmonary artery obstruction due to a metastatic malignant phyllodes tumor of the breast," *General Thoracic and Cardiovascular Surgery*, vol. 58, no. 8, pp. 423–426, 2010.

[19] D. I. Choi, H. S. Chi, S. H. Lee et al., "A rare case of phyllodes tumor metastasis to the stomach presenting as anemia," *Cancer Research and Treatment*, vol. 49, no. 3, pp. 846–849, 2016.

[20] M. A. Bilen, R. Laucirica, M. F. Rimawi, J. R. Nangia, and G. S. Cyprus, "Jejunal intussusception due to malignant phyllodes tumor of the breast," *Clinical Breast Cancer*, vol. 12, no. 3, pp. 219–221, 2012.

[21] B. B. Morcos, B. Baker, and S. A. Hashem, "Ileocaecal intussusception secondary to metastatic phyllodes tumour of the breast," *Annals of the Royal College of Surgeons of England*, vol. 92, no. 6, pp. W29–W30, 2010.

[22] O. Asoglu, H. Karanlik, U. Barbaros et al., "Malignant phyllode tumor metastatic to the duodenum," *World Journal of Gastroenterology*, vol. 12, no. 10, pp. 1649–1651, 2006.

[23] J. Wei, Y.-T. Tan, Y.-C. Cai et al., "Predictive factors for the local recurrence and distant metastasis of phyllodes tumors of the breast: A retrospective analysis of 192 cases at a single center," *Chinese Journal of Cancer*, vol. 33, no. 10, pp. 492–500, 2014.

[24] S. Yoshiba, T. Saotome, T. Mikogami, and T. Shirota, "Metastasis of mammary gland malignant phyllodes tumor to the mandibular region: a case report and review of the literature," *Journal of Oral and Maxillofacial Surgery*, 2016.

[25] R. Sano, E. Sato, T. Watanabe et al., "Phyllodes tumor metastasis to the tonsil with synchronous undifferentiated carcinoma," *International Journal of Surgery Case Reports*, vol. 5, no. 6, pp. 290–293, 2014.

[26] A. Masmoudi, L. Ayadi, and S. Bouassida, "Gingival metastasis in breast phyllodes tumor," *Ann Dermatol Venereol*, vol. 133, no. 5, pp. 449–451, 2006.

[27] G. Deeming, R. Divakaran, D. Butterworth, and M. Foster, "Temporomandibular region metastasis from cystosarcoma phyllodes: a case report and review of the literature," *Journal of Cranio-Maxillo-Facial Surgery*, vol. 31, no. 5, pp. 325–328, 2003.

[28] J. B. Staton, T. H. Costello, F. D. Donovan, and R. E. Laster, "Cystosarcoma phyllodes metastatic to the mandible: report of a rare case and literature review," *Ear, Nose and Throat Journal*, vol. 82, no. 5, pp. 380-381, 2003.

[29] T. Giorgadze, R. M. Ward, Z. W. Baloch, and V. A. LiVolsi, "Phyllodes tumor metastatic to thyroid Hurthle cell adenoma," *Arch Pathol Lab Med*, vol. 126, no. 10, p. 1233, 2002.

[30] B. Karczmarek-Borowska, A. Bukala, K. Syrek-Kaplita, M. Ksiazek, J. Filipowska, and M. Gradalska-Lampart, "A rare case of breast malignant phyllodes tumor with metastases to the kidney," *Medicine (United States)*, vol. 94, no. 33, p. e1312, 2015.

[31] Y. Collin, F. Chagnon, C. J. Mongeau, G. L. Gonzalez-Amaya, and L. Sideris, "Adrenal metastasis of a phyllodes tumor of the breast: case report and review of the literature," *International Journal of Surgery Case Reports*, vol. 4, no. 8, pp. 687–689, 2013.

[32] J. Shan, S. Zhang, Z. Wang, Y. Fu, L. Li, and X. Wang, "Breast malignant phyllodes tumor with rare pelvic metastases and long-term overall survival: a case report and literature review," *Medicine (Baltimore)*, vol. 95, no. 38, Article ID e4942, p. e4942, 2016.

[33] D. L. F. Jardim, A. Conley, and V. Subbiah, "Comprehensive characterization of malignant phyllodes tumor by whole genomic and proteomic analysis: Biological implications for targeted therapy opportunities," *Orphanet Journal of Rare Diseases*, vol. 8, no. 1, article no. 112, 2013.

[34] J. Tan, C. K. Ong, and W. K. Lim, "Genomic landscapes of breast fibroepithelial tumors," *Nature Genetics*, vol. 47, no. 11, pp. 1341–1345, 2015.

[35] W. K. Lim, C. K. Ong, J. Tan et al., "Exome sequencing identifies highly recurrent MED12 somatic mutations in breast fibroadenoma," *Nature Genetics*, vol. 46, no. 8, pp. 877–880, 2014.

[36] N. Yoon, G. E. Bae, S. Y. Kang et al., "Frequency of MED12 mutations in phyllodes tumors: Inverse correlation with histologic grade," *Genes, Chromosomes and Cancer*, vol. 55, no. 6, pp. 495–504, 2016.

[37] M. Laé, S. Gardrat, S. Rondeau et al., "MED12 mutations in breast phyllodes tumors: Evidence of temporal tumoral heterogeneity and identification of associated critical signaling pathways," *Oncotarget*, vol. 7, no. 51, pp. 84428–84438, 2016.

[38] Z. Gatalica, S. Vranic, A. Ghazalpour et al., "Multiplatform molecular profiling identifies potentially targetable biomarkers in malignant phyllodes tumors of the breast," *Oncotarget*, vol. 7, no. 2, pp. 1707–1716, 2016.

42

Daily Vaginal Application of Dienogest (Visanne©) for 3 Months in Symptomatic Deeply Infiltrating Rectovaginal Endometriosis: A Possible New Treatment Approach?

Andreas D. Ebert ⓘ

Praxis für Frauengesundheit, Gynäkologie und Geburtshilfe, Nürnberger Strasse 67, 10787 Berlin, Germany

Correspondence should be addressed to Andreas D. Ebert; adebert@gmx.de

Academic Editor: Maria Grazia Porpora

A 27-year-old patient suffering from deeply infiltrating rectovaginal endometriosis was treated with 2 mg/day dienogest vaginally for 3 months. The therapy was tolerated very well. The patient reported less side effects compared to the oral use of dienogest. After 3 months of dienogest treatment, the rectovaginal gynecological examination identified the visible vaginal part of endometriosis in remission. The firm endometriosis node approximately 3 cm in size and approximately 10 cm ab ano was still palpable, but it was much less painful. The laboratory values for luteinizing hormone (LH) and follicle-stimulating hormone (FSH) were unremarkable, with an LH/FSH quotient of 0.7 during dienogest treatment, while 17-β estradiol and progesterone were suppressed. At palpation and vaginal ultrasonography, there was no change in the findings before and after 3 months of dienogest treatment, but the patient was now de facto asymptomatic. To the best of our knowledge, this is the first report of a vaginal dienogest treatment in symptomatic deeply infiltrating rectovaginal endometriosis. Vaginal administration of dienogest should receive further investigation in pharmacokinetic and clinical studies.

1. Introduction

Symptomatic deeply infiltrating rectovaginal endometriosis with bowel involvement is a diagnostic and therapeutic challenge [1–5].

Oral administration of dienogest (Visanne©) is currently approved in Germany for the treatment of endometriosis alongside subcutaneous application of leuprorelin acetate (Enantone©, Trenantone©). Due to its lower costs and narrower range of side effects, dienogest is currently the drug treatment of choice in comparison with gonadotropin-releasing hormone (GnRH) analogues [6]. In terms of their effects and side effects, the two treatment approaches are equivalent [7–10]. Research studies to date have been carried out with oral administration of dienogest 2 mg/d [11–14]. To the best of our knowledge, there have as yet been no reports on trials of vaginal treatment with 2 mg/d dienogest in patients with symptomatic deeply infiltrating endometriosis.

2. Case Presentation

A 27-year-old woman (gravida I, para I; menarche at age 13) presented on 1 October 2017 due to secondary dysmenorrhea that she was suffering from since the age of 25, dyspareunia with back pain, constipation with perimenstrual tympanites, and contact bleeding in a case of known rectovaginal endometriosis. Her menstrual cycle was regular (27/4). Her visual analogue score for dysmenorrhea ($VAS_{dysmenorrhea}$) was 8. A rectovaginal gynecological examination revealed fresh endometriosis in the posterior fornix, with slight bleeding (Figure 1(a)). The vaginal part of the cervix was unremarkable on colposcopy, cytology, and smear testing. At approximately 10 cm ab ano, palpation identified a typical firm, painful node with a diameter of approximately 3 cm, and poorly displaceable bowel mucosa, which was also clearly visible on vaginal ultrasonography (Figure 2(a)). The bilateral renal ultrasound findings were unremarkable. It was known from

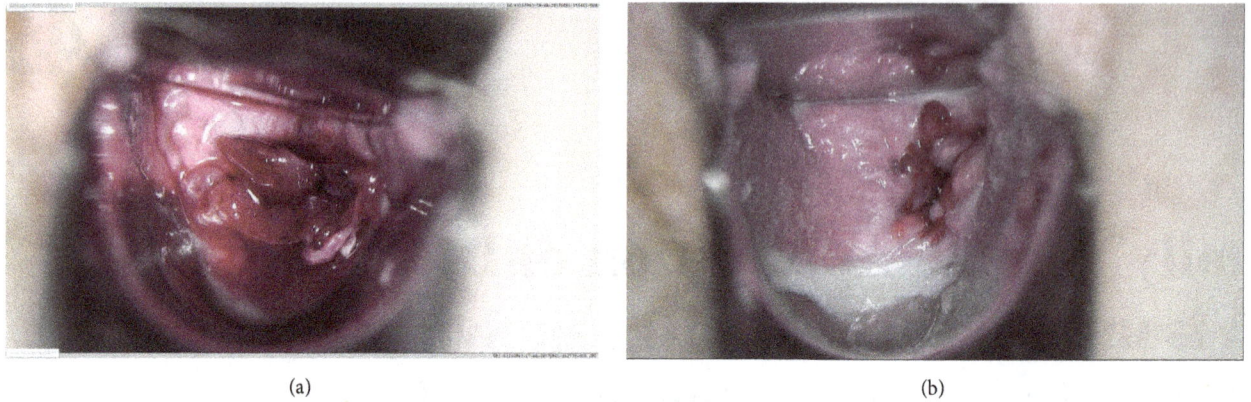

(a)   (b)

FIGURE 1: (a) Fresh, vulnerable, histologically confirmed rectovaginal endometriosis in the posterior fornix (Medivan video colposcope). The visual analogue score for the examination (VAS$_{examination}$) before dienogest therapy was 9. (b) Remission of the same endometriotic lesion in the posterior fornix 3 months later after daily vaginal dienogest application. VAS$_{examination}$ score was now 4.

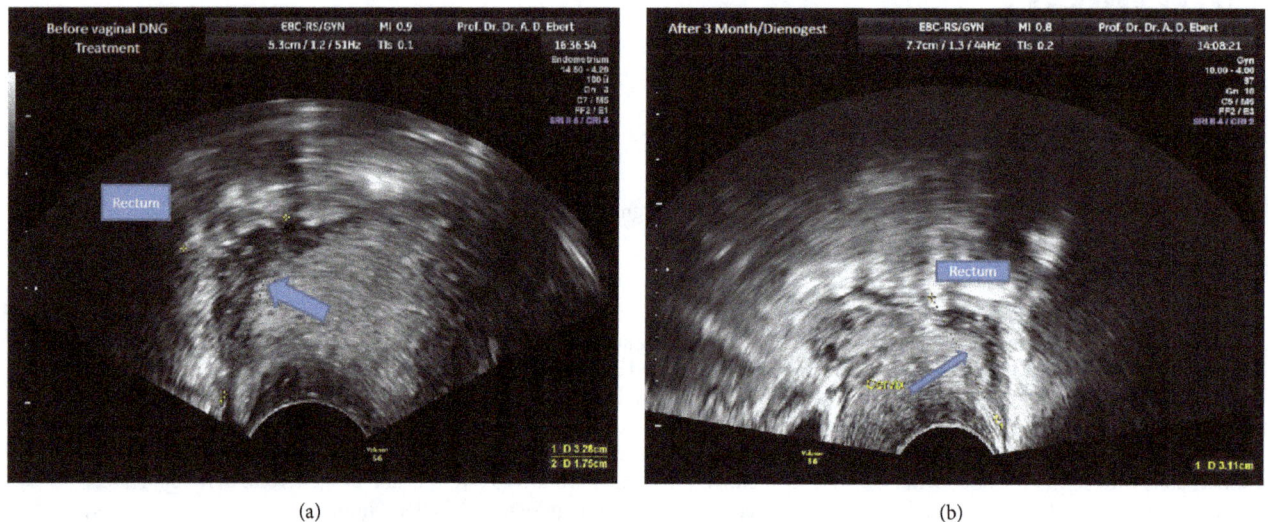

(a)   (b)

FIGURE 2: (a) Vaginal ultrasound appearance of the rectovaginal bowel involvement before the start of treatment in the symptomatic patient. (b) No change in the vaginal ultrasound findings after 3 months of vaginal dienogest administration (2 mg/d) in the patient who was now de facto asymptomatic.

the patient's history that in February 2015 she had undergone a laparoscopy at a different hospital due to symptoms and wanting to have a baby; histology had confirmed deeply infiltrating endometriosis without atypia in the posterior fornix and pouch of Douglas. Adequate removal of the endometriosis was not carried out. The tubes were bilaterally patent. Postoperatively, the patient had taken dienogest (2 mg/d orally) up until August 2015, but she had very poor tolerance for it due to side effects (effluvium, blemished skin, sad mood). She became pregnant in October 2015 and delivered a boy at term in 2016 by emergency cesarean section due to premature placental detachment.

The endometriosis-related symptoms increased postpartum, with progressive deterioration in her quality of life. Despite this, the patient declined surgery due to fear of complications and for family and social reasons. She also declined endocrine treatment options (gonadotropin-releasing hormone antagonists or agonists, progestin-only pills, and oral contraceptives) due to the possible side effects. For this reason, the option of vaginal application of dienogest was discussed with the patient and implemented. The patient presented again after 3 months of vaginal dienogest treatment (2 mg/d vaginally). She reported minor vaginal spotting during the first 4 weeks of the treatment but had been amenorrhoeic for just under 8 weeks. She reported very good satisfaction with the treatment, after transient minimal side effects initially (slight skin blemishes, minimal discharge), and symptomatic freedom from the relevant endometriosis-related symptoms. Slight contact bleeding occurred only during sex. No vaginal infections had occurred during the treatment period. The rectovaginal gynecological examination identified the endometriosis in remission in the posterior fornix (Figure 1(b)). The firm endometriosis node approximately 3 cm in size and approximately 10 cm ab ano was still palpable, but it was much less painful (Figure 2(a)). Bilateral renal ultrasonography was unremarkable. The laboratory values for luteinizing hormone (LH; 5.07 U/L) and follicle-stimulating hormone (FSH; 7.29 U/L) were unremarkable, with an LH/FSH quotient of 0.7 during dienogest treatment, while 17-β estradiol (24.2 pg/mL) and progesterone (<0.05 ng/mL) were suppressed. At palpation and vaginal ultrasonography, there was no change in the findings before and after 3 months of dienogest treatment, but the patient was now de facto asymptomatic. In addition, the vaginal part of endometriosis was clearly in remission as demonstrated by vaginal colposcopy (Figures 1(a) and 1(b)). At her express request, continuation of the vaginal dienogest treatment was agreed.

3. Discussion

In the present case, vaginal dienogest (2 mg/d) was administered for 3 months. During the treatment, remission occurred in the area of the vaginally visible part of the deeply infiltrating endometriosis (Figures 1(a) and 1(b)), while the rectal part showed no significant changes in size on palpation or ultrasonography (Figures 2(a) and 2(b)). Despite this, the patient became free of symptoms apart from contact bleeding—a major therapeutic success. The rectovaginal examination was also significantly less painful after 3 months of dienogest (VAS$_{examination}$ 9 versus VAS$_{examination}$ 4). These findings are in accordance with our own experience and experience reported by others: before the size of the node declines, symptoms initially improve [14]. Despite the higher local dosage of dienogest, a reduction in the size of rectovaginal endometriosis nodes can probably only be observed clinically later on, since rectovaginal endometriosis always represents as *adenomyofibromatous* lesion [15], treatment-related remission of which takes time [16]. Dienogest was effectively resorbed vaginally, leading to therapeutic amenorrhea and the corresponding hormone findings in the present patient.

In principle, vaginal application of dienogest may be able to circumvent the hepatic first-pass effect and achieve higher concentrations of the active agent at the site of effect (e.g., a rectovaginal endometriosis node) with lower side effects than with oral administration [17]. The present patient thus reported that she found the vaginal application of dienogest much more tolerable than oral intake. A reduction in the dosage would also be conceivable with local dienogest administration. Studies with danazol, anastrozole, and contraceptive rings have shown that there is a reduction in lower abdominal pain and particularly in dysmenorrhea. However, a reduction in the size of rectovaginal nodes measured using ultrasound has not been reported by all investigators [17].

With vaginal application of dienogest (or other steroids), higher hormone concentrations can be achieved at the rectovaginal endometriosis node than with oral, intramuscular, or transcutaneous administration [17]. A prerequisite for this is correct placement of the active agents in the upper third of the vagina. For patients with symptomatic rectovaginal endometriosis who decline surgery or other treatment options for various reasons, vaginal dienogest application may thus represent a new approach to treatment, with low side effects. As vaginal application is familiar with other drugs [17], vaginal administration of dienogest (as well as other hormones) should receive further investigation in pharmacokinetic and clinical studies.

References

[1] G. Halis, S. Mechsner, and A. D. Ebert, "The diagnosis and treatment of deep infiltrating endometriosis," *Deutsches Ärzteblatt International*, vol. 107, pp. 446–455, 2010.

[2] N. Berlanda, E. Somigliana, M. P. Frattaruolo, L. Buggio, D. Dridi, and P. Vercellini, "Surgery versus hormonal therapy for deep endometriosis: is it a choice of the physician?" *European Journal of Obstetrics & Gynecology and Reproductive Biology*, vol. 209, pp. 67–71, 2017.

[3] O. Donnez and H. Roman, "Choosing the right surgical technique for deep endometriosis: shaving, disc excision, or bowel resection?" *Fertility and Sterility*, vol. 108, no. 6, pp. 931–942, 2017.

[4] P. Vercellini, L. Buggio, and E. Somigliana, "Role of medical therapy in the management of deep rectovaginal endometriosis," *Fertility and Sterility*, vol. 108, no. 6, pp. 913–930, 2017.

[5] A. Vanhie, C. Meuleman, C. Tomassetti et al., "Consensus on Recording Deep Endometriosis Surgery: The CORDES statement," *Human Reproduction*, vol. 31, no. 6, pp. 1219–1223, 2016.

[6] U. Ulrich, O. Buchweitz, R. Greb et al., "National German Guideline (S2k): Guideline for the diagnosis and treatment of endometriosis," *Geburtshilfe und Frauenheilkunde*, vol. 74, no. 12, pp. 1104–1118, 2014.

[7] T. Strowitzki, J. Marr, C. Gerlinger, T. Faustmann, and C. Seitz, "Dienogest is as effective as leuprolide acetate in treating the painful symptoms of endometriosis: a 24-week, randomized, multicentre, open-label trial," *Human Reproduction*, vol. 25, no. 3, pp. 633–641, 2010.

[8] T. Harada, M. Momoeda, Y. Taketani et al., "Dienogest is as effective as intranasal buserelin acetate for the relief of pain symptoms associated with endometriosis-a randomized, double-blind, multicenter, controlled trial," *Fertility and Sterility*, vol. 91, no. 3, pp. 675–681, 2009.

[9] D.-Y. Lee, J.-Y. Lee, J.-W. Seo, B.-K. Yoon, and D. Choi, "Gonadotropin-releasing hormone agonist with add–back treatment is as effective and tolerable as dienogest in preventing pain recurrence after laparoscopic surgery for endometriosis," *Archives of Gynecology and Obstetrics*, vol. 294, no. 6, pp. 1257–1263, 2016.

[10] M. A. Bedaiwy, C. Allaire, and S. Alfaraj, "Long-term medical management of endometriosis with dienogest and with a gonadotropin-releasing hormone agonist and add-back hormone therapy," *Fertility and Sterility*, vol. 107, no. 3, pp. 537–548, 2017.

[11] M. D. P. Andres, L. A. Lopes, E. C. Baracat, and S. Podgaec, "Dienogest in the treatment of endometriosis: systematic review," *Archives of Gynecology and Obstetrics*, vol. 292, no. 3, pp. 523–529, 2015.

[12] M. Momoeda, T. Harada, N. Terakawa et al., "Long-term use of dienogest for the treatment of endometriosis," *Journal of*

Obstetrics and Gynaecology Research, vol. 35, no. 6, pp. 1069–1076, 2009.

[13] A. Maiorana, D. Incandela, F. Parazzini et al., "Efficacy of dienogest in improving pain in women with endometriosis: a 12-month single-center experience," *Archives of Gynecology and Obstetrics*, vol. 296, no. 3, pp. 429–433, 2017.

[14] J. P. Leonardo-Pinto, C. L. Benetti-Pinto, K. Cursino, and D. A. Yela, "Dienogest and deep infiltrating endometriosis: The remission of symptoms is not related to endometriosis nodule remission," *European Journal of Obstetrics & Gynecology and Reproductive Biology*, vol. 211, pp. 108–111, 2017.

[15] R. Meyer, "Die Pathologie der Bindegewebsgeschwülste und Mischgeschwülste," in *Handbuch der Gynäkologie. 3. Auflage, Band 6, J. F. Bergmann, München*, W. Stoeckel, Ed., pp. 356–615, 1930.

[16] M. Harada, Y. Osuga, G. Izumi et al., "Dienogest, a new conservative strategy for extragenital endometriosis: A pilot study," *Gynecological Endocrinology*, vol. 27, no. 9, pp. 717–720, 2011.

[17] L. Buggio, C. Lazzari, E. Monti, G. Barbara, N. Berlanda, and P. Vercellini, ""Per vaginam" topical use of hormonal drugs in women with symptomatic deep endometriosis: a narrative literature review," *Archives of Gynecology and Obstetrics*, vol. 296, no. 3, pp. 435–444, 2017.

43

Vaginal Angiomyofibroblastoma: A Case Report and Review of Diagnostic Imaging

Sarah Eckhardt [iD],[1] **Renee Rolston,**[1] **Suzanne Palmer,**[2] **and Begum Ozel** [iD][1]

[1]*Division of Female Pelvic Floor and Reconstructive Surgery, Department of Obstetrics and Gynecology,*
 University of Southern California, Los Angeles, CA, USA
[2]*Clinical Radiology and Medicine, Keck Medical Center, University of Southern California, Los Angeles, CA, USA*

Correspondence should be addressed to Sarah Eckhardt; sarah.eckhardt@med.usc.edu

Academic Editor: Maria Grazia Porpora

Background. Angiomyofibroblastoma (AMFB) is a benign mesenchymal tumor most commonly found in the female genital tract of premenopausal women. Although rare, AMFB is an important consideration in the differential diagnosis of vulvar and vaginal masses, as it must be distinguished from aggressive angiomyxoma (AA), a locally recurrent, invasive, and damaging tumor with similar clinical and pathologic findings. *Case.* We describe a patient with a 4 cm vaginal AMFB and the relevant preoperative radiographic imaging findings. *Conclusion.* Preoperative diagnosis of AMFB remains difficult. Common findings on magnetic resonance imaging and transvaginal sonography are described. We conclude that both transvaginal ultrasound and MRI are potentially useful imaging modalities in the preoperative assessment of vulvar and vaginal AMFB, with more data needed to determine superiority of one modality over the other.

1. Introduction

Angiomyofibroblastoma (AMFB) is a rare, indolent mesenchymal tumor that most commonly occurs in the female genital tract in premenopausal women, most frequently in the vulva and vagina. AMFB typically measures less than 5 cm; however, case reports describe tumors of up to 23 cm in size [1]. Few cases have been reported affecting the fallopian tube, ischiorectal fossa, cervix, and bladder, as well as similar tumors in the male spermatic cord, scrotum, and perineum [2–6].

AMFB was first described in the literature by Fletcher et al. in 1992 as an important distinction from aggressive angiomyxoma (AA), which is an infiltrative myxedematous mesenchymal tumor with the potential for local recurrence [7].

Preoperative diagnosis of AMFB and distinction from other soft tissue tumors is often difficult, as there is limited information on characteristic imaging findings. The differential diagnosis for a vaginal or vulvar mass includes Bartholin's gland cyst, epidermal inclusion cyst, Gartner's duct cyst, fibroma, lipoma, hemangioma, leiomyoma, and alternative rare mesenchymal tumors. Here, we describe a case report of a vaginal AMFB and relevant radiologic features to aid in diagnosis and distinction from aggressive angiomyxoma.

2. Case

A 30-year-old gravida 1 para 1 female presented to our Emergency Department complaining of a vaginal mass present since the birth of her child 4 years earlier. At that time, she underwent an uncomplicated vacuum-assisted vaginal delivery and was unaware of significant lacerations or repairs. She felt that the mass had not changed significantly in size since the postpartum period, but she had never been evaluated by a physician. She complained of acutely worsening discharge over the previous month, described as watery yellow to pink and occasionally blood tinged. She denied changes in bowel movements, dysuria, hematuria, fevers, chills, night sweats, changes in appetite, or weight loss. She complained of both entry and deep dyspareunia.

Physical exam was notable for copious serosanguinous fluid within the vaginal vault. A well-circumscribed, smooth cystic structure approximately 4 cm in diameter was noted

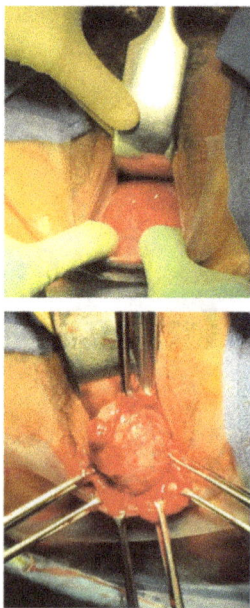

FIGURE 1: Lesion on exam under anesthesia and gross specimen during dissection.

along the posterior vaginal wall. There was also a 0.5x1.0 cm exophytic lesion overlying the mass with serosanguinous drainage (Figure 1). On rectal exam, the mass was noted to be separate from the cervix and within the rectovaginal septum. Rectal involvement was not appreciated.

Tissue biopsies were taken; however, they were of limited diagnostic value, showing fibrous tissue with acute and chronic inflammation and squamous debris, consistent with cyst wall and contents.

A pelvic ultrasound (US) was performed and showed a complex vaginal mass, inseparable from the cervix, measuring 5.1 x 3.8 x 5.4 cm (Figure 2(a)). Color Doppler demonstrated minimal peripheral vascularity (Figure 2(b)). Magnetic resonance imaging (MRI) was subsequently performed for further characterization (Figure 3). The mass measured 4.7 x4.8 x 4.9 cm and appeared to arise from the posterior wall of the vagina, separate from the cervix. The mass was heterogeneously hyperintense on T2-weighted (T2W) images and hypointense on T1-weighted (T1W) images. Postcontrast sequences demonstrated enhancement of the wall, absent internal enhancement superiorly, and bulky, nodular, hyperenhancement inferiorly, consistent with a complex cystic mass.

The patient was taken to the operating room for an uncomplicated surgical excision. Histology was notable for hypocellular edematous myxoid stromal tissue alternating with hypercellular areas of stromal cells clustered around thin walled small to medium-sized vessels, consistent with angiomyofibroblastoma. Stromal cells were noted to be spindled with eosinophilic cytoplasm. Nuclei were round or ovular with fine chromatin (Figure 4). Rare mitotic figures were noted. Immunohistochemical stains were negative for desmin, alpha-smooth muscle actin (α-SMA), and

progesterone receptor but demonstrated focal estrogen receptor positivity.

3. Comment

Although AMFB is a rare diagnosis, it is an important consideration in the premenopausal and perimenopausal patient presenting with a vulvovaginal mass given its predilection for this region of the female genital tract. In a review of the literature in 2015 by Wolf et al., 125 cases of female AMFB had been previously reported, of which 92% were either vulvar (N = 98) or vaginal in origin (N = 17). Median age was 45, and the majority of cases were observed in women less than 60 years of age [8]. Since 2015, there have been 10 additional cases including ours describing AMFB in females, six of which were located in the vulva, one cervical, one in the broad ligament, and one on the patient's foot [2, 9–17]. All women were under the age of 50.

Differential diagnosis for AMFB includes Gartner's duct cyst, epidermal inclusion cyst, leiomyoma, and fibroepithelial polyps among the more common etiologies. It is most important to distinguish AMFB from aggressive angiomyxoma (AA), which can commonly be misdiagnosed based on anatomic and pathologic similarities (Table 1). Although there have been no reports of distant metastasis, AA is known to recur in 33-72% of cases and is locally invasive, often entrapping nerves and mucosal glands [18, 19]. Surgical approach to AA requires wide local excision given the infiltrative nature of the lesion versus simple excision of AMFB; thus, it is important to attempt differentiation between the two prior to surgery.

Diagnostic utility of preoperative imaging for AMFB remains controversial. However, as the number of reported cases increases in the literature, more data exists on common radiographic features (Table 2).

3.1. Ultrasonography. US is typically the first imaging modality used to evaluate vaginal masses due to its intrinsic high resolution, availability, and cost effectiveness. US can be utilized to distinguish vulvar and vaginal AMFB from AA and other mesenchymal tumors [20, 21]. AMFB shows hyperechoic areas with irregular and small hypoechoic cystic areas interspersed within homogenous echogenic stroma [8, 20–23]. Minimal vascularity in AMFB is occasionally noted [8, 22]. Absence of prominent vascularity on color Doppler is consistent histologically with the predominant capillary-like vascular component of AMFB. Echogenic areas have been shown to represent hypocellular stroma on histology, while hypoechogenicity represents hypercellular areas [8, 21]. In our case, US characteristics were similar to those previously described.

In contrast, US appearance of AA is typically a hypoechoic mass with homogenous echogenicity and occasional echogenic septa correlating to fibrous bands on pathology [24, 25]. These fibrous bands can create a layered or swirling appearance similar to that seen on MRI and CT imaging of AA [26]. Vascularity can also be much more prominent on color Doppler of AA than AMFB [26, 27].

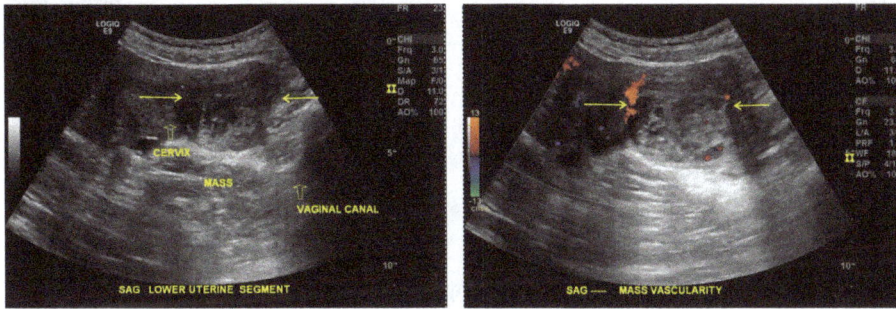

FIGURE 2: Transvaginal ultrasound. (a) Gray scale image shows a mixed echogenicity mass (arrows) with small hypoechoic cystic areas (3.0 MHz) 10 cm. (b) Color Doppler image shows minimal vascularity. Magnitude: 3 MHz.

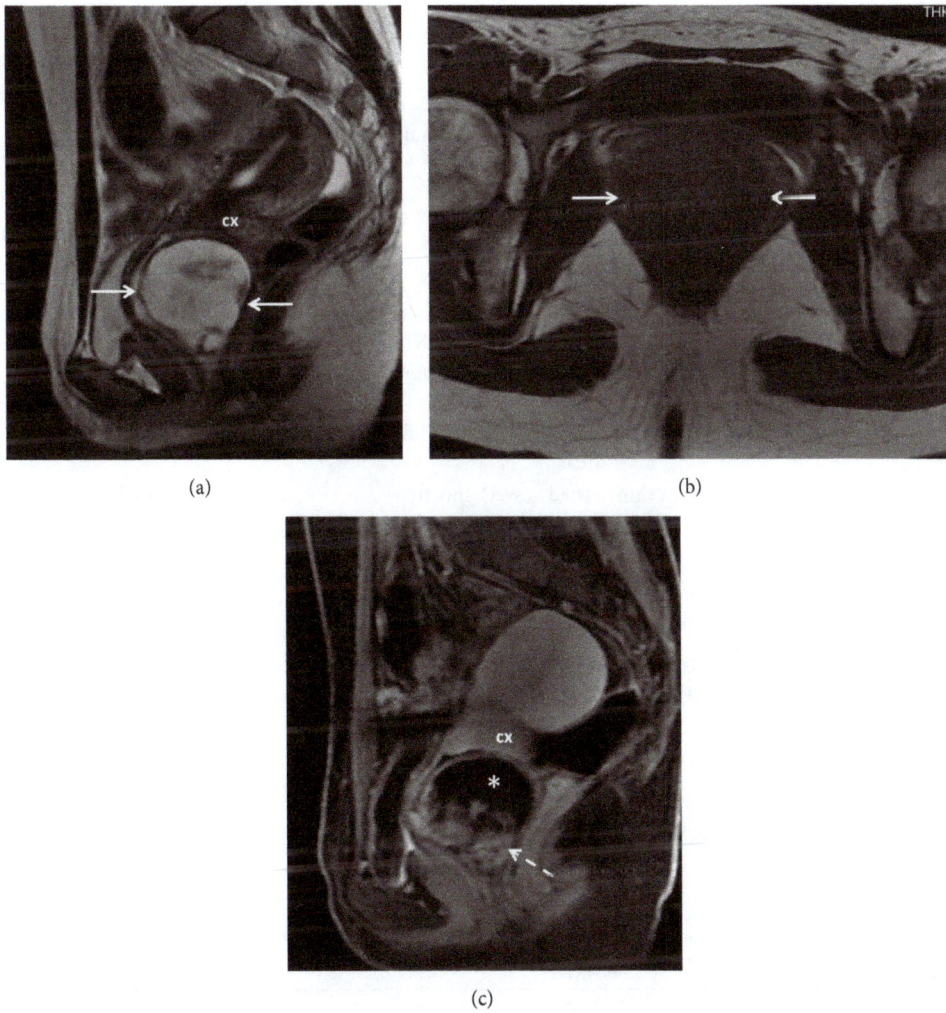

(a)

(b)

(c)

FIGURE 3: (a) Sagittal T2 weighted image shows a predominantly hyperintense mass (arrows) with small central areas of hypointensity. (b) On T1 weighted axial image the mass is homogeneously hypointense (arrows). (c) Sagittal contrast enhanced image demonstrates heterogeneous hyperenhancement inferiorly (dashed arrow) and absent enhancement superiorly (∗). Cervix: cx.

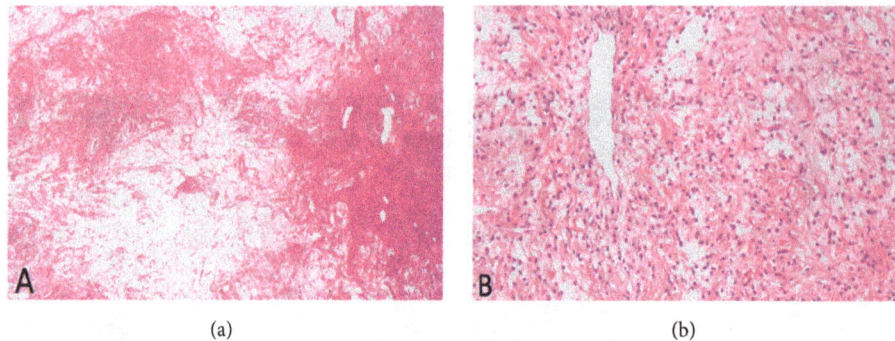

(a)   (b)

FIGURE 4: (a) Mesenchymal lesion with alternating hypercellular and hypocellular areas (4x magnification; hematoxylin and eosin stain). (b) Higher magnification demonstrating ovoid and spindle-shaped cells aggregated around small blood vessel (40x magnification).

TABLE 1: Clinical and pathologic features of AMFB and AA.

	AMFB	AA
Clinical features		
Age (years)	16 – 86 (Median 45)	16 – 70 (Median 37)
Size (cm)	< 5 (0.5 – 23)	>5 (1-60)
Location	Female pelvis and perineum: predominantly vulvar/vaginal	Female pelvis and perineum
Onset	1 month to 8 years	1 month – 5 years
	Predominantly 1-2 years	Predominantly < 1 year
Recurrence	None reported	33-72%
Pathology		
Low-power features	Well-defined	Infiltrative
	No entrapment of mucosal glands or nerve bundles	Entrapped mucosal glands and nerve bundles
	Alternating hypocellular and hypercellular areas	Stromal cells distributed throughout
Vasculature	Abundant thin-walled vessels, mostly capillary-like	Small to medium-sized vessels, mostly thick-walled or hyalinized
	Abundant	Low cellularity
Stromal cells	Spindle, plump spindle, or oval	Thin delicate spindle or stellate
	Perivascular aggregation	Mitotic figures typically absent
	Mitotic figures typically absent	
Stroma	Mucin-poor, containing delicate, wavy collagen fiber	Myxoid, hyaluronic-acid rich
Immunostaining		
Desmin	Positive (50-60%)	Positive (Up to 73%)
α–SMA	Negative (positive in up to 15%)	Positive
S-100	Negative	Negative
Vimentin	Positive	Positive
Estrogen receptor	Positive	Positive
Progesterone receptor	Positive	Positive

To complete the differential diagnosis, vaginal wall cysts are anechoic masses without internal vascularity; vaginal epidermoid cysts are homogeneous hyperechoic masses without internal vascularity; and heterogeneous solid masses are often malignancies or leiomyoma [22].

3.2. *Magnetic Resonance Imaging.* On MRI, AMFB is typically well circumscribed [9]. It is rare to see central necrosis or degeneration but it does not rule out AMFB [9]. AMFB is most often described as hypointense on T1 weighted (T1W) images, similar to that of skeletal muscle, hyperintense on

TABLE 2: Characteristic imaging features of AMFB on MRI and US.

Study	Sex	Age	Size (cm)	Location	MRI	TVUS
Wolf et al.	F	38	9x6x1.5	Vagina	T1 weighted: Homogenous hypointense; T2-weighted: Homogenous hypointense mass	Well-demarcated, homogenous mass, medium echogenicity, few septations; Doppler: several small intralesional vessels
Souza et al.	M	19	2.8	Scrotum	T1-weighted: Central hypointensity Intermediate hyperintensity, capsule; T2-weighted: Intermediate homogenous hyperintensity, Hypointense capsule; Central heterogeneous mixed hypo and hyperintensity	Well-defined, heterogeneous echo texture, small hypoechoic cysts; Doppler: minimal flow
Shoji et al.	F	50	8x7x5	Vulva	T1-weighted: Hypointense mass; GA-T1: Homogenous enhancement, poorly enhanced area at center; T2-weighted: Mildly hyperintense	N/A
Geng et al.	F	46	8.5x6x16	Paravaginal	T1-weighted: signal intensity similar to skeletal muscle; GA-T1: Homogenous hyperintensity; T2-weighted: Hyperintensity, mild hyperintensity mild hypointensity	N/A
Kim et al.	F	40	9x5.5x2.5	Vulva	N/A	Mixed echoic soft tissue mass Hyperechoic areas mixed with irregular hypoechoic areas with tiny hypoechoic components; Doppler: negative
Qiu et al.	F	32	13.2x5.8 x7.8	Posterior cul-de-sac	T1-weighted: N/A	Moderately echoic mass, small hypoechoic area; Doppler: N/A
Kitamura et al.	F	24	3 x 2.8 x 2.8	Urethra	T2 Weighted: homogenous, well-defined, low to moderate hyperintensity	N/A
Lim et al.	F	48	3.8x3.5x2.8	Posterior perivesical space	T1-weighted: Signal intensity similar to skeletal muscle; GA-T1: Strong homogenous enhancement; T2-weighted: well-defined mass heterogeneous intermediate signal intensity, focal nodular and central curvilinear dark signal intensities	N/A
Maruyama et al.	M	72	7.2x5.5x2.2	Scrotum	T1-weighted: Similar to or lower signal intensity than skeletal muscle; GA-T1: strong heterogeneous enhancement; T2-weighted: heterogeneous intermediate to high signal intensity	Mixed echogenicity, with several small hypoechoic cystic areas*

TABLE 2: Continued.

Study	Sex	Age	Size (cm)	Location	MRI	TVUS
Wang et al.	F	N/A	N/A	Anterior vaginal	N/A	Poorly defined, irregularly shaped, hypoechoic, band-like echoes of various width Doppler: positive blood flow
Wang et al.	F	N/A	N/A	Urethral	N/A	Well-defined, hypoechoic cystic solid mass Doppler: positive blood flow
Mortele et al.	F	46	Perineal	2.5x3.5	T1-weighted: hypointense, inhomogeneous mass with small focus of hyperintensity representing fat GA-T1: Strong homogenous uptake T2-weighted: Hyperintense homogenous signal similar to surrounding fat	N/A

T2 weighted (T2W) images, and with homogenous hyperenhancement on gadolinium chelate (Gd-C) enhanced images [1, 9, 23, 28]. Differences in T1W and T2W signal intensity may be attributable to variations in lipid and collagenous content in AMFB [8, 23, 28–31].

Contrast enhanced imaging was only reported in 5 studies. Four showed homogenous hyperenhancement and one demonstrated heterogeneous enhancement [23]. Hyperenhancement is thought to be related to prominent vascularity associated with myofibroblast tumors and AMFB in particular [1, 9, 23, 28, 30–32].

Our case demonstrated heterogeneously high T2 and low T1 signaling intensity on MRI which is consistent with the literature. Postcontrast sequences demonstrated enhancement of the wall, absent internal enhancement superiorly, and bulky nodular enhancement inferiorly, consistent with a complex cystic mass.

When correlated histologically, hyperintensity on T2W and absent enhancement correspond to hypocellular areas with abundant collagenous stroma. Areas of hyperenhancement correspond to areas of hypercellularity and vascularity, with little collagenous stroma and water content. Intermediate intensity on T2W and less avid enhancement are thought to represent areas of intermediate cellularity and collagenous stroma [28].

Data on MRI characteristics of AA is limited. AA has similar findings to AMFB on T1W and T2W images but is thought to be differentiated best by its enhancement characteristics. AA is described as having an intense, swirled or layered pattern. Similar swirling and layered enhancement is also described on contrast enhanced CT [26–28, 33–36]. AMFB does not typically show infiltrative pattern but it can grow around structures. If infiltration and swirled or layered pattern are observed, AA is much more likely than AMFB [28, 34–36].

4. Conclusion

In conclusion, in the patient with a vaginal or vulvar mass, it is important to consider AMFB among the differential diagnoses, particularly because of the importance of distinguishing AMFB from AA for treatment purposes. Postoperative histologic examination is needed for definitive diagnosis; however, we propose that ultrasound and MRI are increasingly useful diagnostic tools, particularly as the number of reported cases increases. Given the cost effectiveness of ultrasound, initiating imaging workup of a solid vaginal or vulvar mass with ultrasonography is suggested.

Additional Points

Precis. Ultrasound and magnetic resonance imaging are useful modalities in the diagnosis of angiomyofibroblastoma, a rare mesenchymal tumor. Teaching Points. (1) AMFB occurs in the vulva and vagina in over 90% of reported cases: AMFB should be considered on the differential diagnosis of benign appearing vulvar and vaginal masses. (2) Transvaginal ultrasound is the recommended first line imaging for AMFB. MRI is recommended as second-line imaging and is preferable to CT. (3) It is important to attempt preoperative distinction from aggressive angiomyxoma in order to optimize surgical approach.

References

[1] K. Nagai, K. Aadachi, and H. Saito, "Huge pedunculated angiomyofibroblastoma of the vulva," *International Journal of Clinical Oncology*, vol. 15, no. 2, pp. 201–205, 2010.

[2] L. Roncati, T. Pusiol, F. Piscioli, G. Barbolini, and A. Maiorana, "Undetermined cervical smear due to angiomyofibroblastoma of the cervix uteri," *Journal of Obstetrics & Gynaecology*, vol. 37, no. 6, pp. 829-830, 2017.

[3] T. Kobayashi, K. Suzuki, T. Arai, and H. Sugimura, "Angiomyofibroblastoma arising from the fallopian tube," *Obstetrics & Gynecology*, vol. 94, no. Supplement, pp. 833-834, 1999.

[4] G. Ding, Y. Yu, M. Jin, J. Xu, and Z. Zhang, "Angiomyofibroblastoma-like tumor of the scrotum: A case report and literature review," *Oncology Letters*, vol. 7, no. 2, pp. 435–438, 2014.

[5] P. M. Deka, J. A. Bagawade, P. Deka, R. Baruah, and N. Shah, "A Rare Case of Intravesical Angiomyofibroblastoma," *Urology*, vol. 106, pp. e15–e18, 2017.

[6] N. E. Tzanakis, G. A. Giannopoulos, S. P. Efstathiou, G. E. Rallis, and N. I. Nikiteas, "Angiomyofibroblastoma of the spermatic cord: a case report," *Journal of Medical Case Reports*, vol. 4, no. 1, 2010.

[7] C. D. M. Fletcher, W. Y. W. Tsang, C. Fisher, K. C. Lee, and J. K. C. Chan, "Angiomyofibroblastoma of the vulva: A benign neoplasm distinct from aggressive angiomyxoma," *The American Journal of Surgical Pathology*, vol. 16, no. 4, pp. 373–382, 1992.

[8] B. Wolf, L.-C. Horn, R. Handzel, and J. Einenkel, "Ultrasound plays a key role in imaging and management of genital angiomyofibroblastoma: A case report," *Journal of Medical Case Reports*, vol. 9, no. 1, article no. 248, 2015.

[9] T. Shoji, R. Takeshita, R. Mukaida, T. Sato, M. Taguchi, and S. Sasou, "Angiomyofibroblastoma of the vulva diagnosed preoperatively: A case report," *Molecular and Clinical Oncology*, vol. 7, no. 3, pp. 407–411, 2017.

[10] H. C. Huang, Y. R. Chen, H. D. Tsai, Y. M. Cheng, and Y. H. Hsiao, "Angiomyofibroblastoma the Broad Ligament: A Case Report," *International Journal of Gynecological Pathology*, vol. 36, no. 5, pp. 471–475, 2017.

[11] Y. P. Wong, G. C. Tan, and P. F. Ng, "Cervical angiomyofibroblastoma: a case report and review of literature," *Journal of Obstetrics and Gynaecology*, vol. 37, no. 5, pp. 681-682, 2017.

[12] A. A. Salunke, Y. Chen, V. K. Lee, and M. E. Puhaindran, "Angiomyofibroblastoma of the Foot: a Rare Soft Tissue Tumor at Unusual Site," *Indian Journal of Surgical Oncology*, vol. 8, no. 2, pp. 210–213, 2017.

[13] S. Oh, D. J. Sung, K. C. Sim et al., "A rare case of vulvar angiomyofibroblastoma: MRI findings and literature review," *Journal of Obstetrics & Gynaecology*, vol. 37, no. 6, pp. 831–833, 2017.

[14] M. Islam, S. Afzal, M. Majeed, F. Monjur, and D. Parowary, "Angiomyofibroblastoma Vulva in a Very Young Adult Female: A Rare Case Report," *Mymensingh Medical Journal*, vol. 26, no. 1, pp. 208–211, 2017.

[15] S. Matsukuma, A. Koga, R. Suematsu, H. Takeo, and K. Sato, "Lipomatous angiomyofibroblastoma of the vulva: A case report and review of the literature," *Molecular and Clinical Oncology*, vol. 6, no. 1, pp. 83–87, 2017.

[16] F. Nili, N. Nicknejad, S. Salarvand, and S. Akhavan, "Lipomatous Angiomyofibroblastoma of the Vulva," *International Journal of Gynecological Pathology*, vol. 36, no. 3, pp. 300–303, 2017.

[17] I. Gelincik, A. Yildirim, I. Sayar, and C. Aktas, "Angiomyofibroblastoma of the right labia major," *Indian Journal of Pathology and Microbiology*, vol. 59, no. 2, p. 257, 2016.

[18] J. F. Fetsch, W. B. Laskin, M. Lefkowitz, L. Kindblom, and J. M. Meis-Kindblom, "Aggressive angiomyxoma: A clinicopathologic study of 29 female patients," *Cancer*, vol. 78, no. 1, pp. 79–90, 1996.

[19] L. R. Bégin, P. B. Clement, M. E. Kirk, S. Jothy, W. T. Elliott McCaughey, and A. Ferenczy, "Aggressive angiomyxoma of pelvic soft parts: a clinicopathologic study of nine cases," *Human Pathology*, vol. 16, no. 6, pp. 621–628, 1985.

[20] P. Qiu, Z. Wang, Y. Li, and G. Cui, "Giant pelvic angiomyofibroblastoma: case report and literature review," *Diagnostic Pathology*, vol. 9, no. 1, p. 106, 2014.

[21] S. W. Kim, J. Lee, J. K. Han, and S. Jeon, "Angiomyofibroblastoma of the Vulva," *Journal of Ultrasound in Medicine*, vol. 28, no. 10, pp. 1417–1420, 2009.

[22] X. Wang, H. Yang, H. Zhang, T. Shi, and W. Ren, "Transvaginal sonographic features of perineal masses in the female lower urogenital tract: A retrospective study of 71 patients," *Ultrasound in Obstetrics & Gynecology*, vol. 43, no. 6, pp. 702–710, 2014.

[23] M. Maruyama, T. Yoshizako, H. Kitagaki, A. Araki, and M. Igawa, "Magnetic resonance imaging features of angiomyofibroblastoma-like tumor of the scrotum with pathologic correlates," *Clinical Imaging*, vol. 36, no. 5, pp. 632–635, 2012.

[24] O. Catalano, "Case report: Aggressive angiomyxoma of the pelvic soft tissues: US and CT findings," *Clinical Radiology*, vol. 53, no. 10, pp. 782-783, 1998.

[25] M. De La Ossa, A. Castellano-Sanchez, E. Alvarez, W. Smoak, and M. J. Robinson, "Sonographic appearance of aggressive angiomyxoma of the scrotum," *Journal of Clinical Ultrasound*, vol. 29, no. 8, pp. 476–478, 2001.

[26] R. Tariq, S. Hasnain, MT. Siddiqui, and R. Ahmed, "Aggressive angiomyxoma: swirled configuration on ultrasound," *Journal of Pakistan Medical Association*, vol. 64, no. 3, pp. 345–348, 2014.

[27] H. Chen, H. Zhao, Y. Xie, and M. Jin, "Clinicopathological features and differential diagnosis of aggressive angiomyxoma of the female pelvis," *Medicine*, vol. 96, no. 20, p. e6820, 2017.

[28] J. Geng, S. Hu, and F. Wang, "Large paravaginal angiomyofibroblastoma: Magnetic resonance imaging findings," *Japanese Journal of Radiology*, vol. 29, no. 2, pp. 152–155, 2011.

[29] W. B. Laskin, J. F. Fetsch, and F. A. Tavassoli, "Angiomyofibroblastoma of the female genital tract: Analysis of 17 cases including a lipomatous variant," *Human Pathology*, vol. 28, no. 9, pp. 1046–1055, 1997.

[30] H. Kitamura, N. Miyao, Y. Sato, M. Matsukawa, T. Tsukamoto, and T. Sato, "Angiomyofibroblastoma of the female urethra," *International Journal of Urology*, vol. 6, no. 5, pp. 268–270, 1999.

[31] J. L. Kyoung, H. M. Jeung, Y. Y. Dae, H. C. Ji, J. L. In, and J. M. Seon, "Angiomyofibroblastoma arising from the posterior perivesical space: A case report with MR findings," *Korean Journal of Radiology*, vol. 9, no. 4, pp. 382–385, 2008.

[32] K. J. Mortele, G. J. Lauwers, P. J. Mergo, and P. R. Ros, "Perineal angiomyofibroblastoma: CT and MR findings with pathologic correlation," *Journal of Computer Assisted Tomography*, vol. 23, no. 5, pp. 687–689, 1999.

[33] X. Li and Z. Ye, "Aggressive angiomyxoma of the pelvis and perineum: a case report and review of the literature," *Abdominal Imaging*, vol. 36, no. 6, pp. 739–741, 2011.

[34] N. N. Jeyadevan, S. A. A. Sohaib, J. M. Thomas, A. Jeyarajah, J. H. Shepherd, and C. Fisher, "Imaging features of aggressive angiomyxoma," *Clinical Radiology*, vol. 58, no. 2, pp. 157–162, 2003.

[35] A. J. Chien, J. A. Freeby, T. T. Win, and K. A. Gadwood, "Aggressive angiomyxoma of the female pelvis: Sonographic, CT, and MR findings," *American Journal of Roentgenology*, vol. 171, no. 2, pp. 530-531, 1998.

[36] S. T. Stewart and S. M. McCarthy, "Case 77: aggressive angiomyxoma.," *Radiology*, vol. 233, no. 3, pp. 697–700, 2004.

44

Uterine Necrosis after Uterine Artery Embolization for Symptomatic Fibroids

Steve Kyende Mutiso ⓘ,[1] **Felix Mwembi Oindi ⓘ,**[1] **Nigel Hacking,**[2,3] **and Timona Obura**[1]

[1]*Department of Obstetrics and Gynaecology, Aga Khan University, Nairobi, Kenya*
[2]*University Hospital Southampton, Southampton, UK*
[3]*Aga Khan University Hospital, Nairobi, Kenya*

Correspondence should be addressed to Steve Kyende Mutiso; steve_mutiso@yahoo.com

Academic Editor: Julio Rosa-e-Silva

Introduction. Uterine artery embolization (UAE) is a minimally invasive intervention that is used in the treatment of fibroids. UAE can lead to complications including postembolization syndrome, postprocedure pain, infection, endometrial atrophy leading to secondary amenorrhea, and uterine necrosis. Uterine necrosis after UAE is very rare and hence poses a clinical dilemma for any clinician in its identification and management. We document a case of uterine necrosis after UAE and conduct a literature review on its causation, clinical features, and management principles. *Case*. A patient presented one month after UAE with abdominal pain and abdominal vaginal discharge. Her work-up revealed features of possible uterine necrosis with sepsis and she was scheduled for a laparotomy and a subtotal hysterectomy was performed. She was subsequently managed with broad spectrum antibiotic and recovered well. *Conclusion*. Uterine necrosis after UAE is a rare occurrence and we hope the documentation of this case will add to the body of knowledge around it. Theories that explain its occurrence include the use of small particles at embolization, the use of Contour-SE a spherical poly-vinyl alcohol, and lack of collateral supply to the uterus. Its symptoms may be nonspecific but unremitting abdominal pain is invariably present. Finally although conservative management may be successful at times, surgical management with hysterectomy will be required in some cases. The prognosis is good after diagnosis and surgical management.

1. Introduction

Uterine artery embolization (UAE) is a minimally invasive intervention that is used in the treatment of fibroids [1]. UAE has been used for reduction of fibroid symptoms especially menorrhagia and offers relief to women not keen on surgical intervention [2, 3]. More so, UAE has been shown to be effective in reduction of fibroid symptoms and is also cost effective when compared to surgical management [4, 5]. Although its cost effectiveness has been disputed recently when compared to surgical interventions for myomas, UAE still remains a viable option for treatment of symptoms of leiomyomas [6, 7]. UAE has contraindications including pregnancy and malignancy, with relative contraindications including existing fertility desires and large myomas that are more than 8–10 centimeters [8].

UAE has various complications associated with it that vary from minor to major [7, 9]. These include postembolization syndrome, postprocedure pain, infection, persistent PV (per vaginam) discharge, fibroid passage PV, endometrial atrophy leading to secondary amenorrhea, nontarget embolization, and uterine necrosis [6]. UAE has also been associated with altered reproductive outcomes due to its associated altered ovarian function and premature ovarian failure in some cases [4, 9]. The rates of these complications vary from around 5.7% for intraprocedural complications, 37.3% for minor complications, and around 5% for major complication within the first year after UAE [7]. These complications may be comparable in rate to the ones of surgical management of fibroids which has a complication rate of 6.3% for intraprocedural complications, 23% for minor complications, and around 7% for major complication within the first year after [6]. However, uterine necrosis after UAE remains one of the rarest complications of UAE with only about 19 cases documented from the advent of UAE [10].

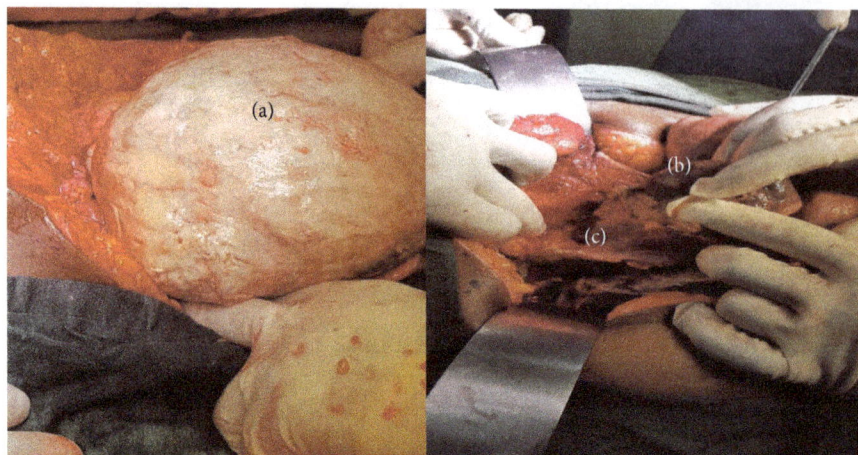

FIGURE 1: Necrosed uterus (a) and matted Necrosed Myomas (b). Serosal adhesions to small and large bowel (c).

Uterine necrosis after UAE poses a clinical dilemma for any clinician in its identification and management [10, 11]. The hypotheses of its pathophysiology include the use of very small particles in UAE (<500 microns) and lack of arterial anastomoses to embolized regions among other theories [10]. The technical risk factors of necrosis also include unselective embolization and embolization till stasis is achieved [8, 10].

Uterine necrosis after UAE has few cases that are documented in literature. Moreover, it offers a diagnostic and management dilemma to clinicians when it occurs hence outlining its clinical significance. We document a case of uterine necrosis after UA and conduct a literature review on its causation, clinical features, and management principles.

2. Case

A 56-year-old African woman presented with symptoms of severe abdominal pain and brownish foul smelling vaginal discharge that had lasted for one month after UAE. She had associated symptoms of nausea and persistent vomiting but reported no fever or any other flu like symptoms. She had an associated nonproductive cough but no other respiratory symptoms.

She had a UAE done a month prior due to symptomatic uterine fibroids with her symptoms being menorrhagia and a feeling of an abdominal mass for a duration of one year. Her Pre-UAE MRi had shown multiple enhancing uterine fibroids numbering around 15 with the largest being around 6.5 centimeters. The UAE had been done with *Spongostan* Gelfoam slurry and she was discharged home after an overnight stay. Her discharge meds after UAE included antibiotics (cefuroxime and clindamycin for a week), analgesics (diclofenac and paracetamol), and metoclopramide as an antiemetic. She had been seen 2 weeks after the UAE with no major complaints with abdominal pain being minimal. This pain worsened afterwards and was associated with a fever that resolved after an antibiotic course (clindamycin and metronidazole).

Her known comorbidities were diabetes mellitus for a duration of 3 years and hypertension for a duration of 5 years for which she was being treated with lorsartan 50 milligrams

once daily. She had not had any prior surgeries and had no other significant history in her past.

On examination she was in good general condition and was oriented in time and place. Her vitals revealed a tachycardia with a pulse of 107 beats per minute with a normal blood pressure of 104/67 millimeters of mercury and a temperature of 36.2 degrees Celsius. Abdominal examination revealed lower abdomen tenderness with a palpable pelvic mass at 14 weeks. The rest of her systems were normal in signs.

Investigations done included a full blood count which revealed a low hemoglobin level at 9.4 grams per deciliter with a normal white cell and platelet count. Her urea, creatinine, and electrolytes were all within normal limits. She had a chest X-ray done that revealed interstitial edema with borderline cardiomegaly and a subsequent computed tomography pulmonary angiogram revealed no evidence of pulmonary embolism.

In view of her worsening condition with first-line treatment and nonremitting abdominal pain, it was decided that a surgical intervention would be appropriate and since she was postmenopausal, a total hysterectomy was advised. She was subsequently scheduled for the surgery which was done on day 2 of admission. Intraoperatively we found a Necrosed uterus with a thin serosal separation that was adhered to small and large bowel (Figure 1). Necrosed Myomas were found as a distinct single matted mass of around 12 myomas (Figure 2). Multiple small pelvic abscesses were also found. A general surgery team was invited to assist in her surgery at this point. The surgery done entailed drainage of the pelvic abscesses, separation of the adhered uterine wall serosa from small bowel, and a subtotal hysterectomy. Peritoneal lavage was done with around 10 liters of 0.9% sodium chloride solution. Bilateral Jackson Pratt drains were left in situ in both pelvic gutters to drain the pelvis.

Postoperatively, she was started on intravenous antibiotics (piperacillin, tazobactam, and clindamycin) and analgesia and thromboprophylaxis with enoxaparin. She required a relook laparotomy on day 4 after surgery due to wound sepsis in which she had abdominal washouts and fascial closure. Her skin incision was left open for subsequent dressing and

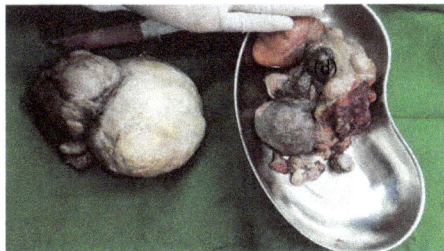

FIGURE 2: Matted Necrosed Myomas and the uterus (d) after extraction from the subtotal hysterectomy.

secondary wound closure. Her wound swab had a positive culture of *Klebsiella pneumoniae* sensitive to Meropenem which she was started on postoperatively. She recovered as an inpatient for a further 10 days and was subsequently discharged after 16 days of admission.

At her follow-up at the clinic 2 weeks afterwards, she reported marked improvement with no major concerns. She underwent subsequent wound dressing and the wound healed well and did not require secondary closure. She was discharged from follow-up care about 3 months after the surgery.

3. Discussion

Uterine necrosis after UAE is a rare complication. The outlined case report documents it and offers insight towards salient feature of its management.

The exact incidence of uterine necrosis after UAE is difficult to ascertain with only a handful of cases reported in literature [6, 10]. The exact pathophysiology of its causation is not well known although there are a few theories that try to explain why it occurs [10]. The first theory postulates that use of fine particles (<500 micrometers) may predispose to post-UAE necrosis since they may embolize even the collateral supply to the uterus provided by the cervicovaginal and utero-ovarian vessels [12]. The other theory postulates that use of a specific spherical poly-vinyl alcohol agent (PVA) as an embolizing agent may also predispose to uterine necrosis [13]. Moreover, patients who do not have good collateral anastomosis between uterine and ovarian arteries at embolization may also be at increased risk of necrosis and hence embolization is avoided if one sees collaterals at the catheter position [14]. Additionally, nonselective embolization during UAE and embolization till stasis also predispose to uterine necrosis and so selective embolization is also a key factor in trying to prevent necrosis [8, 10]. Lastly other theories that exist include the lack of antibiotic prophylaxis after UAE and the existence of sepsis [15]. The current patient had gelatin used for her embolization and the size of the particles was larger than 500 micrometers; she also had collateral anastomosis to the uterus and we used antibiotic prophylaxis after UAE and hence none of the postulated theories seem to explain the occurrence of uterine necrosis in her.

The symptoms of uterine necrosis may be nonspecific. Most commonly the reported clinical picture includes abdominal pain, fever, leucorrhea, and menorrhagia at times [10]. Patients may also present with symptoms of sepsis if concurrent infection is present [7]. The current patient had most of the above symptoms with abdominal pain and abnormal discharge; she was however not septic at presentation. Other symptoms may occur with nontarget embolization leading to concurrent necrosis of adjacent organs such as the bladder, adnexa, vagina, or even the labia which have all been reported in literature [14, 16]. The current patient had no other concurrent organs involved and hence did not have target symptoms of these organs. Clinical acumen and ultrasound may be sufficient in the diagnosis of uterine necrosis after UAE although additional imaging such as a computed tomography scan and magnetic resonance imaging may help in its diagnosis [10, 16]. The current patient did not have any preoperative scans and a clinical diagnosis was sufficient.

The treatment of uterine necrosis usually involves either removal of the Necrosed portion of the uterus and myomas or a hysterectomy [15, 17]. Conservative management has also been described in literature as an option for a handful of patients [18]. The choice of the option of treatment largely depends upon the severity of symptoms of necrosis and associated complications [11, 15]. The current patient had severe abdominal pain and also had failed conservative management with antibiotics and oral analgesics, hence the decision for surgery and hysterectomy. Additional measures that seem to aid in the good outcome of such patients are the treatment of concurrent infection with broad spectrum antibiotic and multidisciplinary management in cases of adjacent organ involvement [15, 16]. The current patient had concurrent antibiotics after the surgery due to sepsis and also had a surgical team involved in her treatment and subsequently seemed to recover well.

In conclusion, uterine necrosis after UAE is a rare occurrence and we hope the documentation of this case will add to the body of knowledge around it. Theories that explain its occurrence include the use of small particles at embolization, the use of Contour-SE a spherical poly-vinyl alcohol, and lack of collateral supply to the uterus. Its symptoms may be nonspecific but unremitting abdominal pain is invariably present. Finally although conservative management may be successful at times, surgical management with hysterectomy will be required in some cases. The prognosis is good after diagnosis and surgical management.

References

[1] L. H. Greenwood, M. G. Glickman, P. E. Schwartz, S. S. Morse, and D. F. Denny, "Obstetric and nonmalignant gynecologic bleeding: Treatment with angiographic embolization," *Radiology*, vol. 164, no. 1, pp. 155–159, 1987.

[2] S. C. Goodwin, S. Vedantham, B. McLucas, A. E. Forno, and R. Perrella, "Preliminary experience with uterine artery

embolization for uterine fibroids," *Journal of Vascular and Interventional Radiology*, vol. 8, no. 4, pp. 517–526, 1997.

[3] J. H. Ravina, J. M. Bouret, N. Ciraru-Vigneron, D. Repiquet, D. Herbreteau, A. Aymard et al., "Recourse to particular arterial embolization in the treatment of some uterine leiomyoma," *Bulletin de l'Academie nationale de medecine*, vol. 181, no. 2, pp. 233–243, 1997.

[4] J. B. Spies, "The EMMY trial of uterine artery embolization for the treatment of symptomatic uterine fibroid tumors: Randomized, yes, but a flawed trial nonetheless," *Journal of Vascular and Interventional Radiology*, vol. 17, no. 3, pp. 413–415, 2006.

[5] A. Hirst, S. Dutton, O. Wu et al., "A multi-centre retrospective cohort study comparing the efficacy, safety and cost-effectiveness of hysterectomy and uterine artery embolisation for the treatment of symptomatic uterine fibroids. The HOPEFUL study.," *Health Technology Assessment*, vol. 12, no. 5, pp. 1–248, 2008.

[6] J. K. Gupta, A. Sinha, M. A. Lumsden, and M. Hickey, "Uterine artery embolization for symptomatic uterine fibroids," *Cochrane Database of Systematic Reviews*, vol. 12, p. CD005073, 2014.

[7] M. C. M. Fonseca, R. Castro, M. Machado, T. Conte, and M. J. B. C. Girao, "Uterine Artery Embolization and Surgical Methods for the Treatment of Symptomatic Uterine Leiomyomas: A Systemic Review and Meta-analysis Followed by Indirect Treatment Comparison," *Clinical Therapeutics*, vol. 39, no. 7, pp. 1438–1455.e2, 2017.

[8] H. van Overhagen and J. A. Reekers, "Uterine Artery Embolization for Symptomatic Leiomyomata," *CardioVascular and Interventional Radiology*, vol. 38, no. 3, pp. 536–542, 2015.

[9] A. Khaund and M. A. Lumsden, "Impact of fibroids on reproductive function," *Best Practice & Research Clinical Obstetrics & Gynaecology*, vol. 22, no. 4, pp. 749–760, 2008.

[10] O. Poujade, P. F. Ceccaldi, C. Davitian et al., "Uterine necrosis following pelvic arterial embolization for post-partum hemorrhage: Review of the literature," *European Journal of Obstetrics & Gynecology and Reproductive Biology*, vol. 170, no. 2, pp. 309–314, 2013.

[11] J. P. Pelage, W. J. Walker, and O. Le Dref, "Uterine Necrosis After Uterine Artery Embolization for Leiomyoma," *Obstetrics & Gynecology*, vol. 99, no. 4, pp. 676-677, 2002.

[12] L. Coulange, N. Butori, R. Loffroy et al., "Uterine necrosis following selective embolization for postpartum hemorrhage using absorbable material," *Acta Obstetricia et Gynecologica Scandinavica*, vol. 88, no. 2, pp. 238–240, 2009.

[13] I. Repa, G. P. Moradian, L. P. Dehner et al., "Mortalities associated with use of a commercial suspension of polyvinyl alcohol," *Radiology*, vol. 170, no. 2, pp. 395–399, 1989.

[14] G. Porcu, V. Roger, A. Jacquier et al., "Uterus and bladder necrosis after uterine artery embolisation for postpartum haemorrhage," *BJOG: An International Journal of Obstetrics & Gynaecology*, vol. 112, no. 1, pp. 122-123, 2005.

[15] B. Courbiere, C. Jauffret, M. Provansal et al., "Failure of conservative management in postpartum haemorrhage: Uterine necrosis and hysterectomy after angiographic selective embolization with gelfoam," *European Journal of Obstetrics & Gynecology and Reproductive Biology*, vol. 140, no. 2, pp. 291–293, 2008.

[16] L. Löwenstein, I. Solt, E. Siegler, N. Raz, and A. Amit, "Focal cervical and vaginal necrosis following uterine artery embolisation," *European Journal of Obstetrics & Gynecology and Reproductive Biology*, vol. 116, no. 2, pp. 250-251, 2004.

[17] L. Sabatini, W. Atiomo, and A. Magos, "Successful myomectomy following infected ischaemic necrosis of uterine fibroids after uterine artery embolisation," *BJOG: An International Journal of Obstetrics & Gynaecology*, vol. 110, no. 7, pp. 704–706, 2003.

[18] M. Rohilla, P. Singh, J. Kaur, G. R. V. Prasad, V. Jain, and A. Lal, "Uterine necrosis and lumbosacral-plexopathy following pelvic vessel embolization for postpartum haemorrhage: report of two cases and review of literature," *Archives of Gynecology and Obstetrics*, vol. 290, no. 4, pp. 819–823, 2014.

45

Uterine Sarcoma Presenting with Sepsis from *Clostridium perfringens* Endometritis in a Postmenopausal Woman

Mary J. Kao ⓘ,[1] **Madhuchhanda Roy,**[2] **Josephine Harter,**[2] **and Ryan J. Spencer** ⓘ[3]

[1]*Department of Obstetrics and Gynecology, University of Wisconsin School of Medicine and Public Health, Madison, WI 53792, USA*
[2]*Department of Pathology and Laboratory Medicine, University of Wisconsin School of Medicine and Public Health, Madison, WI 53792, USA*
[3]*Division of Gynecologic Oncology, University of Wisconsin School of Medicine and Public Health, Madison, WI 53792, USA*

Correspondence should be addressed to Ryan J. Spencer; rjspencer2@wisc.edu

Academic Editor: Julio Rosa-e-Silva

Clostridium perfringens is an anaerobic gram positive rod that is found in normal vaginal and cervical flora in 1–10% of healthy women. Uterine infection with *Clostridium perfringens* is seen rarely but is often related to underlying uterine pathology and can progress quickly to sepsis. Early recognition of sepsis, prompt treatment with antibiotics, and source control with surgical management allow for optimal chance of recovery. We present a case of a postmenopausal woman who presented with sepsis, vaginal bleeding, and back pain who was found to have *Clostridium perfringens* infection in the setting of undifferentiated uterine sarcoma.

1. Introduction

Uterine sarcomas are stromal neoplasms that arise from dividing cells within the myometrium or from connective tissue elements within the endometrium. Uterine sarcoma accounts for 3 to 5% of all uterine malignancies [1]. Like other uterine malignancies, uterine sarcomas generally present with postmenopausal or abnormal uterine bleeding, abdominal pain, or pelvic pressure symptoms.

The prognosis for uterine sarcomas is generally poor compared to uterine carcinomas due to the aggressive nature of the tumor. The five-year survival rate ranges from 17 to 54% depending on the histopathological subtype [1]. We review a case of undifferentiated uterine sarcoma in a postmenopausal woman that initially presented as *Clostridium perfringens* sepsis, with the source of sepsis being endometritis in the setting of a large, necrotic tumor.

2. Case

This case involves a 79-year-old female G5P3023 who presented with *Clostridium perfringens* sepsis. She was in her usual state of health until two days prior to admission to an outside hospital with mental status changes and low back pain. She had fevers and her family reported that she seemed confused and was slow in response. She reported postmenopausal bleeding and lower abdominal pain that began a few days prior to admission. Her past medical history included history of deep venous thrombosis of her left lower extremity on lifelong anticoagulation, hypertension, hyperlipidemia, insulin resistance, hiatal hernia, and early stages of dementia. Her past surgical history was noncontributory. Her obstetrical history was significant for five pregnancies with three vaginal deliveries, a stillbirth, and a spontaneous abortion.

On admission to the outside hospital, the patient was febrile to 103°F and white blood cell count (WBC) was 12,500 cells/μL. A urinalysis was suggestive of a urinary tract infection so she was started empirically on vancomycin and ceftriaxone. Initial blood cultures grew gram positive bacilli, so metronidazole was added. CT of the abdomen and pelvis demonstrated an enlarged uterus with endometrial canal thickening and endometrial canal air with surrounding

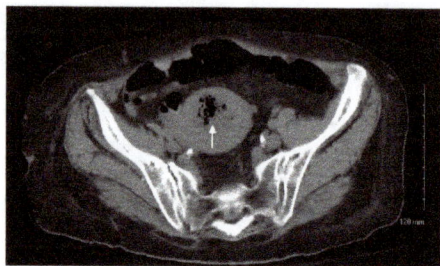

FIGURE 1: Axial CT image showing enlarged uterus with endometrial canal thickening and endometrial canal air (arrow) with surrounding inflammatory stranding, suggestive of endometritis.

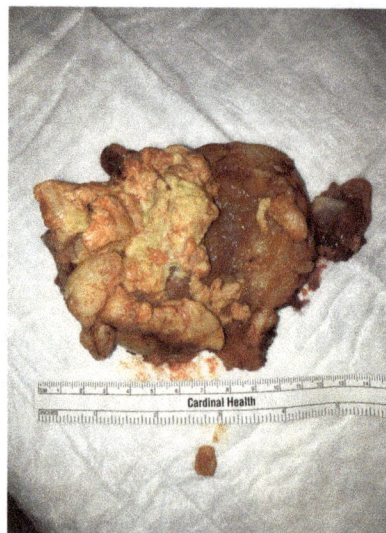

FIGURE 2: Gross specimen, bisected uterus and cervix, fallopian tubes, and ovaries, showing an exophytic, friable endometrial mass.

inflammatory stranding, suggestive of endometritis (Figure 1). Final blood cultures returned on HD3 as *Clostridium perfringens*, with the source presumed to be endometritis. Her antibiotics were changed to IV ertapenem. Follow-up blood cultures on HD2 and HD3 showed clearance of her bacteremia. She underwent dilation and curettage with an endometrial culture. Pathology revealed fragments of adenocarcinoma in a background of necrosis and the endometrial culture also grew *Clostridium perfringens*, *Bacteroides uniformis*, and scant *Peptoniphilus asaccharolyticus*. The patient was clinically stable and was transferred to our tertiary care center for management of her adenocarcinoma in the setting of *Clostridium perfringens* endometritis and septicemia after seven days at the outside hospital and seven days on IV antibiotics. Over time at the outside institution, her mental status improved and was clinically stable.

On evaluation after transfer, the patient felt well and denied pain or nausea. She was tolerating oral intake, voiding, having regular bowel movements, and ambulating. On exam, her vitals were normal and her BMI was 28.68 kg/m^2. Her abdomen was soft, nondistended, and nontender with no rebound or guarding. Her extremities were warm and well perfused with significant venous stasis changes on bilateral lower extremities with associated skin breakdown. Her neurological exam was grossly intact. On pelvic exam, she had a smooth cervix and small 6-week sized mobile uterus, and no adnexal masses were appreciated. No purulent discharge was noted.

On admission to our institution (HD 7), laboratory values were significant for normal electrolytes, INR of 3.4, and white blood cell count of 10,000 cells/μL. The IV ertapenem was continued. CT scan of the chest, abdomen, and pelvis was repeated, which showed a decrease in the gas component compared to the previous exam seven days earlier. The patient was clinically stable so preoperative planning was undertaken and included reversal of therapeutic anticoagulation. She received vitamin K on HD 7 with a repeat INR of 2.1. She was then given two units of fresh frozen plasma on HD 8 prior to surgery.

On HD 8, she underwent a total laparoscopic hysterectomy and bilateral salpingo-oophorectomy. Given her recent clinical condition, decision was made prior to surgery to forego lymphadenectomy which was discussed with patient. Intraoperative findings revealed purulence draining from the cervical os. The uterus was enlarged and globular, but mobile. Her fallopian tubes and ovaries were normal in appearance. There were no adnexal masses or evidence of metastatic disease. The procedure was uncomplicated and estimated blood loss was 300 cc. Intraoperatively, she received one unit of packed red blood cells due to acute blood loss superimposed on chronic anemia. Her preoperative hemoglobin was 8.2. After the procedure, she was transitioned from IV ertapenem to IV ceftriaxone and oral clindamycin per infectious disease consultant recommendations to provide excellent coverage for clostridial bacteremia and enteric gram negative rods in the immediate postoperative setting. Postoperative course was uncomplicated and she was discharged to a skilled nursing facility on HD 10/POD 2. She was discharged on oral ciprofloxacin with a plan for three additional days of treatment and oral clindamycin for fourteen additional days.

A picture of the bisected gross specimen is shown in Figure 2. The cervix is directly over the 8-9 cm marker of the ruler; the left tube and ovary are clearly visualized with the right tube visible at approximately 10 o'clock behind the necrotic intrauterine mass. Pathology revealed an undifferentiated uterine sarcoma mainly in the endometrium with invasion into the inner half of the myometrium. On gross examination, the endometrial cavity revealed an exophytic and friable mass (6.2 × 5.4 × 2.3 cm) located 2.2 cm from the lower uterine segment. Additional detached fragments of loose pink-tank, friable tumor mass (5.5 × 5.0 × 2.0 cm) were also submitted for histologic examination. The cervix, bilateral ovaries, and fallopian tubes were not grossly involved.

Microscopically, the tumor was centered in the endometrium and was composed entirely of spindled to oval cells (Figures 3(a)–3(c)). Mitoses were readily identified (Figure 3(c), circles). There were large areas of necrosis. Differential diagnostic considerations included carcinosarcoma (malignant mixed Müllerian tumor/MMMT), endometrial stromal sarcoma (both low and high grade

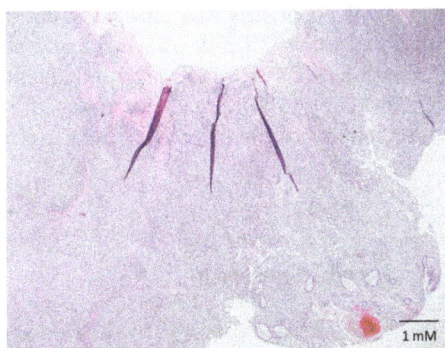

(a) Microscopic tumor with spindled to oval cells and large areas of necrosis

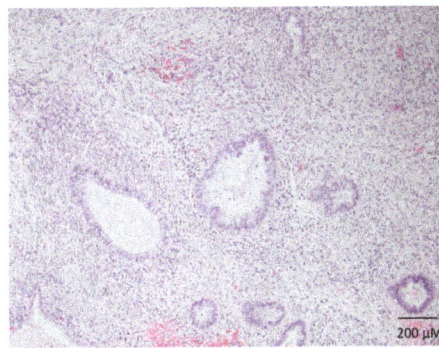

(b) Microscopic tumor with a few mildly atypical glandular epithelial elements but no overtly carcinomatous component identified

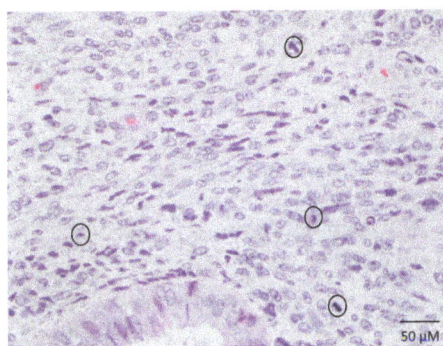

(c) Microscopic tumor with mitotic figures

FIGURE 3

variants), adenosarcoma with sarcomatous overgrowth, and leiomyosarcoma. While there were a few mildly atypical glandular epithelial elements, no overtly carcinomatous component was identified, militating against the diagnosis of carcinosarcoma (Figures 3(a) and 3(b)).

Immunohistochemically, the malignant cells demonstrated patchy positivity for cytokeratin AE1/AE3, ER (estrogen receptor), PR (progesterone receptor), CD10, cyclin D1, h-caldesmon, desmin, and SMA (smooth muscle actin) and were negative for myogenin, ALK, and DOG-1 (not shown). Fluorescence in situ hybridization (FISH) testing for *JAZF1*, *PHF1*, and *YWHAE* rearrangements was negative.

The pathology slides of the dilation and curettage from the outside hospital were reviewed and compared to the hysterectomy specimen. While specimens did contain some mildly atypical glandular epithelial elements, they were detached and did not have an overtly malignant morphology. When evaluated in the context of the hysterectomy specimen, which contained no carcinomatous component, we interpreted that glandular component as fragments of benign cervix/endometrium.

The patient was followed up in the office 5 weeks after surgery and had recovered well although still requiring intermittent nursing care at home. Adjuvant chemotherapy with gemcitabine and docetaxel was recommended at that time and arrangements were made to see a medical oncologist closer to her home. Ultimately, she was diagnosed with a second primary lung cancer a short time after her recovery which was not apparent on her imaging for this hospital admission. A few months later she died from what was thought to be diffuse metastatic disease with multiple lung masses by the physicians caring for her at that time.

3. Discussion

Clostridium species are anaerobic gram positive rods and are commonly found in nature in soil and marine sediments due to their ability to form endospores. *Clostridium* soft tissue infections are seen in wound contamination, anaerobic cellulitis, myonecrosis, and necrotizing fasciitis [2]. Clostridial myonecrosis, also known as clostridial gas gangrene, is a life-threatening muscle infection that often develops contiguously from an area of trauma or from hematogenous spread from the gastrointestinal tract with muscle seeding.

Clostridium species produce extracellular toxins known as alpha and theta toxins. Alpha toxins cause the absence of tissue inflammatory response by potently stimulating platelet aggregation and upregulating adherence molecules on polymorphonuclear leukocytes and endothelial cells. This causes a decline in muscle blood flow and ischemic necrosis due to the formation of occlusive intravascular aggregates composed of activated platelets, leukocytes, and fibrin. Theta toxin causes reduced systemic vascular resistance and increased cardiac output via induction of endogenous mediators such as prostacyclin and platelet activating factor that caused vasodilation [3, 4].

Clostridium myonecrosis progresses rapidly, often presenting with sudden onset severe pain at the site of infection with a mean incubation period of less than 24 hours. Signs of systemic infection include tachycardia, fever, shock, and multiorgan failure. Other complications of clostridial myonecrosis include jaundice, renal failure, hypotension, and liver necrosis. This was the case for our patient, who was in her usual state of health until two days prior to presentation when she started having lower back and abdominal pain. She had also been experiencing fevers in the 24 hours prior to admission and presented with altered mental status secondary to sepsis. Treatment includes early recognition of infection, surgical debridement, antibiotic therapy, and supportive measures [5]. Antibiotic therapy should include penicillin plus clindamycin or tetracycline. Our patient received antibiotics promptly and once the source of the infection was confirmed, prompt surgical removal of the infected organ was performed upon arrival to our institution. Prognosis is worse in patients who are already in shock at the time of diagnosis. In a series of 139 patients treated with antibiotics, surgery, and hyperbaric oxygen, 67 were in shock at admission, and all deaths (27 patients) occurred in this subset. Overall survival was 81% [6].

Clostridial myonecrosis is most commonly seen in wartime injuries or among victims of natural disasters due to delayed treatment of injuries. Less commonly, *Clostridium* infection is also seen in obstetrics, associated with abortion, retained placenta, intrauterine fetal demise, or prolonged rupture of membranes. *C. perfringens* is considered normal vaginal flora, found in the vagina and cervix in 1–10% of healthy women [7]. In the absence of infection, *C. perfringens* has no clinical significance and causes clinical illness in only about 5% of isolates [7]. *C. perfringens* uterine infection, while rare, is most commonly associated with uterine instrumentation during procedures such as dilation and curettage or during the postpartum period—neither of which preceded this infection.

We were able to identify only six other cases of clostridial sepsis in postmenopausal women in the literature. These women also had underlying uterine pathology, including four cases with uterine endometrial adenocarcinoma [8–10] and two cases with degenerating uterine leiomyoma [11, 12]. Of the cases with endometrial adenocarcinoma, two were being treated with intrauterine radiocesium and the infection is thought to have been transmitted from one patient to the next. The third case was a spontaneous case of clostridial infection, who presented with sepsis similar to our patient but had progressed to the point of uterine perforation and was treated with emergency surgery.

In the current case, the underlying uterine sarcoma likely made the uterus more susceptible to infection, resulting in a quick progression to septicemia. The tumor had large areas of necrosis into the myometrium and vascular insufficiency, likely predisposing the site to infection. Clinically, sepsis was identified promptly and the patient was started on broad-spectrum antibiotics while the source of infection was investigated. Although surgical exploration and removal of the involved organs was ultimately undertaken, it was not until eight days after diagnosis. Ideally, surgery would have been undertaken immediately upon diagnosis or suspicion of a necrotizing soft tissue infection as source control is critical to patient outcome and optimizing antimicrobial therapy.

Acknowledgments

The research was supported by the Department of Obstetrics and Gynecology at the University of Wisconsin School of Medicine and Public Health.

References

[1] C. G. Tropé, V. M. Abeler, and G. B. Kristensen, "Diagnosis and treatment of sarcoma of the uterus. A review," *Acta Oncologica*, vol. 51, no. 6, pp. 694–705, 2012.

[2] M. M. Awad, A. E. Bryant, D. L. Stevens, and J. I. Rood, "Virulence studies on chromosomal α-toxin and Θ-toxin mutants constructed by allelic exchange provide genetic evidence for the essential role of α-toxin in Clostridium perfringens-mediated gas gangrene," *Molecular Microbiology*, vol. 15, no. 2, pp. 191–202, 1995.

[3] D. L. Stevens, J. Mitten, and C. Henry, "Effects of α and θ Toxins from Clostridium Perfringens on Human Polymorphonuclear Leukocytes," *The Journal of Infectious Diseases*, vol. 156, no. 2, pp. 324–333, 1987.

[4] D. L. Stevens, R. W. Titball, M. Jepson, C. R. Bayer, S. M. Hayes-Schroer, and A. E. Bryant, "Immunization with the C-domain of α-toxin prevents lethal infection, localizes tissue injury, and promotes host response to challenge with Clostridium perfringens," *The Journal of Infectious Diseases*, vol. 190, no. 4, pp. 767–773, 2004.

[5] I. Brook, "Microbiology and management of soft tissue and muscle infections," *International Journal of Surgery*, vol. 6, no. 4, pp. 328–338, 2008.

[6] G. B. Hart, R. C. Lamb, and M. B. Strauss, "Gas gangrene: I. A collective review," *Journal of Trauma - Injury Infection and Critical Care*, vol. 23, no. 11, pp. 991–1000, 1983.

[7] T. F. Halpin and J. A. Molinari, "Diagnosis and management of Clostridium perfringens sepsis and uterine gas gangrene," *Obstetrical & Gynecological Survey*, vol. 57, no. 1, pp. 53–57, 2002.

[8] R. P. Symonds and A. G. Robertson, "Clostridium welchii septicaemia after intrauterine caesium insertion," *British Medical Journal*, vol. 1, no. 6115, pp. 754-755, 1978.

[9] R. Kurashina, H. Shimada, T. Matsushima, D. Doi, H. Asakura, and T. Takeshita, "Spontaneous uterine perforation due to clostridial gas gangrene associated with endometrial carcinoma," *Journal of Nippon Medical School*, vol. 77, no. 3, pp. 166–169, 2010.

[10] J. Braverman, A. Adachi, M. Lev-Gur et al., "Spontaneous clostridia gas gangrene of uterus associated with endometrial malignancy," *American Journal of Obstetrics & Gynecology*, vol. 156, no. 5, pp. 1205–1207, 1987.

[11] C. S. Bryant, L. Perry, J. P. Shah, S. Kumar, and G. Deppe, "Life-threatening clostridial sepsis in a postmenopausal patient with degenerating uterine leiomyoma," *Case Reports in Medicine*, vol. 2010, Article ID 541959, 2010.

[12] B. M. Kaufmann, J. M. Cooper, and P. Cookson, "Clostridium perfringens septicemia complicating degenerating uterine leiomyomas," *American Journal of Obstetrics & Gynecology*, vol. 118, no. 6, pp. 877-878, 1974.

46

Epithelioid Angiosarcoma Arising from a Huge Leiomyoma: A Case Report and a Literature Review

Takeya Hara [ID]**, Ai Miyoshi, Yuji Kamei, Nao Wakui, Akiko Fujishiro, Serika Kanao, Hirokazu Naoi, Hirofumi Otsuka, and Takeshi Yokoi**

Department of Obstetrics and Gynecology, Kaizuka City Hospital, Osaka, Japan

Correspondence should be addressed to Takeya Hara; tttake.0303@gmail.com

Academic Editor: Giampiero Capobianco

Uterine mesenchymal tumors other than leiomyosarcoma, carcinosarcoma, and endometrial stromal sarcomas are extremely uncommon. We describe a case of epithelioid angiosarcoma of the uterus and review previous literature on such rare tumors. A 48-year-old woman presented with a 1-year history of abdominal fullness and 10kg weight loss. Pelvic magnetic resonance imaging (MRI) revealed a huge (30×18cm) uterus accompanied by degeneration and necrosis. She underwent supracervical hysterectomy and right salpingo-oophorectomy. We postoperatively diagnosed the mass as an epithelioid angiosarcoma arising from a leiomyoma. Vasodilatation was observed within the range of 2 cm × several mm in the leiomyoma, and proliferation of atypical cells was observed covering the surface of the luminal side. The tumor showed a partly fine vascular structure and was associated with obvious nuclear atypia and mitotic figures. She received 6 courses of adjuvant chemotherapy with paclitaxel, epirubicin, and carboplatin, and there have been no signs of recurrence for 10 months.

1. Introduction

Angiosarcoma is defined as a tumor of the endothelial cells presenting in blood vessels. Microscopically, the tumor is composed of anastomosing vascular tubes, having endothelial cells in larger numbers than needed to line the vessels [1]. Angiosarcoma accounts for less than 1% of all soft tissue sarcomas. It is an aggressive and malignant soft tissue neoplasm [2]. Although angiosarcoma can arise in any region of the body, most occur in the skin or superficial soft tissue in the elderly [3]. Uterine mesenchymal tumors other than leiomyosarcoma, carcinosarcoma, and endometrial stromal sarcomas are uncommon. Primary uterine epithelioid angiosarcoma is an extremely rare malignant tumor with a poor prognosis. We report here a new case of epithelioid angiosarcoma arising in a leiomyoma of the uterus and we include a literature review concerning the previous similar cases in the past 50 years.

2. Case Presentation

A 48-year-old woman, gravida 1, para 1, visited the internal medicine department at another hospital with a complaint of abdominal fullness and weight loss of 10kg during the last year. A huge abdominal mass was palpated, and she was referred to the gynecology department to search for a tumor of uterine origin. She was premenopausal and had no significant past medical history. Physical findings revealed a large elastic hard mass extending from the xiphoid to the pubic bone. The magnetic resonance imaging (MRI) examination revealed a huge tumor on the uterine corpus, and a number of dilated vessels were observed between the tumor and the myometrium. Therefore, the tumor was suspected to derive from the uterus. The tumor showed an uneven signal on T2-weighted sagittal section (Figure 1), and the enhanced MRI study showed that the tumor edge but not the center was enhanced (Figure 2). As such, necrosis was suspected to have occurred in the center of the tumor. Uterine sarcoma was primarily suspected due to the large size, degeneration, and necrosis on MRI imaging. Computed tomography (CT) examination showed no lymph node swelling or distant metastasis. Preoperative laboratory testing revealed anemia (hemoglobin level, 5.6g/dl). We transfused 18 units of RCC before surgery. CT examination and ultrasonography on lower extremities indicated an

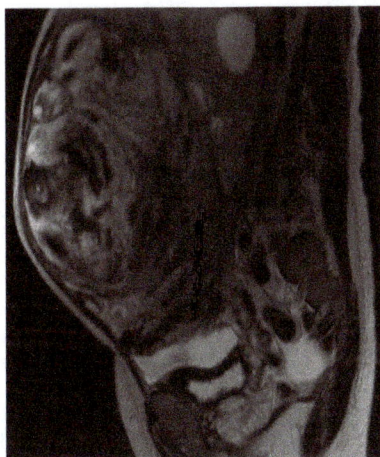

FIGURE 1: MRI image of a T2-weighted sagittal section. A huge abdominal tumor derived from the uterus, presenting with uneven intratumor signal.

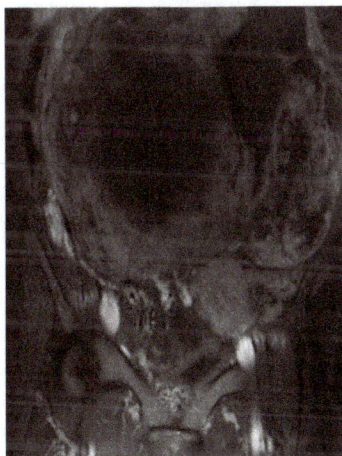

FIGURE 2: MRI image of a Gadolinium enhanced T1-weighted coronal section. The center of the abdominal tumor was not enhanced, implicating a suspicion of necrosis in the center.

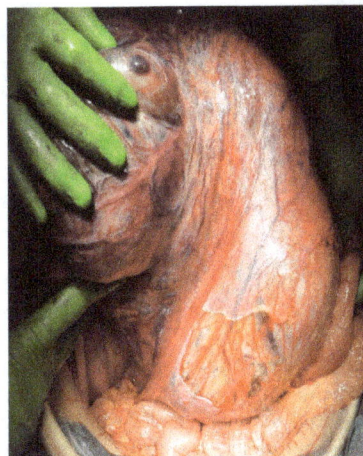

FIGURE 3: Intraoperative findings of the abdominal tumor. The surgery revealed a huge tumor occupying the space from the pelvis to the diaphragm. The tumor surface was smooth and hard with many dilated veins.

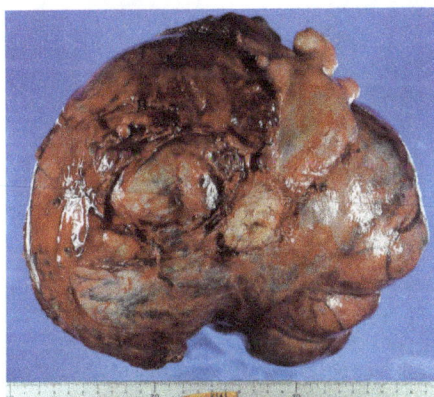

FIGURE 4: Gross findings of the excised tumor. The size of the tumor was 28 × 23 cm and the weight was 7600g. The tumor showed continuity with the posterior wall of the uterus.

absence of thrombosis. Preoperative serum levels of CEA, CA 19-9, CA 125, and LDH were within normal limits. A biopsy of the endometrium was not collected as the sounding examination of the endometrium was unsuccessful due to a deviated uterine cervix. At this point, preoperatively, we suspected the tumor was a leiomyosarcoma or leiomyoma with degeneration.

The patient underwent laparotomy, where we identified a huge tumor occupying a space from the pelvis to the diaphragm. The tumor surface was smooth and hard with many dilated veins (Figure 3). A massive tumor with a diameter of 30 cm was observed arising from the posterior uterine wall with a smooth contour and invaded the retroperitoneal cavity under the mesentery. The tumor was firmly adhered to both the mesentery and right ovary. There were no findings of extra-uterine dissemination. The intraoperative frozen section report for the uterine tumor

was of degenerated myoma with no findings indicating malignancy. A total abdominal hysterectomy (TAH) and right salpingo-oophorectomy (RSO) were performed. The operation duration and blood loss were approximately 216 minutes and 1000 ml, respectively. The excised specimen weighed 7600 g.

Macroscopic findings of the tumor revealed a well-circumscribed tumor showing extensive continuity with the posterior wall of the uterus, measuring 28 × 23 cm (Figure 4). On the sliced surface of the tumor, an obvious heterogeneous pattern was recognized within the mixture of a whitish homogeneous area, suggesting benign uterine fibroids, and a vulnerable area, due to bleeding and necrosis (Figure 5).

For the intraoperative frozen section, we examined three areas, namely, a white homogenous part, a necrotic part, and a cystic part, of which all were findings of a leiomyoma. In the permanent histological examination, 10 additional sections were collected from the tumor. The basic histological findings of all the sections were the same. The tumor was

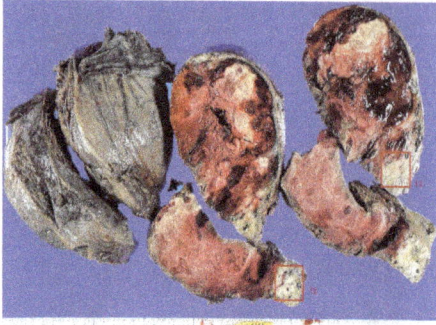

FIGURE 5: Macroscopic findings of sections of the tumor. On the sliced surface of the tumor, an obvious heterogeneous pattern was recognized within the mixture of a white homogeneous area, suggesting benign uterine fibroids, and a vulnerable part, due to bleeding and necrosis.

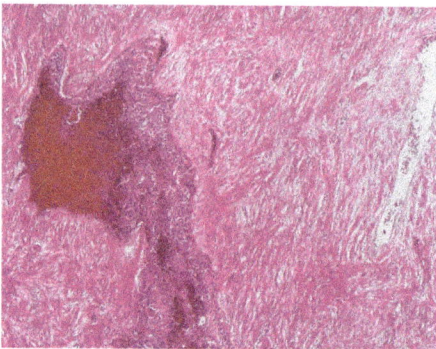

FIGURE 6: Microscopic findings of the tumor (H.E. stain; original magnification X40). The tumor was mostly composed of spindle-shaped cells, consistent with degenerated leiomyoma. Enlargement of blood vessels was observed within an area of about 2 cm × several mm, and proliferation of atypical cells showing a fine meshwork microvascular structure was observed in the blood vessel cavity.

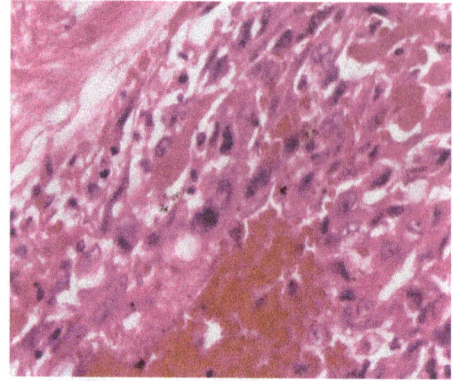

FIGURE 7: Microscopic findings of the tumor (H.E. stain; original magnification X400). These atypical cells consisted of various contours, such as cubic, polygonal, and short spindle shape. The nucleus was circular with a high degree of vacuolar enlargement and pleomorphism. Abnormal mitotic figures were also interspersed.

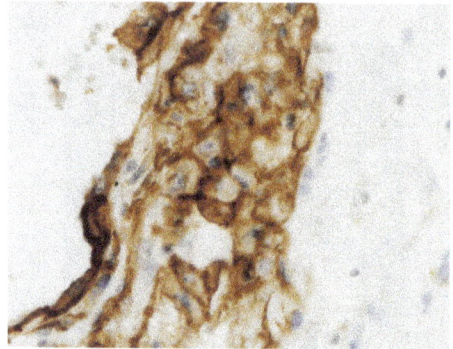

FIGURE 8: Immunohistochemical findings of the tumor (ERG; original magnification X400). The cytoplasm of the tumor cells was strongly positive for ERG stains.

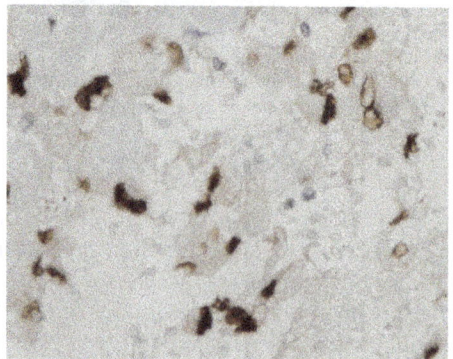

FIGURE 9: Immunohistochemical findings of the tumor (CD31; original magnification X400). The cytoplasm of the tumor cells was diffusely positive for CD31 stains.

comprised of spindle-shaped cells, homologous to smooth muscle cells, which were arranged in bundles with areas of hyalinization, consistent with a degenerated leiomyoma. The tumor was mostly comprised of degenerated uterine leiomyoma. However, enlarged blood vessels were observed within an area of approximately 2 cm × several mm, and proliferation of atypical cells showing a fine meshwork microvascular structure was observed in the blood vessel cavity (Figure 6). These atypical cells consisted of various contours, such as cubic, polygonal, and short spindle shape. The nucleus was circular with a high degree of vacuolar enlargement and pleomorphism. Abnormal mitotic figures were also interspersed (Figure 7). A tumor derived from a blood vessel was thus considered, and malignancy was suggested by the presence of nuclear atypia and abnormal mitosis.

Immunohistochemical analysis revealed the atypical tumor cells to be positive for ERG, CD31, and AE1/3 (Figures 8 and 9), partially positive for Factor VIII, and negative for α-SMA, desmin, H-caldesmon, EMA, CD34, and D2-40. From the above, the atypical tumor cells were of epithelial origin and the final diagnosis was epithelioid angiosarcoma arising in a degenerated uterine leiomyoma.

The efficacy of postoperative adjuvant therapy for angiosarcoma has not been demonstrated and there is currently no established chemotherapy regimen. In this case, because the atypical tumor was observed in the blood vessel cavity, we thought it could have been spread hematogenously throughout the body. Hence, we selected adjuvant chemotherapy rather than adjuvant radiotherapy. Six courses of combination adjuvant chemotherapy with paclitaxel (150mg/m2), epirubicin (50mg/m2), and carboplatin (area under the curve = 4) were administered in the present case, following referral to previous reported cases. No recurrence has been observed 10 months after the primary surgery.

3. Discussion

Soft tissue sarcoma accounts for less than 1 percent of all adult malignancies [4]. Less than 1% of all soft tissue sarcoma are angiosarcoma [2]. It can occur in any region of the body. Approximately half of the angiosarcomas occur in the skin, followed by breast and soft tissues. These account for 75% of angiosarcomas [5]. Chronic lymphedema and radiation are the most widely recognized predisposing factors for angiosarcoma of the skin and soft tissue. In general, angiosarcoma has an overall 5-year survival of approximately 35% [6]. Even with localized disease and optimal surgery conditions, only 60% of patients survive for more than 5 years. In advanced cases, the prognosis is poor with a median survival of 7 months [7].

Although angiosarcoma rarely occurs in the female genital tract [6], it has been reported to originate from the uterus, cervix, fallopian tube, ovary, uterine parametrium, broad ligament, and vagina [8]. To our knowledge, only 22 cases have been reported to date [8–25], as summarized in Table 1. Here we report the 23rd case in the literature.

Uterine angiosarcoma can occur in both premenopausal and postmenopausal women, although most women who develop uterine epithelioid angiosarcoma are postmenopausal. The most common symptom is vaginal bleeding, and in some cases patients come to the hospital with anemia or weight loss. The median age of the 23 patients was 61 years (range, 17-81 years). The uterus was characteristically large for almost all those women. It is clearly described with image inspection such as ultrasound, CT, and MRI. Our case also had a large uterus, but the patient was premenopausal. As such, this is considered a very rare case of angiosarcoma.

There are characteristic pathological findings, both grossly and microscopically. Grossly, the tumor is composed of whitish or grayish hemorrhagic tissue with areas of necrosis or calcification. It may have a lobulated pattern [10, 11, 13]. Our case had similar macroscopic findings and angiosarcoma was detected from whitish hemorrhagic tissue.

The histological features can vary and as such, distinguishing angiosarcoma from a benign proliferative or inflammatory lesion with light microscopy is often difficult. Microscopically, the tumors contain irregular rudimentary vascular significant pleomorphism and nuclear hyperchromatism, with frequent mitotic figures. In addition, there are numerous solid areas composed of cells that have eosinophilic cytoplasm with occasional vacuolization and round nuclei. Binucleated and multinucleated giant tumor cells are also present [11, 15].

Angiosarcomas are typically positive for endothelial markers including CD31, CD34, and Factor VIII. Muscle markers such as actin, desmin, and S-100 protein are usually negative. Concerning the epithelial marker AE 1/3, such tumors are often negative but were positive in the present case [15]. Immunohistochemical analysis is therefore important in confirming the diagnosis.

There is a lack of consensus on the optimal treatment and factors influencing the prognosis for angiosarcoma of the uterus. Most published reports of angiosarcoma treatment are retrospective case series. Wide resections are often required because of the invasive and multifocal nature of angiosarcoma.

In the past 50 years, all patients were initially treated by TAH with bilateral salpingo-oophorectomy (BSO). The limited information available in the literature does not support a routine pelvic and/or para-aortic lymphadenectomy.

Some patients who underwent postoperative adjuvant chemotherapy and radiotherapy have survived for more than 4 years but are limited. Chemotherapy is also performed in various combinations, but there is no established regimen. Paclitaxel is currently the most commonly used drug for angiosarcoma [26]. In one report, eight of nine patients with scalp angiosarcoma experienced a major response, four with partial responses and four clinically complete responses with paclitaxel [7]. However, the largest study of adjuvant chemotherapy in soft tissue sarcoma has failed to demonstrate any survival advantage [27]. High dose adjuvant radiotherapy (>50 Gy) and wide treatment field are recommended due to the high risk of local recurrence. No formal radiotherapy trials have been done, but retrospective studies suggest that it improves local control and overall survival [28]. There is no compelling evidence for adjuvant chemotherapy and radiotherapy. We administered combined chemotherapy, including paclitaxel as adjuvant chemotherapy, with reference to previous case reports

Uterine angiosarcoma often recurs within a few months, and its prognosis is very poor (Table 1). However, there are 4 cases with no recurrence for more than 3 years following surgical treatment alone. In three cases, the lesion was as small as 5 cm or less, and invasion of the uterine myometrium was less than half [13, 17, 23]. Based on these findings, if the tumor diameter is 5 cm or less with less than half of the myometrium being invaded, it may be possible to extend the prognosis with only wide resection surgery.

Among the 23 cases, there are only six cases of epithelioid angiosarcoma arising in the leiomyoma of the uterus. It suggests that the increased vascular proliferation secondary to a mechanical pressure effect of adjacent leiomyomas might have induced the endothelial neoplastic transformation [16]. However, most uterine angiosarcomas were not associated with uterine leiomyoma. This finding suggests that whereas uterine angiosarcoma can arise in association with uterine leiomyomas, it more commonly develops de novo [21].

Recently, laparoscopic treatment has been widely conducted in the gynecological field. Petrillo et al. reported cases of low grade endometrial stromal sarcoma occurred in the site of trocar placement five years after laparoscopic myomectomy with intraabdominal morcellation. Therefore,

TABLE 1: **Summary of the uterine epithelioid angiosarcomas in literature review**. TAH: total abdominal hysterectomy, BSO: bilateral salpingo-oophorectomy, LSO: left salpingo-oophorectomy, RSO: right salpingo-oophorectomy, POM: partial omentectomy, PLN: pelvic lymphadenectomy, PAN: para-aortic lymphadenectomy, NED: no evidence of disease, DOD: dead of disease.

Case No.	Author (Year)	Age	size	Presentation	Treatment	Outcome (months)
1	Purola and Strandell (1967)	57	–	Vaginal bleeding	TAH, BSO appendectomy, RT	NED, 18mo
2	Ehrmann and Griffiths (1979)	17	9	Vaginal bleeding	TAH, LSO, CT, RT	DOD, 84mo
3	Ongkasuwan (1982)	70	11	Malaise weight loss	TAH, BSO	NED, 5mo
4	Witkin (1987)	71	15×17×7	Vaginal bleeding	TAH, BSO, RT	Reccurence 6mo
5	Milne (1990)	76	18	Vaginal bleeding urinary retention	TAH, BSO	DOD, 6mo
6	Quinonez (1991)	65	8	Vaginal bleeding	TAH, BSO, PLN CT, RT	NED, 48mo
7	Lack (1991)	71	–	Vaginal bleeding	TAH, BSO, RT	DOD, 2mo
8	Tallini (1993)	56	30×24	Vaginal bleeding	TAH, BSO, POM PAN, appendectomy,	DOD, 7mo
9	Drachenberg (1994)	58	12	Vaginal bleeding	TAH, BSO, CT, RT	DOD, 2mo
10	Schammel (1998)	49	29×29×19	Vaginal mass	TAH, BSO	DOD, 3mo
11	Schammel (1998)	58	12	Vaginal bleeding	TAH, BSO, CT, RT	DOD, 2mo
12	Schammel (1998)	70	5×3×3	Vaginal bleeding	TAH, BSO	NED, 37mo
13	Schammel (1998)	75	6×6×5	Vaginal bleeding	TAH, BSO	DOD, 7mo
14	Mendez (1999)	59	12-wk-size uterus	Vaginal bleeding	TAH, BSO	DOD, 2.5mo
15	Konishi (2007)	62	17×15×7.5	Anemia	TAH, BSO, CT	NED, 2mo
16	Cardinale (2008)	81	8×7×5	Lower abdominal pain anemia	TAH, BSO	DOD, 6mo
17	Cardinale (2008)	35	25	Shortness of breath dry cough	TAH, BSO	No information
18	Olawaiye (2008)	54	11×6	Enlarged uterus	TAH, BSO	NED,12mo
19	Hwang and Lim (2013)	61	12×10×9	Vaginal bleeding	TAH, BSO, PAN, RT	No information
20	Suzuki (2014)	64	7.5×5.5×3.5	Vaginal bleeding	TAH, BSO	DOD, 50mo
21	Yankun Liu (2015)	56	11×8×7	Anemia	TAH, BSO	No information
22	Strickland (2017)	67	21×18×15	Fatigue, weight loss	TAH, BSO	DOD, 2mo

we propose that laparoscopic procedure should be avoided when treating leiomyoma with potential malignant tumors [29].

Suzuki et al. identified breakages at three loci, i.e., YWHAE (17p13), FAM22A (10q23), and FAM22B (10q22) in the case of uterine angiosarcoma. These findings suggest that an abnormality in the loci of YWHAE, FAM22A, and

FAM22B may contribute to the development of uterine angiosarcoma [23].

We described a patient with a primary angiosarcoma arising from a leiomyoma that was treated initially by surgery and adjuvant chemotherapy. If the tumor diameter is 5 cm or less with less than half of the muscle layer being infiltrated, it may be possible to extend the prognosis by performing wide resection it. Moreover, in the presence of a huge uterus, angiosarcoma may be contained within. Consequently, detailed histological diagnosis for whitish or grayish hemorrhagic tissue with areas of necrosis or calcification is required.

References

[1] A. P. Stout, "Hemangio-endothelioma: atumor of blood vessels featuring vascular endothelial cells," *Annals of Surgery*, vol. 118, no. 3, pp. 445–464, 1943.

[2] S. W. Weiss and J. R. Goldblum, *Enzinger and Weiss's Soft Tissue Tumors*, 5th edition, 2008.

[3] J. C. Maddox and H. L. Evans, "Angiosarcoma of skin and soft tissue: a study of forty-four cases," *Cancer*, vol. 48, no. 8, pp. 1907–1921, 1981.

[4] R. L. Siegel, K. D. Miller, and A. Jemal, "Cancer statistics, 2017," *CA: A Cancer Journal for Clinicians*, vol. 67, no. 1, pp. 7–30, 2017.

[5] G. Lahat, A. R. Dhuka, H. Hallevi et al., "Angiosarcoma: clinical and molecular insights," *Annals of Surgery*, vol. 251, no. 6, pp. 1098–1106, 2010.

[6] R. J. Young, N. J. Brown, M. W. Reed, D. Hughes, and P. J. Woll, "Angiosarcoma," *The Lancet Oncology*, vol. 11, no. 10, pp. 983–991, 2010.

[7] F. Fata, E. O'Reilly, D. Ilson et al., "Paclitaxel in the treatment of patients with angiosarcoma of the scalp or face," *Cancer*, vol. 86, no. 10, pp. 2034–2037, 1999.

[8] G. B. Witkin, F. B. Askin, J. D. Geratz, and R. L. Reddick, "Angiosarcoma of the uterus: A light microscopic immunohistochemical and ultrastructural study," *International Journal of Gynecological Pathology*, vol. 6, pp. 176–184, 1987.

[9] E. Purola and R. Strandell, "Haemangioendothelioma of the uterus," *Annales Chirurgiae Et Gynaecologiae Fenniae*, vol. 56, no. 1, pp. 102–104, 1967.

[10] R. L. Ehrmann and C. T. Griffiths, "Malignant hemangioendothelioma of the uterus," *Gynecologic Oncology*, vol. 8, no. 3, pp. 376–383, 1979.

[11] C. Ongkasuwan, J. E. Taylor, C. K. Tang, and T. Prempree, "Angiosarcomas of the uterus and ovary: clinicopathologic report," *Cancer*, vol. 49, no. 7, pp. 1469–1475, 1982.

[12] D. S. Milne, K. Hinshaw, A. J. Malcolm, and P. Hilton, "Primary angiosarcoma of the uterus: a case report," *Histopathology*, vol. 16, no. 2, pp. 203–205, 1990.

[13] G. E. Quinonez, M. P. Paraskevas, M. S. Diocee, and S. M. Lorimer, "Angiosarcoma of the uterus: A case report," *American Journal of Obstetrics & Gynecology*, vol. 164, no. 1, pp. 90–92, 1991.

[14] E. E. Lack, P. Bitterman, and J. T. Sundeen, "Müllerian adenosarcoma of the uterus with pure angiosarcoma: Case report," *Human Pathology*, vol. 22, no. 12, pp. 1289–1291, 1991.

[15] G. Tallini, F. V. Price, and M. L. Carcangiu, "Epithelioid angiosarcoma arising in uterine leiomyomas," *American Journal of Clinical Pathology*, vol. 100, no. 5, pp. 514–518, 1993.

[16] C. B. Drachenberg, F. J. Faust, A. Borkowski, and J. C. Papadimitriou, "Epithelioid angiosarcoma of the uterus arising in a leiomyoma with associated ovarian and tubal angiomatosis,"

American Journal of Clinical Pathology, vol. 102, no. 3, pp. 388-388, 1994.

[17] D. P. Schammel and F. A. Tavassoli, "Uterine angiosarcomas: A morphologic and immunohistochemical study of four cases," *The American Journal of Surgical Pathology*, vol. 22, no. 2, pp. 246–250, 1998.

[18] L. E. Mendez, S. Joy, R. Angioli, R. Estape, and M. Penalver, "Primary uterine angiosarcoma," *Gynecologic Oncology*, vol. 75, no. 2, pp. 272–276, 1999.

[19] Y. Konishi, H. Sato, H. Fujimoto, H. Tanaka, O. Takahashi, and T. Tanaka, "A case of primary uterine angiosarcoma: Magnetic resonance imaging and computed tomography findings," *International Journal of Gynecological Cancer*, vol. 17, no. 1, pp. 280–284, 2007.

[20] L. Cardinale, M. Mirra, C. Galli, J. R. Goldblum, S. Pizzolitto, and G. Falconieri, "Angiosarcoma of the Uterus: Report of 2 New Cases With Deviant Clinicopathologic Features and Review of the Literature," *Annals of Diagnostic Pathology*, vol. 12, no. 3, pp. 217–221, 2008.

[21] A. B. Olawaiye, J. A. Morgan, A. Goodman, A. F. Fuller Jr., and R. T. Penson, "Epithelioid angiosarcoma of the uterus: A review of management," *Archives of Gynecology and Obstetrics*, vol. 278, no. 5, pp. 401–404, 2008.

[22] J. P. Hwang and S. M. Lim, "Uterine epithelioid angiosarcoma on F-18 FDG PET/CT," *Nuclear Medicine and Molecular Imaging*, vol. 47, no. 2, pp. 134–137, 2013.

[23] S. Suzuki, F. Tanioka, H. Minato, A. Ayhan, M. Kasami, and H. Sugimura, "Breakages at YWHAE, FAM22A, and FAM22B loci in uterine angiosarcoma: A case report with immunohistochemical and genetic analysis," *Pathology - Research and Practice*, vol. 210, no. 2, pp. 130–134, 2014.

[24] Y. Liu, S. Guo, L. Wang, S. Suzuki, H. Sugimura, and Y. Li, "Uterine angiosarcoma: A case report and literature review," *International Journal of Gynecological Pathology*, vol. 35, no. 3, pp. 264–268, 2016.

[25] S. V. Strickland, M. R. Kilgore, E. J. Simons, and M. H. Rendi, "Epithelioid angiosarcoma arising in a uterine leiomyoma with associated elevated CA-125: A case report," *Gynecologic Oncology Reports*, vol. 21, pp. 1–4, 2017.

[26] M. G. Fury, C. R. Antonescu, K. J. Van Zee, M. F. Brennan, and R. G. Maki, "A 14-year retrospective review of angiosarcoma: clinical characteristics, prognostic factors, and treatment outcomes with surgery and chemotherapy," *Cancer Journal*, vol. 11, no. 3, pp. 241–247, 2005.

[27] P. J. Woll, M. van Glabbeke, P. Hohenberger et al., "Adjuvant chemotherapy (CT) with doxorubicin and ifosfamide in resected soft tissue sarcoma (STS): interim analysis of a randomised phase III trial," in *Proceedings of the ASCO Annual Meeting*, vol. 25, 2007.

[28] J. A. Abraham, F. J. Hornicek, A. M. Kaufman et al., "Treatment and outcome of 82 patients with angiosarcoma," *Annals of Surgical Oncology*, vol. 14, no. 6, pp. 1953–1967, 2007.

[29] M. Petrillo, M. Dessole, and V. Chiantera, "Peritoneal sarcomatosis 5 years after laparoscopic morcellation of uterine leiomyoma," *American Journal of Obstetrics & Gynecology*, vol. 218, no. 6, p. 626, 2018.

47

A Vaginal Angiomyofibroblastoma as a Rare Cause of a Prolapsing Vaginal Mass: A Case Report and Review of the Literature

Harriet Calvert ⓘ,[1,2] **Supuni Kapurubandara,**[3,4,5] **Yogesh Nikam,**[3,4,5] **Raghwa Sharma,**[5,6,7] **and Anita Achan**[6]

[1]Department of Obstetrics and Gynaecology, The Maitland Hospital, Maitland, NSW, Australia
[2]Department of Obstetrics and Gynaecology, John Hunter Hospital, Newcastle, NSW, Australia
[3]Department of Obstetrics and Gynaecology, Westmead Hospital, Sydney, NSW, Australia
[4]Sydney West Advanced Pelvic Surgery (SWAPS), Sydney, NSW, Australia
[5]University of Sydney, Sydney, NSW, Australia
[6]Department of Tissue Pathology and Diagnostic Oncology, Institute of Clinical Pathology and Medical Research, Westmead Hospital, Sydney, NSW, Australia
[7]Western Sydney University, Sydney, NSW, Australia

Correspondence should be addressed to Harriet Calvert; harriet.calvert@hnehealth.nsw.gov.au

Academic Editor: Yoshio Yoshida

Introduction. Angiomyofibroblastoma (AMFB) is a rare, benign, mesenchymal cell tumour which presents as a slow-growing mass. It is most commonly seen in the vulva and is often mistaken for Bartholin's abscess. It is histologically diagnosed by the presence of stromal cells intermingled with small blood vessels. It is morphologically similar to cellular angiofibroma and aggressive angiomyxoma, the latter of which is locally invasive and has a possibility of metastasis and a high risk of local recurrence. There is one reported case of an AMFB undergoing sarcomatous transformation. *Case Report.* We report a case of a multiparous, 36-year-old woman with an anterior vaginal mass which was inappropriately treated as a vaginal prolapse prior to definitive surgical management. This is only the second reported case of an AMFB presenting as a prolapsing mass.

1. Introduction

Angiomyofibroblastoma (AMFB) is a rare, benign, mesenchymal tumour that most commonly occurs as a slow-growing mass in the vulva, first described in 1992 [1]. It is often misdiagnosed as Bartholin's gland cyst [1, 2].

This type of solid tumour has also less commonly been described in the vagina and the inguinoscrotal region of men.

It is most prevalent in women in the reproductive age group with a mean age of 45 and varies in size (from 0.5 to 23 cm) but is usually less than 5 cm [1–4].

Histologically, it has a defined border and is characterised by alternating hypo- and hypercellular areas with numerous blood vessels [1, 5].

2. Case Report

We describe a case of a 36-year-old multiparous (G3P2) woman who presented with an acute episode of pelvic pain. She was referred to a general gynaecological clinic after ultrasound findings revealed a 4.1 cm complex left ovarian cyst suggestive of an endometrioma.

She also reported a 2-year history of a bulge that protruded from her vagina and was associated with discomfort and dyspareunia and occasionally required digital reduction especially with tampon use. She had been diagnosed with a vaginal prolapse by a gynaecology clinic at another institution.

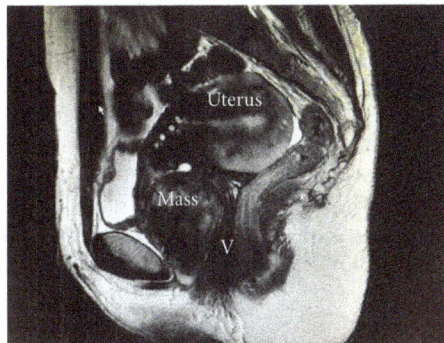

FIGURE 1: Sagittal section of MRI showing the 45 mm × 50 mm solid mass in the vesicovaginal septum in relation to the uterus, mass, and vagina (V).

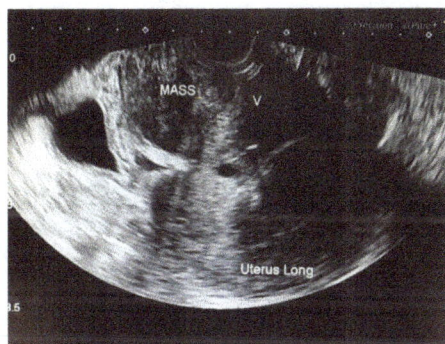

FIGURE 2: Ultrasound scan showing relation of mass to uterus and vagina.

Her past medical history consisted of migraines with aura, exercise induced asthma, and a family history of breast cancer (half-sister). She had never had a PAP smear.

On bimanual examination, a well-delineated solid mass was found on the anterior vaginal wall in the midline, measuring 5 cm by 5 cm. There was no evidence of pelvic organ prolapse with good support of the uterus, posterior wall, and anterior wall above the mass. The cervix was visualised anteriorly and there was no evidence of cervical excitation. A routine PAP smear was performed with difficulty secondary to the vaginal mass.

With respect to investigations, Ca 125 was 29 U/mL giving a low relative malignancy index. A repeat ultrasound scan demonstrated a 2.9 cm left ovarian cyst, suggestive of an endometrioma and a solid mass inferior to the uterus and anterior to the vagina, displacing the bladder (Figure 2).

On Magnetic Resonance Imaging, a 45 mm × 50 mm solid mass in the vesicovaginal septum with a well-defined margin was demonstrated (Figure 1). The mass was displacing the bladder anteriorly and displacing the urethra towards the left of the midline. T2 imaging showed a predominantly hypointense, heterogenous signal with areas of hyperintensity. There was mild enhancement after gadolinium injection. Close to the external urethral orifice, the interface between the mass and the urethra was ill defined. Evidence of a left ovarian endometrioma and endometriosis deposits were seen elsewhere in the pelvis.

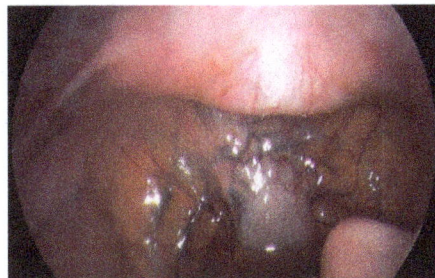

FIGURE 3: View of mass on diagnostic laparoscopy; uterus anteverted.

These MRI findings suggested that the mass was either endometriosis with surrounding reactive fibrous and smooth muscle proliferation, neoplasm, or an infection relating to a urethral diverticulum. After a multidisciplinary meeting with a urogynaecologist, the patient underwent an examination under anaesthesia, diagnostic laparoscopy, cystoscopy, excision of endometriosis, and excision of the vaginal mass.

The vaginal mass was removed with laparoscopic assessment via a midline incision on the anterior vaginal wall with lateral dissection around the cystic structure (Figures 3–6). A cystoscopy and urethroscopy suggested no involvement and the cyst was enucleated. Multiple haemostatic sutures were needed with surgical snow to achieve haemostasis and the defect was closed. A repeat cystoscopy and urethroscopy showed no injury.

Histopathological macroscopic assessment of the mass showed pale tan tissue surrounded by a thin capsule and on sectioning a homogeneous whorled tan tissue (Figure 6). Microscopically the low power photomicrographs showed a well-circumscribed border. It comprised collagenised areas of epithelioid to spindled cells with small to thin walled arborizing vessels. Aggregation of cells around vessels was noted and there were no atypical mitoses, necrosis, or atypia (Figures 7 and 8).

The immunohistochemistry showed positive desmin, SMA, CD34, and vimentin. The cells displayed high intensity nuclear positivity for progesterone and oestrogen receptors. These findings were consistent with a diagnosis of angiomyofibroblastoma.

3. Discussion

AMFB is a very rare benign, mesenchymal tumour with less than 100 cases previously having been reported in the literature. There has been a reported age range of 17–86 with a mean age at presentation of 45 [2, 6, 7].

It commonly presents as a painless, slow-growing, vulval mass and is most commonly diagnosed as Bartholin's cyst or abscess (46%) or a lipoma (15%) [2]. There is only one other reported case of it presenting as a prolapsing vaginal mass [8]. There is often a delay in diagnosis with a mean duration of 29 months between initial symptoms and diagnosis [2, 6].

AMFB is morphologically similar to other invasive mesenchymal cell tumours such as aggressive angiomyxoma (AAM) and cellular angiofibroma and they share many

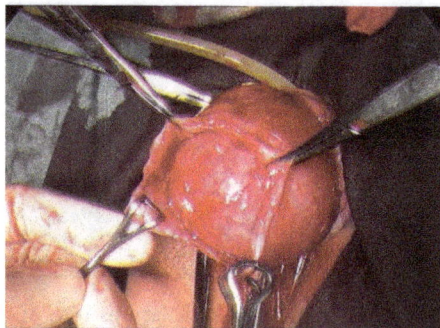

FIGURE 4: Marsupialisation of vaginal mass from anterior vaginal wall.

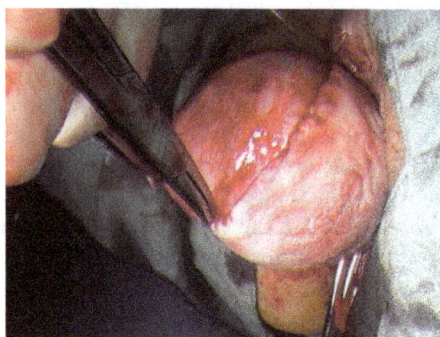

FIGURE 5: Excision of vaginal mass from anterior vaginal wall.

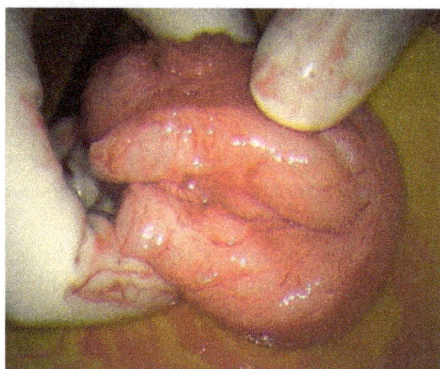

FIGURE 6: Cut surface of mass.

overlapping immunohistochemical and structural features [9, 10].

It is diagnostically challenging to differentiate between AMFB and AAM but important due to the latter's locally invasive nature, the possibility of metastasis, and the high risk of local recurrence [11, 12]. AMFB can be diagnosed by a higher cellularity, distinct border, plump stromal cells, increased presence of small blood vessels, and a lesser degree of stromal myxoid change [6]. Other differential diagnoses include cellular angiofibroma and vulvovaginal myofibroblastoma. Cellular angiofibromas are uniformly cellular with thick-walled, hyalinised blood vessels without surrounding aggregation of epithelioid or plasmacytoid cells. Adipocytes

are often found in the periphery [10]. Vulvovaginal myofibroblastomas characteristically contain ovoid, spindle, or stellate cells in a variety of architectural patterns. They also do not have the perivascular aggregates seen in AMFB [10]. Both cellular angiofibromas and myofibroblastomas exhibit the loss of RB1 and FOXO1A1 genes due to the deletion of the 13q14 chromosomal region. This typical loss of genetic material is not found in AMFB [13].

Immunohistologically, AMFB tumours have been found to be strongly positive for vimentin, positive for desmin, and to a lesser degree alpha-smooth muscle actin. Staining is rarely useful in differentiating between tumour types [13]. The stromal cells are characteristically positive for oestrogen and progesterone receptors, suggesting a hormonal role in the development of the tumour [14].

There have only been 5 previous reports of MRI findings of an AMFB. All report a mass with well-defined margins and as in our case they have been found to appear as a heterogeneous signal intensity on T2-weighted MRI. All other cases reported fast and persistent enhancement on dynamic gadolinium-enhanced MRI whereas ours showed only mild enhancement [15, 16].

The other studies found a mass with homogeneous intermediate signal intensity on T2 weighted MRI [7, 17, 18].

Ultrasound has been reported to be useful in assessing heterogeneity, vascularity, and delineating infiltration and relation to surrounding structures [7, 19].

It is widely accepted that AMFB can be treated with wide local excision with clear margins. There has only been one case report of a benign local recurrence. This was a pedunculated mass 5 × 3 cm arising from the vaginal vault which was excised with clear margins. Upon follow-up 14 months later 3 small, nodular growths were found close to the site of excision on the anterior and posterior vaginal walls which, when excised, showed the same features as the previous tumour with no transformation [8].

There has also been reported one case of previously diagnosed AMFB undergoing sarcomatous change. A 13 cm vulval mass was resected which showed many accepted features of an AMFB however did show focal sarcomatous change at the resected margin. At 2 years, the mass had recurred at the same site and resection demonstrated a 14 cm mass comprised of only the high-grade sarcomatous component with vascular invasion that was not previously present [20].

Another reported case of a locally invasive recurrence of AMFB at 2 years after resection was due to a misdiagnosed AAM on the original specimen [21]. The local recurrence rate of AAM after clear margin resection has been reported to be up to 47% [22–25].

4. Conclusion

The majority of AMFB occur in the vulva, most commonly presenting as a painless mass.

Vaginal AMFB are rarer and may present later with dyspareunia, awareness of a vaginal mass, or an incidental finding on exam [26–28]. Wide local excision is the recommended treatment, with enough surrounding tissue to enable

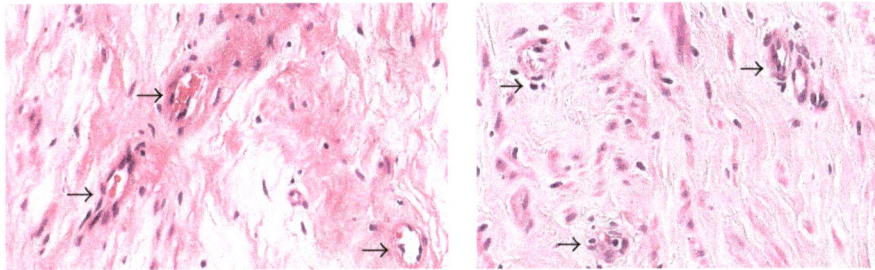

(a) Low power photomicrographs of the angiomy-ofibroblastoma with prominent thin walled vessels surrounded by clusters of epithelioid to spindle shaped cells (arrows)

(b) Low power photomicrographs of the angiomy-ofibroblastoma with prominent thin walled vessels surrounded by clusters of epithelioid to spindle shaped cells (arrows)

FIGURE 7

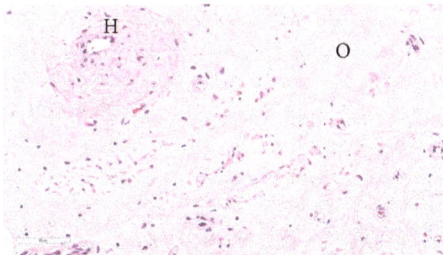

FIGURE 8: Cross section showing alternating hypercellular areas around blood vessels (H) and hypocellular (O) areas containing slender collagen fibrils with no evidence of necrosis.

the pathologist to differentiate between AMFB and the locally infiltrative AAM.

MRI and US can be useful imaging modalities depending on location of the tumour. Due to the rarity of cases, there are no recommendations on long-term monitoring but due to the reported instances of tumour recurrence and sarcomatous transformation we suggest that follow-up should be considered until at least 2 years postoperatively [8, 20].

References

[1] C. D. M. Fletcher, W. Y. W. Tsang, C. Fisher, K. C. Lee, and J. K. C. Chan, "Angiomyofibroblastoma of the vulva: A benign neoplasm distinct from aggressive angiomyxoma," *The American Journal of Surgical Pathology*, vol. 16, no. 4, pp. 373–382, 1992.

[2] S. M. Sims, K. Stinson, F. W. McLean, J. D. Davis, and E. J. Wilkinson, "Angiomyofibroblastoma of the vulva: A case report of a pedunculated variant and review of the literature," *Journal of Lower Genital Tract Disease*, vol. 16, no. 2, pp. 149–154, 2012.

[3] J. Seo, K. Lee, N. Yoon, J. Lee, B. Kim, and D. Bae, "Angiomyofibroblastoma of the vulva," *Obstetrics & Gynecology Science*, vol. 56, no. 5, pp. 349–351, 2013.

[4] K. Nagai, K. Aadachi, and H. Saito, "Huge pedunculated angiomyofibroblastoma of the vulva," *International Journal of Clinical Oncology*, vol. 15, no. 2, pp. 201–205, 2010.

[5] M. R. Nucci and C. D. M. Fletcher, "Vulvovaginal soft tissue tumours: update and review," *Histopathology*, vol. 36, no. 2, pp. 97–108, 2000.

[6] G. P. Nielsen and R. H. Young, "Mesenchymal tumors and tumor-like lesions of the female genital tract: a selective review with emphasis on recently described entities," *International Journal of Gynecological Pathology*, vol. 20, no. 2, pp. 105–127, 2001.

[7] B. Wolf, L.-C. Horn, R. Handzel, and J. Einenkel, "Ultrasound plays a key role in imaging and management of genital angiomy-ofibroblastoma: A case report," *Journal of Medical Case Reports*, vol. 9, no. 1, article no. 248, 2015.

[8] M. M. Saleh, A. H. Yassin, and M. S. Zaklama, "Recurrent angiomyofibroblastoma of the vagina: a case report," *Eur J Gynaecol Oncol*, vol. 28, no. 4, p. 324, 2007.

[9] F. Alameda, A. Munné, T. Baró et al., "Vulvar angiomyxoma, aggressive angiomyxoma, and angiomyofibroblastoma: An immunohistochemical and ultrastructural study," *Ultrastructural Pathology*, vol. 30, no. 3, pp. 193–205, 2006.

[10] W. G. McCluggage, "A review and update of morphologically bland vulvovaginal mesenchymal lesions," *Int J Gynecol Pathol*, vol. 24, no. 1, pp. 26–38, 2005.

[11] R. M. Siassi, T. Papadopoulos, and K. E. Matzel, "Metastasizing aggressive angiomyxoma," *The New England Journal of Medicine*, vol. 341, no. 23, article 1772, 1999.

[12] S. Blandamura, J. Cruz, L. Faure Vergara, I. M. Puerto, and V. Ninfo, "Aggressive angiomyxoma: a second case of metastasis with patient's death," *Human Pathology*, vol. 34, no. 10, pp. 1072–1074, 2003.

[13] G. Magro, A. Righi, R. Caltabiano, L. Casorzo, and M. Michal, "Vulvovaginal angiomyofibroblastomas: Morphologic, immunohistochemical, and fluorescence in situ hybridization analysis for deletion of 13q14 region," *Human Pathology*, vol. 45, no. 8, pp. 1647–1655, 2014.

[14] W. G. McCluggage and R. G. White, "Angiomyofibroblastoma of the vagina," *J Clin Pathol*, pp. 53–803, 2000.

[15] J. Geng, S. Hu, and F. Wang, "Large paravaginal angiomyofibroblastoma: Magnetic resonance imaging findings," *Japanese Journal of Radiology*, vol. 29, no. 2, pp. 152–155, 2011.

[16] J. L. Kyoung, H. M. Jeung, Y. Y. Dae, H. C. Ji, J. L. In, and J. M. Seon, "Angiomyofibroblastoma arising from the posterior

perivesical space: A case report with MR findings," *Korean Journal of Radiology*, vol. 9, no. 4, pp. 382–385, 2008.

[17] H. Kitamura, N. Miyao, Y. Sato, M. Matsukawa, T. Tsukamoto, and T. Sato, "Angiomyofibroblastoma of the female urethra," *International Journal of Urology*, vol. 6, no. 5, pp. 268–270, 1999.

[18] K. J. Mortele, G. J. Lauwers, P. J. Mergo, and P. R. Ros, "Perineal angiomyofibroblastoma: CT and MR findings with pathologic correlation," *Journal of Computer Assisted Tomography*, vol. 23, no. 5, pp. 687–689, 1999.

[19] X. Wang, H. Yang, H. Zhang, T. Shi, and W. Ren, "Transvaginal sonographic features of perineal masses in the female lower urogenital tract: A retrospective study of 71 patients," *Ultrasound in Obstetrics & Gynecology*, vol. 43, no. 6, pp. 702–710, 2014.

[20] G. P. Nielsen, R. H. Young, G. R. Dickersin, and A. E. Rosenberg, "Angiomyofibroblastoma of the vulva with sarcomatoms transformation ('angiomyofibrosarcoma')," *The American Journal of Surgical Pathology*, vol. 21, no. 9, pp. 1104–1108, 1997.

[21] Y.-F. Wang, H.-L. Qian, and H.-M. Jin, "Local recurrent vaginal aggressive angiomyxoma misdiagnosed as cellular angiomyofibroblastoma: A case report," *Experimental and Therapeutic Medicine*, vol. 11, no. 5, pp. 1893–1895, 2016.

[22] J. F. Fetsch, W. B. Laskin, M. Lefkowitz, L.-G. Kindblom, and J. M. Meis-Kindblom, "Aggressive angiomyxoma: a clinicopathologic study of 29 female patients," *Cancer*, vol. 78, no. 1, pp. 79–90, 1996.

[23] L. R. Bégin, P. B. Clement, M. E. Kirk, S. Jothy, W. T. Elliott McCaughey, and A. Ferenczy, "Aggressive angiomyxoma of pelvic soft parts: a clinicopathologic study of nine cases," *Human Pathology*, vol. 16, no. 6, pp. 621–628, 1985.

[24] B. J. Sutton and J. Laudadio, "Aggressive angiomyxoma," *Archives of Pathology & Laboratory Medicine*, vol. 136, no. 2, pp. 217–221, 2012.

[25] I. M. Chan, E. Hon, S. W. Ngai, T. Y. Ng, and L. C. Wong, "Aggressive angiomyxoma in females: is radical resection the only option?" *Acta Obstetricia et Gynecologica Scandinavica*, vol. 79, no. 3, pp. 216–220, 2000.

[26] R. Laiyemo, S. Disu, G. Vijaya, and B. Wise, "Post-menopausal vaginal angiomyofibroblastoma: A case report," *Archives of Gynecology and Obstetrics*, vol. 273, no. 2, pp. 129-130, 2005.

[27] Z. N. Kavak, A. Başgül, F. Eren, and N. Ceyhan, "Angiomyofibroblastoma of the vulva: A rare but distinct entity," *Acta Obstetricia et Gynecologica Scandinavica*, vol. 79, no. 7, pp. 612-613, 2000.

[28] K. Banerjee, S. D. Gupta, and S. R. Mathur, "Vaginal angiomyofibroblastoma," *Archives of Gynecology and Obstetrics*, vol. 270, no. 2, pp. 124-125, 2004.

48

Pitfall in the Diagnosis of Diabetes Insipidus and Pregnancy

Melissa Sum,[1] Jessica B. Fleischer,[1] Alexander G. Khandji,[2] and Sharon L. Wardlaw[1]

[1]*Department of Medicine, College of Physicians and Surgeons, Columbia University, New York, NY, USA*
[2]*Department of Radiology, College of Physicians and Surgeons, Columbia University, New York, NY, USA*

Correspondence should be addressed to Melissa Sum; ms2452@columbia.edu

Academic Editor: Akihide Ohkuchi

Diabetes insipidus (DI) during pregnancy and the perinatal period is an uncommon medical problem characterized by polyuria and excessive thirst. Diagnosis of DI may be overlooked in the setting of pregnancy, a time when increased water intake and urine output are commonly reported. We report two cases: one of transient DI in a young woman during her third trimester of twin pregnancy in association with acute fatty liver and hypertension and one of postpartum DI secondary to Sheehan syndrome from rupture of a splenic artery aneurysm. These cases illustrate the spectrum with which DI related to pregnancy and delivery can present and highlight the difficulty in making the diagnosis since the symptoms are often initially overlooked.

1. Introduction

Diabetes insipidus (DI) during pregnancy is an uncommon medical problem estimated to occur in two to six of 100,000 pregnancies [1]. One possible explanation is release of vasopressinase, a cysteine aminopeptidase, from the placenta leading to a fourfold increase in the rate of breakdown of arginine vasopressin (AVP) [2]. AVP regulates water reabsorption in the kidney and a decreased level leads to water loss. Other cases have been caused by uncommon hypothalamic-pituitary disorders leading to deficient secretion of AVP [3–5]. Timely diagnosis can be challenging because symptoms of polyuria, defined as a urine output exceeding 3 liters per day, and polydipsia may be attributed to the state of pregnancy. We present a case of transient DI in a woman during her third trimester of twin pregnancy and a second case of postpartum DI secondary to Sheehan syndrome to illustrate two different causes of DI associated with pregnancy and to highlight the difficulty in making a diagnosis of DI in the peri- and postpartum states.

2. Case 1

A 28-year-old para 1 woman was admitted in the 33rd week of gestation for hypertension and elevated liver enzymes. Concern for acute fatty liver of pregnancy or early preeclampsia prompted Cesarean section, which yielded two viable female infants. Her prenatal course was uncomplicated until week 25, when she developed polyuria and polydipsia leading to intake of 12 liters of water daily. The quantity and significance of the polyuria were initially not recognized and attributed to the gestational state.

On examination, her temperature was 37.1°C, blood pressure was 128/76 mmHg, and pulse was 90 beats per minute with normal skin turgor and no peripheral edema. Admission laboratory data included elevated liver enzymes and normal serum sodium that increased to 154 mmol/L after C-section (Table 1). Postpartum she had polyuria up to 1000 mL/h, 24-hour fluid intake was 9.5 liters, and urine output was 10.6 liters. She exhibited severe thirst, ongoing dilute polyuria, and elevated serum osmolality during her water deprivation test unresponsive to 8-arginine vasopressin (Pitressin) but responsive to 1-deamino-8-D-arginine-vasopressin (DDAVP), which provided the patient with substantial relief (Table 2). Liver function tests improved at five days postpartum, but DI persisted, requiring DDAVP 10 μg intranasally twice a day. Brain MRI (Figures 1(a) and 1(b)) showed loss of the normal hyperintense posterior pituitary signal consistent with AVP depletion. By eighteen days postpartum, her polyuria and polydipsia resolved, and DDAVP was discontinued. Urine osmolality was 687 mOsm/kg. Four months postpartum, repeat MRI (Figures 1(c) and 1(d))

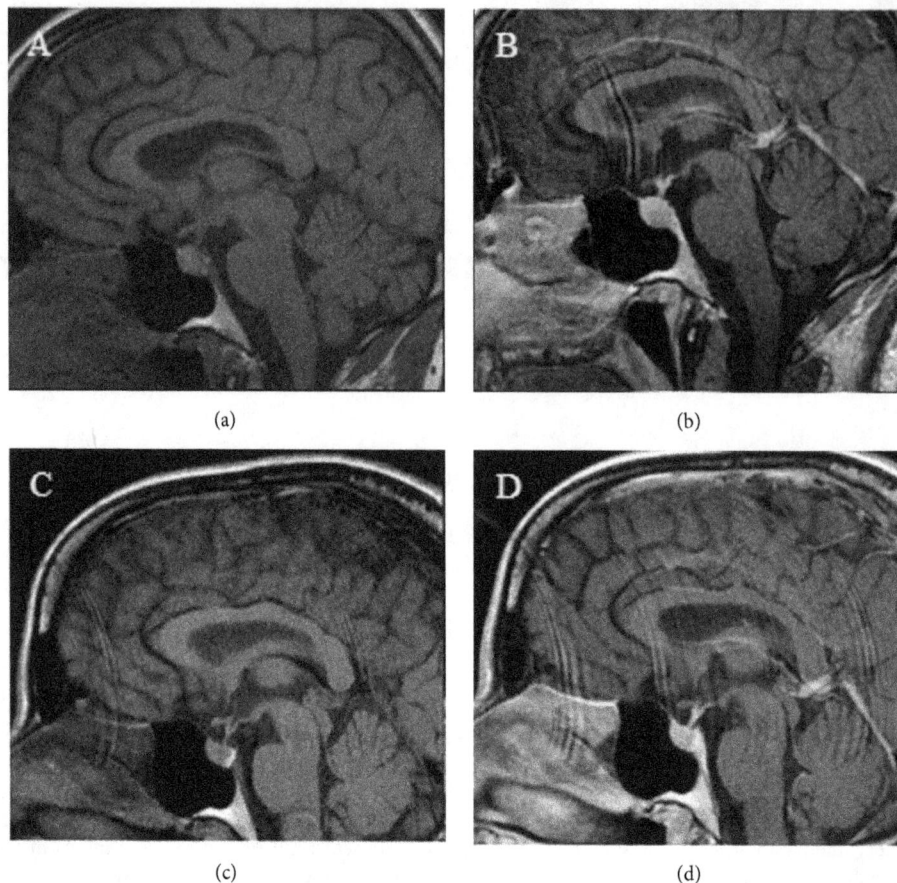

FIGURE 1: (a, b) Pre- and postcontrast brain MRI images of case 1 show that posterior pituitary bright spot is not visualized. (c, d) Pre- and postcontrast brain MRI images of case 1 at four months postpartum show return of posterior pituitary bright spot.

TABLE 1: Laboratory data for Case 1.

Laboratory data on admission		Laboratory data, 1 day postpartum	
Sodium [135–145 mmol/L]	137	Sodium	147
BUN [7–20 mg/dL]	17	Serum osmolality [275–295 mOsm/kg]	328
Creatinine [0.5–0.9 mg/dL]	1.0	Urine osmolality [500–800 mOsm/kg]	116
AST [7–41 U/L]	1337	TSH [0.34–4.25 U/mL]	0.79
ALT [12–38 U/L]	1359	Free T4 [0.8–1.8 ng/dL]	1.1
Total bilirubin [0.30–1.3 mg/dL]	3.4	Prolactin [1–25 ng/mL]	135
Alkaline phosphatase [33–96 U/L]	496	Cortisol [6.2–19.4 μg/dL]	12.1

showed return of the hyperintense posterior pituitary signal, consistent with AVP repletion.

3. Case 2

A 35-year-old nulliparous woman in her 29th week of an uncomplicated gestation presented for severe, generalized abdominal pain. Ultrasound was concerning for pelvic free fluid. She subsequently decompensated and was rushed to the emergency room for resuscitation. She required fluid boluses, pressors, intubation, and emergent C-section. Hemorrhage ensued, and she underwent an exploratory laparotomy where her ruptured splenic artery aneurysm was ligated and spleen was removed, resulting in hemostasis. She required 18 units of transfused packed red blood cells. The baby did not survive.

Her past medical history was notable for polycystic kidney disease diagnosed in adulthood and a family history of polycystic kidney disease in her mother and brother. Postoperatively, her exam was notable for a soft abdomen and closed midline incision. Ten days afterwards while still in-house, she noted onset of polyuria and polydipsia initially attributed to fluid shifts from her resuscitation, postpartum, and postoperative state. However, those symptoms worsened upon discharge. She reported strong desire for cold fluids and polyuria that interrupted sleep. Four weeks later, she was admitted for wound infection and noted to have up to 450 mL/hr of urine output with osmolality 101 mOsm/kg and elevated serum osmolality 297 mOsm/kg. She responded well

TABLE 2: Pitressin and DDAVP challenge for Case 1.

	Time	Urine output	Urine specific gravity	Urine osm [mOsm/kg]	Serum osm [mOsm/kg]	Sodium [mmol/L]
5 units of SQ Pitressin	1400 h	500 mL		116	328	
	1600 h	600 mL		87	301	
	1700 h	600 mL	1.005			141
	1800 h	150 mL	1.005		301	144
	1900 h	350 mL				
10 μg of intranasal DDAVP	2100 h					
	2200 h	700 mL				135
	0000 h					
	0200 h	75 mL				
	0400 h	60 mL				
	0600 h	60 mL	1.020			131

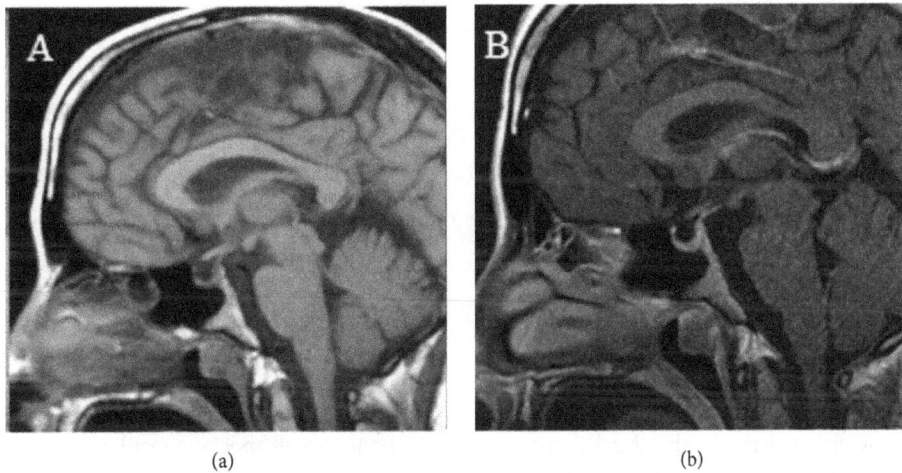

(a)   (b)

FIGURE 2: (a, b) Pre- and postcontrast brain MRI images of case 2 show that posterior pituitary bright spot is not visualized and that the anterior pituitary appears small for age and postpartum state.

to DDAVP 10 μg intranasally with concentration of her urine and relief of symptoms. She was subsequently maintained on nightly intranasal DDAVP. She denied headache or vision problems. Results of her pituitary hormone panel included TSH 4.05 U/mL, free T4 0.9 ng/dL, PRL 25 ng/mL, FSH 1.1 [<15.0 mIU/mL], LH 0.5 [<15.0 mIU/mL], estradiol 121 [100–400 pg/mL], and cortisol 7.9 μg/dL. She had no symptoms suggesting hypothyroidism or adrenal insufficiency. Brain MRI (Figures 2(a) and 2(b)) showed lack of normal hyperintense posterior pituitary signal and small pituitary size for age and postpartum state. Repeat morning cortisol was 17.3 μg/dL. She had eventual resumption of menses. Two years later, she had a spontaneous pregnancy and uneventful delivery of a full-term healthy baby boy. Her DI has persisted and remains controlled on DDAVP.

4. Discussion

Diabetes insipidus is characterized by polyuria and polydipsia. Since these symptoms are nonspecific and may be attributed to the gestational state, DI during pregnancy is often overlooked and diagnosis is delayed. Indeed, in normotensive healthy human pregnant subjects, the osmotic threshold for AVP release and thirst perception is decreased compared to nonpregnant subjects [6]. The change in osmotic threshold may be mediated by human chorionic gonadotropin (hCG), as administration of hCG to women during the menstrual luteal phase has been shown to induce similar threshold changes for ADH release and thirst [7, 8]. As a result of these set point changes, plasma osmolality in normal pregnancy decreases to about 270 mosmol/kg and plasma sodium concentration decreases 4 to 5 meq/L below nonpregnancy levels [9]. In addition to a physiologic decrease in threshold for thirst perception, urinary frequency, defined as voiding more than 7 times per day, and nocturia, defined as voiding more than or equal to 2 times per night, are common and can affect 80–95% of pregnant women [10–12]. Yet in DI, the polyuria is generally of rapid onset and defined by abnormally high volumes of dilute urine exceeding three liters per day and the thirst can be intense.

In general, the evaluation of patients with suspected DI begins with a detailed history including rate of onset of polyuria, appearance of urine, and measurement of fluid intake and urine output. Typical findings include increased serum osmolality though, notably, the osmolality may be comparable to that of a nonpregnant woman in light of the decreased physiologic set point that occurs in pregnancy, elevated serum sodium concentration, and decreased urine osmolality when fluid is restricted. An increase in urine osmolality of at least 50% in response to DDAVP is consistent with central versus nephrogenic DI. The water restriction test must be performed in a monitored setting because potentially severe volume depletion and hypernatremia can occur in patients with significant polyuria. During pregnancy, the test is generally not recommended or must be undertaken with significant caution and low threshold to terminate since dehydration can lead to uteroplacental insufficiency.

DI associated with pregnancy can result from decreased AVP production associated with pathological processes involving the hypothalamus and pituitary such as lymphocytic hypophysitis and infundibulitis or postpartum hemorrhage or from increased AVP destruction secondary to increased vasopressinase activity by means of enhanced placental production or decreased clearance in the setting of liver dysfunction. Patients with prepregnancy mild subclinical central DI that may have been present due to prior hypothalamic/pituitary disease experience worsening of symptoms which are unmasked by the increased vasopressinase activity during gestation. Furthermore, the marked increase in glomerular filtration rate during pregnancy may worsen preexisting subclinical nephrogenic DI.

Transient DI of pregnancy attributed to increased vasopressinase activity typically presents in the third trimester. Loss of the hyperintense posterior pituitary signal indicating a decrease in AVP reserves has been reported [13]. Our first case also documents return of the hyperintense posterior pituitary signal following resolution of gestational DI. There appears to be an association with hepatic abnormalities perhaps because liver dysfunction results in decreased hepatic degradation of vasopressinase [14]. Prior gestational history may also be notable for occurrence of polyuria and polydipsia [13]. In our first patient, twin pregnancy with an extra placenta likely contributed to increased vasopressinase production while hepatic abnormalities hindered its clearance, leading to DI. Her diagnosis was delayed until the postpartum setting when her urine output was quantified. The water deprivation test might not have been needed since the patient was already hypernatremic and a vasopressin challenge could have been done. But notably, during the deprivation test, our patient had better response to DDAVP than AVP, consistent with involvement of vasopressinase in the pathogenesis of her DI, as vasopressinase cleaves the N-terminus of AVP and oxytocin and DDAVP lacks an amino group, thereby protecting it from degradation.

Our second case is the first report of isolated DI secondary to Sheehan syndrome from rupture of a splenic artery aneurysm. Sheehan syndrome is a well-known complication of postpartum hemorrhage that typically manifests with anterior pituitary hormone deficiencies including lactation failure and amenorrhea. Rare cases of DI in the setting of Sheehan syndrome have been reported, nearly all of which involved anterior pituitary hypofunction; we found only one case with isolated DI [3]. Only one reported case of Sheehan syndrome was secondary to ruptured splenic artery aneurysm [15]. Our patient's history of polycystic kidney disease may have predisposed her to aneurysm development [16]. Despite a known history of large volume blood loss placing her at risk of Sheehan syndrome, her diagnosis of DI was delayed until her readmission for a wound infection when the amount of polyuria was recorded.

These cases illustrate the spectrum with which DI related to pregnancy and delivery can present and highlight the difficulty of making the diagnosis. This report does not illustrate the full range of etiologies of DI and pregnancy reported in literature but does highlight 2 important causes including one case of decreased AVP in the setting of likely increased vasopressinase release and decreased hepatic degradation and a second case of deficient AVP secretion. The patient courses described here are also consistent with other reports of delayed diagnoses, as the diagnosis of DI is often not considered since urinary frequency is common during gestation. In both cases reported here, quantification of urine output was helpful in alerting physicians about the presence of true polyuria. The treatment of choice for DI is DDAVP. Recognition and treatment of DI are important to prevent dehydration, hypernatremia, and oligohydramnios and to alleviate the distress associated with unrelenting polyuria and polydipsia. Furthermore, for pregnant patients on DDAVP receiving parenteral fluids in the peripartum period, recognition of the risk of hyponatremia and avoidance of hypotonic fluids are important. As such, the diagnosis and treatment of DI during pregnancy merit special consideration.

References

[1] J. A. Durr, "Diabetes insipidus in pregnancy," *American Journal of Kidney Diseases*, vol. 9, no. 4, pp. 276–283, 1987.

[2] J. M. Davison, E. A. Sheills, P. R. Philips, W. M. Barron, and M. D. Lindheimer, "Metabolic clearance of vasopressin and an analogue resistant to vasopressinase in human pregnancy," *American Journal of Physiology*, vol. 264, no. 2, part 2, pp. F348–F353, 1993.

[3] M. L. Collins, P. O'Brien, and A. Cline, "Diabetes insipidus following obstetric shock," *Obstet Gynecol*, vol. 53, no. 3, supplement, pp. 16S–17S, 1979.

[4] S. Kumar, D. Burrows, S. Dang, and D. Simmons, "Sheehan syndrome presenting as central diabetes insipidus: a rare presentation of an uncommon disorder," *Endocrine Practice*, vol. 17, no. 1, pp. 108–114, 2011.

[5] T. Tulandi, N. Yusuf, and B. I. Posner, "Diabetes insipidus: a postpartum complication," *Obstet Gynecol*, vol. 70, no. 3, part 2, pp. 492–495, 1987.

[6] J. M. Davison, E. A. Gilmore, J. Durr, G. L. Robertson, and M. D. Lindhemier, "Altered osmotic thresholds for vasopressin secretion and thirst in human pregnancy," *American Journal of Physiology*, vol. 246, no. 1, part 2, pp. F105–F109, 1984.

[7] J. M. Davison, E. A. Shiells, P. R. Philips, and M. D. Lindheimer, "Serial evaluation of vasopressin release and thirst in human pregnancy. Role of human chorionic gonadotrophin in the osmoregulatory changes of gestation," *Journal of Clinical Investigation*, vol. 81, no. 3, pp. 798–806, 1988.

[8] J. M. Davison, E. A. Shiells, P. R. Philips, and M. D. Lindhemier, "Influence of humoral and volume factors on altered osmoregulation of normal human pregnancy," *American Journal of Physiology*, vol. 258, no. 4, part 2, pp. F900–F907, 1990.

[9] M. D. Lindheimer, W. M. Barron, and J. M. Davison, "Osmoregulation of thirst and vasopressin release in pregnancy," *American Journal of Physiology*, vol. 257, no. 2, part 2, pp. F159–F169, 1989.

[10] W. J. Francis, "Disturbances of bladder function in relation to pregnancy," *The Journal of Obstetrics and Gynaecology of the British Empire*, vol. 67, pp. 353–366, 1960.

[11] S. L. Stanton, R. Kerr-Wilson, and V. Grant Harris, "The incidence of urological symptoms in normal pregnancy," *The British Journal of Obstetrics and Gynaecology*, vol. 87, no. 10, pp. 897–900, 1980.

[12] H. J. van Brummen, H. W. Bruinse, J. G. van der Bom, A. P. M. Heintz, and C. H. van der Vaart, "How do the prevalences of urogenital symptoms change during pregnancy?" *Neurourology and Urodynamics*, vol. 25, no. 2, pp. 135–139, 2006.

[13] I. Kalelioglu, A. K. Uzum, A. Yildirim, T. Ozkan, F. Gungor, and R. Has, "Transient gestational diabetes insipidus diagnosed in successive pregnancies: review of pathophysiology, diagnosis, treatment, and management of delivery," *Pituitary*, vol. 10, no. 1, pp. 87–93, 2007.

[14] Y. Yamanaka, K. Takeuchi, E. Konda et al., "Transient postpartum diabetes insipidus in twin pregnancy associated with HELLP syndrome," *Journal of Perinatal Medicine*, vol. 30, no. 3, pp. 273–275, 2002.

[15] G. Agostinis, "Sheehan's syndrome due to very grave hemorrhagic shock caused by rupture of the splenic artery in pregnancy: pathogenetic and resuscitational therapeutic considerations," *Acta anaesthesiologica*, vol. 20, no. 1, pp. 187–193, 1969.

[16] N. S. Kanagasundaram, E. P. Perry, and J. H. Turney, "Aneurysm of the splenic artery in a patient with autosomal dominant polycystic kidney disease," *Nephrology Dialysis Transplantation*, vol. 14, no. 1, pp. 183-184, 1999.

Permissions

List of Contributors

Yuki Fukutani, Yoshitsugu Chigusa, Eiji Kondoh, Kaoru Kawasaki, Shingo Io and Noriomi Matsumura
Department of Gynecology and Obstetrics, Kyoto University, 54 Shogoin Kawahara-cho, Sakyo-ku, Kyoto 606-8507, Japan

Matthew J. Bicocca
Department of Obstetrics and Gynecology, Houston Methodist Hospital, Houston, TX, USA

Andrea R. Gilbert
Department of Pathology and Genomic Medicine, Houston Methodist Hospital, Houston, TX, USA

Saeed S. Sadrameli
Department of Neurosurgery, Houston Methodist Hospital, Houston, TX, USA

Michael L. Pirics
Department of Obstetrics and Gynecology, Houston Methodist Hospital, Houston, TX, USA
Department of Obstetrics and Gynecology, Weill Cornell Medical College, New York, NY, USA

Gieta Bhikha-kori, Marieke Sueters and Johanna M. Middeldorp
Fetal Therapy, Department of Obstetrics, Leiden University Medical Center, Leiden, Netherlands

Jessica Parrott and Cecily Clark-Ganheart
Division of Maternal Fetal Medicine, Department of Obstetrics and Gynecology, University of Kansas School of Medicine, 3901 Rainbow Boulevard, Kansas City, KS 66160, USA

Mitch Tener and Matthew Sharpe
Department of Pulmonary and Critical Care Medicine, University of Kansas School of Medicine, 3901 Rainbow Boulevard, Kansas City, KS 66160, USA

Katie Dennis
Department of Pathology and Laboratory Medicine, University of Kansas School of Medicine, 3901 Rainbow Boulevard, Kansas City, KS 66160, USA

Shuhei Terada, Takashi Suzuki, Akihiro Hasegawa, Satoru Nakayama and Hiroshi Adachi
Department of Gynecology, Seirei Hamamatsu General Hospital, 2-12-12 Sumiyoshi, Naka-ku, Hamamatsu, Shizuoka 430-8558, Japan

Franco Pepe
U.O.C. Ostetricia e Ginecologia e PS, Ospedale Santo Bambino, Catania, Italy

Mariagrazia Stracquadanio
Istituto di Patologia Ostetrica e Ginecologica, Ospedale Santo Bambino, Catania, Italy

Francesco De Luca and Agata Privitera
U.O. Cardiologia Pediatrica, Ospedale Santo Bambino, Catania, Italy

Elisabetta Sanalitro and Puccio Scarpinati
Modulo Dipartimentale Anestesia Ostetrica, Ospedale Santo Bambino, Catania, Italy

Fernando Augusto Rozário Garcia and Vanessa Pereira Gaigher
Medical Resident, Department of Obstetrics and Gynecology, Hospital Santa Casa de Misericórdia de Vitória, Vitória, ES, Brazil

Rodrigo Neves Ferreira
Pathologist, Hospital Santa Casa de Misericórdia de Vitória, Vitória, ES, Brazil

Antônio Chambô Filho
MD, PhD, Full Professor, Department of Obstetrics and Gynecology, Escola Superior de Ciências, Santa Casa de Misericórdia de Vitória, ES, Brazil
Head of the Department of Obstetrics and Gynecology, Hospital Santa Casa de Misericórdia de Vitória, Vitória, ES, Brazil

Haruhisa Konishi, Iemasa Koh, Yukie Kidani, Satoshi Urabe, Norifumi Tanaka, Eiji Hirata and Yoshiki Kudo
Department of Obstetrics and Gynecology, Graduate School of Biomedical Science, Hiroshima University, Japan

Noriyuki Shiroma and Koji Arihiro
Department of Anatomical Pathology, Hiroshima University Hospital, Japan

Lawrence Hsu Lin, Koji Fushida, Eliane Azeka Hase, Laysa Manatta Tenorio and Rossana Pulcineli Vieira Francisco
University of Sao Paulo Trophoblastic Disease Center, University of Sao Paulo Medical School, Sao Paulo, SP, Brazil

Regina Schultz
Department of Pathology, University of Sao Paulo Medical School, Sao Paulo, SP, Brazil

Fabricia Andrea Rosa Madia, Evelin Aline Zanardo and Leslie Domenici Kulikowski
Cytogenomic Laboratory, Department of Pathology, University of Sao Paulo Medical School, Sao Paulo, SP, Brazil

I-Ting Peng and Ching-Chung Lin
Department of Obstetrics and Gynecology, Chi Mei Medical Center, Taiwan

Ming-Ting Chung
Department of Obstetrics and Gynecology, Chi Mei Medical Center, Taiwan
Chia Nan University of Pharmacy and Science, Taiwan

Helen J. Trihia, Maria Papazian and Natasa Novkovic
Department of Pathology, "Metaxas" Cancer Hospital, 18537 Piraeus, Greece

John Provatas
Department of Cytology, "Metaxas" Cancer Hospital, 18537 Piraeus, Greece

Sotiria Tsangouri and Dimitrios C. Papatheodorou
Department of Gynaecology, "Metaxas" Cancer Hospital, 18537 Piraeus, Greece

Terumi Tanigawa, Shintaro Morisaki, Hisanobu Fukuda, Shuichiro Yoshimura, Hisayoshi Nakajima and Kohei Kotera
Department of Obstetrics and Gynecology, Nagasaki Harbor Medical Center City Hospital, 6-39 Shinchimachi, Nagasaki-shi, Nagasaki 850-8555, Japan

Mariko Jitsumori and Toshiya Yamamoto
Department of Obstetrics and Gynecology, Sakai City Medical Center, Sakai, Japan

Satoru Munakata
Department of Pathology, Sakai City Medical Center, Sakai, Japan

T. Hockertz and M. Velickovic
Department of Orthopedic Surgery, Sports Traumatology and Trauma Surgery, Städtisches Klinikum Wolfenbüttel, Alter Weg 80, 38302Wolfenbüttel, Germany

Layan Alrahmani and Carl H. Rose
Mayo Clinic, Division of Maternal-Fetal Medicine, Department of Obstetrics and Gynecology, 200 First St. SW, Rochester, MN 55905, USA

Jaclyn Rivington
Metrohealth Medical Center, Department of Internal Medicine, 2500 Metrohealth Dr., Cleveland, OH 44109, USA

Masafumi Yamamoto, Mio Takami, Ryosuke Shindo, Michi Kasai and Shigeru Aoki
Perinatal Center for Maternity and Neonate, Yokohama City University Medical Center, Yokohama, Japan

Nobue Kojima, Yui Yamasaki, Houu Koh and Hiroki Morita
Department of Obstetrics and Gynecology, Rokko Island Konan Hospital, Kobe, Japan

Masaru Miyashita
Department of Surgery, Konan Hospital, Kobe, Japan

Süleyman Salman, Fatma Ketenci Gencer, Bülent BabaoLlu, Melih Bestel, Serkan Kumbasar, Guray Tuna, Esra Güzel, Durkadın Elif Yıldız, Tuba Kotancı, Ali Selçuk Yeniocak, and Özlem Söğüt
Gaziosmanpaşa Taksim Eğitim ve Araştırma Hastahanesi, Kadın Hastalıkları ve Doğum Bölümü, İstanbul, Turkey

Nishat Fatema and Muna Mubarak Al Badi
Department of Gynaecology and Obstetric, Ibri Regional Hospital, Ministry of Health, Ibri, Oman

Cynthia O'Sullivan
Department of Urology, Wellington Hospital, Wellington, New Zealand

Shankari Arulkumaran, Lorin Lakasing and Karl Murphy
Department of Obstetrics and Gynaecology, St. Mary's Hospital, Imperial College London NHS Trust, Praed Street, London W2 1NY, UK

Eric Jauniaux
Academic Department of Obstetrics and Gynaecology, Institute for Women's Health, University College London, 86-96 Chenies Mews, LondonWC1E 6HX, UK

Simone Garzon, Giovanni Zanconato, Nicoletta Zatti and Massimo Franchi
Department of Surgical, Odontostomatological and Maternal and Child Sciences, University of Verona, Piazzale L.A. Scuro 10, 37134 Verona, Italy

Giuseppe Chiarioni
Department of Medicine and Gastroenterology, University of Verona, Piazzale L.A. Scuro 10, 37134 Verona, Italy

Annachiara Basso, Mariana Rita Catalano, Giuseppe Loverro, Serena Nocera, Edoardo Di Naro, Matteo Loverro and Salvatore Andrea Mastrolia
Department of Obstetrics and Gynecology, Azienda Ospedaliera Universitaria Policlinico di Bari, School of Medicine, Università degli Studi di Bari "Aldo Moro", Bari, Italy

Mariateresa Natrella
School of Nursing, Azienda Ospedaliera Universitaria Policlinico di Bari, School of Medicine, Università degli Studi di Bari "Aldo Moro", Bari, Italy

Kenji Horie, Hironori Takahashi, Yosuke Baba, Akihide Ohkuchi and Shigeki Matsubara
Department of Obstetrics and Gynecology, Jichi Medical University, Japan

Daisuke Matsubara and Koichi Kataoka
Department of Pediatrics, Jichi Medical University, Japan

Rieko Furukawa
Department of Radiology, Jichi Medical University, Japan

Connie D. Cao
Rutgers Robert Wood Johnson Medical School, Rutgers University, New Brunswick, NJ, USA

Lena Merjanian and Adrian Balica
Department of Obstetrics, Gynecology, and Reproductive Sciences, Rutgers Robert Wood Johnson Medical School, Rutgers University, New Brunswick, NJ, USA

Joelle Pierre
Department of Surgery, Rutgers Robert Wood Johnson Medical School, Rutgers University, New Brunswick, NJ, USA

Yuko Sonan, Shigeru Aoki, Kimiko Enomoto and Kazuo Seki
Perinatal Maternity and Neonatal Center of Yokohama City University Medical Center, Yokohama, Japan

Etsuko Miyagi
Department of Obstetrics and Gynecology, Yokohama City University Hospital, Yokohama, Japan

Shariska S. Petersen and Raminder Khangura
Department of Women's Health Services, Henry Ford Hospital, Detroit, MI 48202, USA

Dmitry Davydov
Wayne State University School of Medicine, Detroit, MI 48202, USA

Ziying Zhang
Department of Pathology, Cytopathology Laboratory, Henry Ford Hospital, Detroit, MI 48202, USA

Roopina Sangha
Department of Women's Health Services, Henry Ford Hospital, Detroit, MI 48202, USA
Wayne State University School of Medicine, Detroit, MI 48202, USA

Nicole Sahasrabudhe, Nickolas Teigen and Diana S. Wolfe
Department of Obstetrics and Gynecology, Albert Einstein College of Medicine, Bronx, NY, USA

Cynthia Taub
Department of Cardiology, Albert Einstein College of Medicine, Bronx, NY, USA

Shannon Armstrong-Kempter
Department of Women's and Newborn Health, Westmead Hospital, Westmead, NSW2145, Australia
Western Sydney University, Campbelltown, NSW 2560, Australia

Supuni Kapurubandara
Department of Women's and Newborn Health, Westmead Hospital, Westmead, NSW2145, Australia
University of Sydney, Camperdown, NSW2006, Australia
Sydney West Advanced Pelvic Surgery Unit, NSW, Australia

Brian Trudinger
University of Sydney, Camperdown, NSW2006, Australia

Noel Young
Western Sydney University, Campbelltown, NSW 2560, Australia
Department of Radiology, Westmead Hospital, Westmead, NSW2145, Australia

Naim Arrage
Department of Women's and Newborn Health, Westmead Hospital, Westmead, NSW2145, Australia
SydneyWest Advanced Pelvic Surgery Unit, NSW, Australia

Matthew J. Blitz and Adiel Fleischer
Division of Maternal-Fetal Medicine, Department of Obstetrics and Gynecology, Long Island Jewish Medical Center, Donald and Barbara Zucker School of Medicine at Hofstra/Northwell, New Hyde Park, NY, USA

Lilian Yukari Miura, Monica Tessmann Zomer, Reitan Ribeiro and William Kondo
Vita Batel Hospital, Rua Alferes Angelo Sampaio, 1896 Curitiba, PR, Brazil

Miriam Anyury Daquin Maure
Complejo Hospitalario Metropolitano, Via Simon Bolivar, Panama City, Panama

Teresa Cristina Santos Cavalcanti
Citolab, Rua Vicente Machado 1192 Curitiba, PR, Brazil

Stephanie C. Tardieu and Elizabeth Schmidt
Department of Obstetrics and Gynecology, Hofstra Northwell School of Medicine, Hofstra University, North Shore-LIJ University Hospital, 270-05 76th Avenue, New Hyde Park, NY 11040, USA

Emanuelle J. Best
Maternity and Gynaecology, John Hunter Hospital, New Lambton Heights, NSW, Australia

Cecelia M. O'Brien, Wendy Carseldine and Felicity Park
Maternity and Gynaecology, John Hunter Hospital, New Lambton Heights, NSW, Australia
Maternal Fetal Medicine Unit, John Hunter Hospital, New Lambton Heights, NSW, Australia

Aniruddh Deshpande
Department of Paediatric Surgery, John Hunter Children's Hospital, New Lambton Heights, NSW, Australia

Rebecca Glover
Neonatal Intensive Care Unit, John Hunter Children's Hospital, New Lambton Heights, NSW, Australia

Houda Nasser Al Yaqoubi and Nishat Fatema
Department of Obstetrics and Gynaecology, Ibri Regional Hospital, Ministry of Health, Ibri, Oman

Jennifer Hartley, Muhammad Akhtar and Edmond Edi-Osagie
Saint Mary's Hospital, Central Manchester University Hospitals NHS Foundation Trust, Oxford Road, Manchester M13 9WL, UK

Nikolina P. Docheva, Emily D. Slutsky, Roger Sandelin and James W. Van Hook
Department of Obstetrics and Gynecology, University of Toledo, Toledo, OH, USA

Rawan Bajis
King Edward Memorial Hospital, Australia

Gregg Eloundou
Joondalup Health Campus, Australia

Marianna Politou, Giorgos Dryllis, Maria Efstathopoulou, Serena Valsami and Faidra-Evangelia Triantafyllou
Department of Hematology and Blood Transfusion Unit, Aretaieion Hospital, School of Medicine, National and Kapodistrian University of Athens, Greece

Athanasia Tsaroucha
Anesthesiology Clinic, Aretaieion General Hospital, School of Medicine, University of Athens, National and Kapodistrian University of Athens, Greece

Antonios Kattamis
Second Department of Obstetrics and Gynecology, Aretaieion General Hospital, School of Medicine, National and Kapodistrian University of Athens, Greece

Nikos F. Vlahos
First Department of Pediatrics, University General Hospital "Attikon", School of Medicine, National and Kapodistrian University of Athens, Greece

Yui Kinjo, Hitoshi Masamoto, Hayase Nitta, Tadatsugu Kinjo and Yoichi Aoki
Department of Obstetrics and Gynecology, Graduate School of Medicine, University of the Ryukyus, Okinawa, Japan

Tomoko Tamaki and Naoki Yoshimi
Department of Pathology and Oncology, Graduate School of Medicine, University of the Ryukyus, Okinawa, Japan

Nikolina Docheva, Emily D. Slutsky, James W. Van Hook and Sonyoung Seo-Patel
Department of Obstetrics and Gynecology, University of Toledo, Toledo, Ohio, USA

Nicolette Borella
Mercyhurst University, Department of Biology, Eerie, Pennsylvania, USA

Renee Mason
Promedica Physicians Obstetrics-Gynecology, Maumee, Ohio, USA

Rauf Melekoglu and Hasim Kural
Department of Obstetrics and Gynecology, Faculty of Medicine, The University of Inonu, 44280 Malatya, Turkey

Ebru Celik
Department of Obstetrics and Gynecology, Faculty of Medicine, The University of Koc, 34010 İstanbul, Turkey

Tiphaine de Foucher and Myriam Deloménie
Department of Breast and Gynecological Surgical Oncology, Hôpital Européen Georges Pompidou, AP-HP, Paris, France

Hélène Roussel
Department of Pathology, Hôpital Européen Georges Pompidou, AP-HP, Paris, France

Mikael Hivelin
Department of Plastic and Reconstructive Surgery, Hôpital Européen Georges Pompidou, AP-HP, Paris, France
Paris Descartes University, Sorbonne Paris Cité, Paris, France

Léa Rossi, Caroline Cornou, Anne-Sophie Bats, Fabrice Lécuru and Charlotte Ngô
Department of Breast and Gynecological Surgical Oncology, Hôpital Européen Georges Pompidou, AP-HP, Paris, France
Paris Descartes University, Sorbonne Paris Cité, Paris, France

Andreas D. Ebert
Praxis für Frauengesundheit, Gynäkologie und Geburtshilfe, Nürnberger Strasse 67, 10787 Berlin, Germany

Sarah Eckhardt, Renee Rolston and Begum Ozel
Division of Female Pelvic Floor and Reconstructive Surgery, Department of Obstetrics and Gynecology, University of Southern California, Los Angeles, CA, USA

Suzanne Palmer
Clinical Radiology and Medicine, Keck Medical Center, University of Southern California, Los Angeles, CA, USA

Steve Kyende Mutiso, Felix Mwembi Oindi and Timona Obura
Department of Obstetrics and Gynaecology, Aga Khan University, Nairobi, Kenya

Nigel Hacking
University Hospital Southampton, Southampton, UK
Aga Khan University Hospital, Nairobi, Kenya

Mary J. Kao
Department of Obstetrics and Gynecology, University of Wisconsin School of Medicine and Public Health, Madison, WI 53792, USA

Madhuchhanda Roy and Josephine Harter
Department of Pathology and Laboratory Medicine, University of Wisconsin School of Medicine and Public Health, Madison, WI 53792, USA

Ryan J. Spencer
Division of Gynecologic Oncology, University of Wisconsin School of Medicine and Public Health, Madison, WI 53792, USA

Takeya Hara, Ai Miyoshi, Yuji Kamei, Nao Wakui, Akiko Fujishiro, Serika Kanao, Hirokazu Naoi, Hirofumi Otsuka and Takeshi Yokoi
Department of Obstetrics and Gynecology, Kaizuka City Hospital, Osaka, Japan

Harriet Calvert
Department of Obstetrics and Gynaecology, The Maitland Hospital, Maitland, NSW, Australia
Department of Obstetrics and Gynaecology, John Hunter Hospital, Newcastle, NSW, Australia

Supuni Kapurubandara and Yogesh Nikam
Department of Obstetrics and Gynaecology, Westmead Hospital, Sydney, NSW, Australia
Sydney West Advanced Pelvic Surgery (SWAPS), Sydney, NSW, Australia
University of Sydney, Sydney, NSW, Australia

Raghwa Sharma
University of Sydney, Sydney, NSW, Australia
Department of Tissue Pathology and Diagnostic Oncology, Institute of Clinical Pathology and Medical Research, Westmead Hospital, Sydney, NSW, Australia
Western Sydney University, Sydney, NSW, Australia

Anita Achan
Department of Tissue Pathology and Diagnostic Oncology, Institute of Clinical Pathology and Medical Research, Westmead Hospital, Sydney, NSW, Australia

Melissa Sum, Jessica B. Fleischer and Sharon L. Wardlaw
Department of Medicine, College of Physicians and Surgeons, Columbia University, New York, NY, USA

Index